50% OFF Online NCLEX-RN Prep Course!

Dear Customer,

We consider it an honor and a privilege that you chose our NCLEX-RN Study Guide. As a way of showing our appreciation and to help us better serve you, we have partnered with Mometrix Test Preparation to offer **50% off their online NCLEX-RN Prep Course.** Many NCLEX-RN courses are needlessly expensive and don't deliver enough value. With our course, you get access to the best NCLEX-RN prep material, and you only pay half price.

Mometrix has structured their online course to perfectly complement your printed study guide. The NCLEX-RN Prep Course contains **over 300 lessons** that cover all the most important topics, **40+ video reviews** that explain difficult concepts, **over 700 practice questions** to ensure you feel prepared, and **digital flashcards**, so you can fit some studying in while you're on the go.

Online NCLEX-RN Prep Course

Topics Covered:

- Management of Care
    - *Case Management*
    - *Collaborative Care Management*
    - *Ethical Practices*
- Safety and Infection Control
    - *Accident, Error, and Injury Prevention*
    - *Emergency Response*
    - *Infectious Diseases and Infection Control*
- Health Promotion and Maintenance
    - *Developmental Stages and Transitions*
    - *Disease Prevention*
    - *Health Screening*

Course Features:

- NCLEX-RN Study Guide
    - Get content that complements our best-selling study guide.
- 6 Full-Length Practice Tests
    - With over 700 practice questions, you can test yourself again and again.
- Mobile Friendly
    - If you need to study on-the-go, the course is easily accessible from your mobile device.
- NCLEX-RN Flashcards
    - The course includes a flashcard mode consisting of over 600 content cards to help you study.

To receive this discount, simply head to their website: www.mometrix.com/university/courses/nclex and add the course to your cart. At the checkout page, enter the discount code: **TPBNCLEX50**

If you have any questions or concerns, please don't hesitate to contact Mometrix at universityhelp@mometrix.com.

Sincerely,

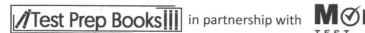 in partnership with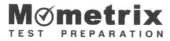

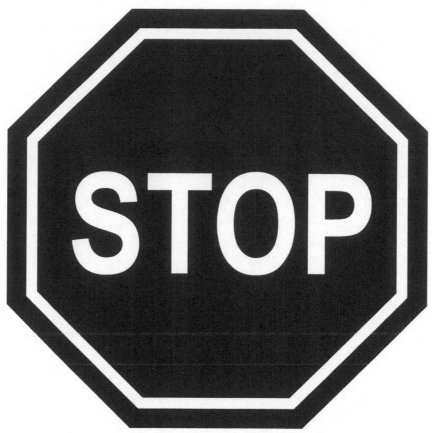

FREE Test Taking Tips DVD Offer

To help us better serve you, we have developed a Test Taking Tips DVD that we would like to give you for FREE. **This DVD covers world-class test taking tips that you can use to be even more successful when you are taking your test.**

All that we ask is that you email us your feedback about your study guide. Please let us know what you thought about it – whether that is good, bad or indifferent.

To get your **FREE Test Taking Tips DVD**, email freedvd@studyguideteam.com with "FREE DVD" in the subject line and the following information in the body of the email:

a. The title of your study guide.

b. Your product rating on a scale of 1-5, with 5 being the highest rating.

c. Your feedback about the study guide. What did you think of it?

d. Your full name and shipping address to send your free DVD.

If you have any questions or concerns, please don't hesitate to contact us at freedvd@studyguideteam.com.

Thanks again!

NCLEX RN 2019 & 2020 Study Guide

NCLEX RN Examination Test Prep & Practice Test
Questions for the National Council Licensure Examination
for Registered Nurses [Updated for the NEW 2019 Outline]

Test Prep Books

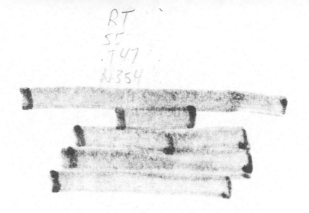

Written and edited by Test Prep Books.

Interested in buying more than 10 copies of our product? Contact us about bulk discounts:
bulkorders@studyguideteam.com

ISBN 13: 9781628456363
ISBN 10: 1628456361

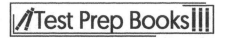

Table of Contents

50% OFF Online NCLEX-RN Prep Course! ---------------------- 1

Quick Overview -- 1

Test-Taking Strategies --- 2

FREE DVD OFFER --- 6

Introduction to the NCLEX-RN Exam -------------------------- 7

Management of Care -- 9

Safety and Infection Control -----------------------------------30

Health Promotion and Maintenance ---------------------------49

Psychosocial Integrity ---57

Basic Care and Comfort -- 80

Pharmacological and Parenteral Therapies --------------------96

Reduction of Risk Potential ------------------------------------109

Physiological Adaptation --------------------------------------138

NCLEX Practice Test #1 ---------------------------------------161

NCLEX Answer Explanations #1 -------------------------------177

NCLEX Practice Test #2 ---------------------------------------190

NCLEX Answer Explanations #2 ------------------------------224

Index ---248

Quick Overview

As you draw closer to taking your exam, effective preparation becomes more and more important. Thankfully, you have this study guide to help you get ready. Use this guide to help keep your studying on track and refer to it often.

This study guide contains several key sections that will help you be successful on your exam. The guide contains tips for what you should do the night before and the day of the test. Also included are test-taking tips. Knowing the right information is not always enough. Many well-prepared test takers struggle with exams. These tips will help equip you to accurately read, assess, and answer test questions.

A large part of the guide is devoted to showing you what content to expect on the exam and to helping you better understand that content. In this guide are practice test questions so that you can see how well you have grasped the content. Then, answer explanations are provided so that you can understand why you missed certain questions.

Don't try to cram the night before you take your exam. This is not a wise strategy for a few reasons. First, your retention of the information will be low. Your time would be better used by reviewing information you already know rather than trying to learn a lot of new information. Second, you will likely become stressed as you try to gain a large amount of knowledge in a short amount of time. Third, you will be depriving yourself of sleep. So be sure to go to bed at a reasonable time the night before. Being well-rested helps you focus and remain calm.

Be sure to eat a substantial breakfast the morning of the exam. If you are taking the exam in the afternoon, be sure to have a good lunch as well. Being hungry is distracting and can make it difficult to focus. You have hopefully spent lots of time preparing for the exam. Don't let an empty stomach get in the way of success!

When travelling to the testing center, leave earlier than needed. That way, you have a buffer in case you experience any delays. This will help you remain calm and will keep you from missing your appointment time at the testing center.

Be sure to pace yourself during the exam. Don't try to rush through the exam. There is no need to risk performing poorly on the exam just so you can leave the testing center early. Allow yourself to use all of the allotted time if needed.

Remain positive while taking the exam even if you feel like you are performing poorly. Thinking about the content you should have mastered will not help you perform better on the exam.

Once the exam is complete, take some time to relax. Even if you feel that you need to take the exam again, you will be well served by some down time before you begin studying again. It's often easier to convince yourself to study if you know that it will come with a reward!

Test-Taking Strategies

1. Predicting the Answer

When you feel confident in your preparation for a multiple-choice test, try predicting the answer before reading the answer choices. This is especially useful on questions that test objective factual knowledge. By predicting the answer before reading the available choices, you eliminate the possibility that you will be distracted or led astray by an incorrect answer choice. You will feel more confident in your selection if you read the question, predict the answer, and then find your prediction among the answer choices. After using this strategy, be sure to still read all of the answer choices carefully and completely. If you feel unprepared, you should not attempt to predict the answers. This would be a waste of time and an opportunity for your mind to wander in the wrong direction.

2. Reading the Whole Question

Too often, test takers scan a multiple-choice question, recognize a few familiar words, and immediately jump to the answer choices. Test authors are aware of this common impatience, and they will sometimes prey upon it. For instance, a test author might subtly turn the question into a negative, or he or she might redirect the focus of the question right at the end. The only way to avoid falling into these traps is to read the entirety of the question carefully before reading the answer choices.

3. Looking for Wrong Answers

Long and complicated multiple-choice questions can be intimidating. One way to simplify a difficult multiple-choice question is to eliminate all of the answer choices that are clearly wrong. In most sets of answers, there will be at least one selection that can be dismissed right away. If the test is administered on paper, the test taker could draw a line through it to indicate that it may be ignored; otherwise, the test taker will have to perform this operation mentally or on scratch paper. In either case, once the obviously incorrect answers have been eliminated, the remaining choices may be considered. Sometimes identifying the clearly wrong answers will give the test taker some information about the correct answer. For instance, if one of the remaining answer choices is a direct opposite of one of the eliminated answer choices, it may well be the correct answer. The opposite of obviously wrong is obviously right! Of course, this is not always the case. Some answers are obviously incorrect simply because they are irrelevant to the question being asked. Still, identifying and eliminating some incorrect answer choices is a good way to simplify a multiple-choice question.

4. Don't Overanalyze

Anxious test takers often overanalyze questions. When you are nervous, your brain will often run wild, causing you to make associations and discover clues that don't actually exist. If you feel that this may be a problem for you, do whatever you can to slow down during the test. Try taking a deep breath or counting to ten. As you read and consider the question, restrict yourself to the particular words used by the author. Avoid thought tangents about what the author *really* meant, or what he or she was *trying* to say. The only things that matter on a multiple-choice test are the words that are actually in the question. You must avoid reading too much into a multiple-choice question, or supposing that the writer meant something other than what he or she wrote.

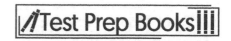

5. No Need for Panic

It is wise to learn as many strategies as possible before taking a multiple-choice test, but it is likely that you will come across a few questions for which you simply don't know the answer. In this situation, avoid panicking. Because most multiple-choice tests include dozens of questions, the relative value of a single wrong answer is small. As much as possible, you should compartmentalize each question on a multiple-choice test. In other words, you should not allow your feelings about one question to affect your success on the others. When you find a question that you either don't understand or don't know how to answer, just take a deep breath and do your best. Read the entire question slowly and carefully. Try rephrasing the question a couple of different ways. Then, read all of the answer choices carefully. After eliminating obviously wrong answers, make a selection and move on to the next question.

6. Confusing Answer Choices

When working on a difficult multiple-choice question, there may be a tendency to focus on the answer choices that are the easiest to understand. Many people, whether consciously or not, gravitate to the answer choices that require the least concentration, knowledge, and memory. This is a mistake. When you come across an answer choice that is confusing, you should give it extra attention. A question might be confusing because you do not know the subject matter to which it refers. If this is the case, don't eliminate the answer before you have affirmatively settled on another. When you come across an answer choice of this type, set it aside as you look at the remaining choices. If you can confidently assert that one of the other choices is correct, you can leave the confusing answer aside. Otherwise, you will need to take a moment to try to better understand the confusing answer choice. Rephrasing is one way to tease out the sense of a confusing answer choice.

7. Your First Instinct

Many people struggle with multiple-choice tests because they overthink the questions. If you have studied sufficiently for the test, you should be prepared to trust your first instinct once you have carefully and completely read the question and all of the answer choices. There is a great deal of research suggesting that the mind can come to the correct conclusion very quickly once it has obtained all of the relevant information. At times, it may seem to you as if your intuition is working faster even than your reasoning mind. This may in fact be true. The knowledge you obtain while studying may be retrieved from your subconscious before you have a chance to work out the associations that support it. Verify your instinct by working out the reasons that it should be trusted.

8. Key Words

Many test takers struggle with multiple-choice questions because they have poor reading comprehension skills. Quickly reading and understanding a multiple-choice question requires a mixture of skill and experience. To help with this, try jotting down a few key words and phrases on a piece of scrap paper. Doing this concentrates the process of reading and forces the mind to weigh the relative importance of the question's parts. In selecting words and phrases to write down, the test taker thinks about the question more deeply and carefully. This is especially true for multiple-choice questions that are preceded by a long prompt.

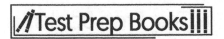

9. Subtle Negatives

One of the oldest tricks in the multiple-choice test writer's book is to subtly reverse the meaning of a question with a word like *not* or *except*. If you are not paying attention to each word in the question, you can easily be led astray by this trick. For instance, a common question format is, "Which of the following is...?" Obviously, if the question instead is, "Which of the following is not...?," then the answer will be quite different. Even worse, the test makers are aware of the potential for this mistake and will include one answer choice that would be correct if the question were not negated or reversed. A test taker who misses the reversal will find what he or she believes to be a correct answer and will be so confident that he or she will fail to reread the question and discover the original error. The only way to avoid this is to practice a wide variety of multiple-choice questions and to pay close attention to each and every word.

10. Reading Every Answer Choice

It may seem obvious, but you should always read every one of the answer choices! Too many test takers fall into the habit of scanning the question and assuming that they understand the question because they recognize a few key words. From there, they pick the first answer choice that answers the question they believe they have read. Test takers who read all of the answer choices might discover that one of the latter answer choices is actually *more* correct. Moreover, reading all of the answer choices can remind you of facts related to the question that can help you arrive at the correct answer. Sometimes, a misstatement or incorrect detail in one of the latter answer choices will trigger your memory of the subject and will enable you to find the right answer. Failing to read all of the answer choices is like not reading all of the items on a restaurant menu: you might miss out on the perfect choice.

11. Spot the Hedges

One of the keys to success on multiple-choice tests is paying close attention to every word. This is never truer than with words like almost, most, some, and sometimes. These words are called "hedges" because they indicate that a statement is not totally true or not true in every place and time. An absolute statement will contain no hedges, but in many subjects, the answers are not always straightforward or absolute. There are always exceptions to the rules in these subjects. For this reason, you should favor those multiple-choice questions that contain hedging language. The presence of qualifying words indicates that the author is taking special care with his or her words, which is certainly important when composing the right answer. After all, there are many ways to be wrong, but there is only one way to be right! For this reason, it is wise to avoid answers that are absolute when taking a multiple-choice test. An absolute answer is one that says things are either all one way or all another. They often include words like *every*, *always*, *best*, and *never*. If you are taking a multiple-choice test in a subject that doesn't lend itself to absolute answers, be on your guard if you see any of these words.

12. Long Answers

In many subject areas, the answers are not simple. As already mentioned, the right answer often requires hedges. Another common feature of the answers to a complex or subjective question are qualifying clauses, which are groups of words that subtly modify the meaning of the sentence. If the question or answer choice describes a rule to which there are exceptions or the subject matter is complicated, ambiguous, or confusing, the correct answer will require many words in order to be expressed clearly and accurately. In essence, you should not be deterred by answer choices that seem excessively long. Oftentimes, the author of the text will not be able to write the correct answer without

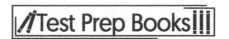

offering some qualifications and modifications. Your job is to read the answer choices thoroughly and completely and to select the one that most accurately and precisely answers the question.

13. Restating to Understand

Sometimes, a question on a multiple-choice test is difficult not because of what it asks but because of how it is written. If this is the case, restate the question or answer choice in different words. This process serves a couple of important purposes. First, it forces you to concentrate on the core of the question. In order to rephrase the question accurately, you have to understand it well. Rephrasing the question will concentrate your mind on the key words and ideas. Second, it will present the information to your mind in a fresh way. This process may trigger your memory and render some useful scrap of information picked up while studying.

14. True Statements

Sometimes an answer choice will be true in itself, but it does not answer the question. This is one of the main reasons why it is essential to read the question carefully and completely before proceeding to the answer choices. Too often, test takers skip ahead to the answer choices and look for true statements. Having found one of these, they are content to select it without reference to the question above. Obviously, this provides an easy way for test makers to play tricks. The savvy test taker will always read the entire question before turning to the answer choices. Then, having settled on a correct answer choice, he or she will refer to the original question and ensure that the selected answer is relevant. The mistake of choosing a correct-but-irrelevant answer choice is especially common on questions related to specific pieces of objective knowledge. A prepared test taker will have a wealth of factual knowledge at his or her disposal, and should not be careless in its application.

15. No Patterns

One of the more dangerous ideas that circulates about multiple-choice tests is that the correct answers tend to fall into patterns. These erroneous ideas range from a belief that B and C are the most common right answers, to the idea that an unprepared test-taker should answer "A-B-A-C-A-D-A-B-A." It cannot be emphasized enough that pattern-seeking of this type is exactly the WRONG way to approach a multiple-choice test. To begin with, it is highly unlikely that the test maker will plot the correct answers according to some predetermined pattern. The questions are scrambled and delivered in a random order. Furthermore, even if the test maker was following a pattern in the assignation of correct answers, there is no reason why the test taker would know which pattern he or she was using. Any attempt to discern a pattern in the answer choices is a waste of time and a distraction from the real work of taking the test. A test taker would be much better served by extra preparation before the test than by reliance on a pattern in the answers.

FREE DVD OFFER

Don't forget that doing well on your exam includes both understanding the test content and understanding how to use what you know to do well on the test. We offer a completely FREE Test Taking Tips DVD that covers world class test taking tips that you can use to be even more successful when you are taking your test.

All that we ask is that you email us your feedback about your study guide. To get your **FREE Test Taking Tips DVD**, email freedvd@studyguideteam.com with "FREE DVD" in the subject line and the following information in the body of the email:

- The title of your study guide.
- Your product rating on a scale of 1-5, with 5 being the highest rating.
- Your feedback about the study guide. What did you think of it?
- Your full name and shipping address to send your free DVD.

Introduction to the NCLEX-RN Exam

Function of the Test

The National Council Licensure Examination (NCLEX) is a standardized test reviewed by the state board of nursing to determine whether or not the test taker is ready to begin entry-level nursing practice. Those who take the NCLEX exam should already have a nursing degree from an accredited university and should also apply for a license from their state board of nursing before taking the exam. The board of nursing will determine eligibility for taking the test after the test taker has applied. In 2017, those professionals who held a baccalaureate degree had a passing rate of 90.04% for the total year to date.

Test Administration

To schedule an appointment to take the NCLEX exam, it is suggested that you go through the Pearson VUE online website, keeping in mind that you've received your Authorization to Test (ATT) in the mail. When scheduling your exam via Pearson VUE, you will have to create a username and password and then you will be given the option to request a preference for your testing time, date, and location. The NCLEX is also offered at international testing centers.

Those who wish to retake the exam are able to do so 45 days after administration of the exam. Those who have applied for licensure with the nursing board are allowed to take the NCLEX eight times a year, no more than once in a 45-day time frame.

Requests for accommodations are handled by the individual testing program. There are request forms for accommodations on the Pearson VUE website.

Test Format

For the NCLEX exam on test day, you should arrive at the testing center 30 minutes before the test begins. Electronics will be stored in plastic bags provided by the testing site. You will need an ID and a palm scan of your hand before entering the testing site. You will also be required to leave any personal belongings outside the testing area. Any large jewelry, hats, or scarves must be removed, although allowances can be made for religious apparel. A note board will be provided for you in the test room, and you will have six hours to complete the test. This time includes a short tutorial and two scheduled breaks.

For the structure of the NCLEX exam, RN candidates take a maximum of 265 questions and LPN candidates take a maximum of 205 questions, but the number of questions may vary.

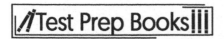

The following table depicts what kind of content is on the NCLEX exam:

Subject	Percentage on Test
Physiological Adaptation	14%
Reduction of Risk Potential	12%
Pharmacological and Parenteral Therapies	15%
Basic Care and Comfort	9%
Management of Care	20%
Safety and Infection Control	12%
Health Promotion and Maintenance	9%
Psychosocial Integrity	9%

Scoring

The NCLEX is a computer-based exam. No questions can be skipped on the NCLEX—candidates must answer a question before moving onto the next one. The NCLEX uses computerized adaptive testing, which means that the number of questions a candidate is given depends on their answers to the previous questions. When it can be determined with a 95% confidence that a candidate is either below or above the passing standard, then the exam will end.

Recent/Future Developments

In July 2017, the NCSBN presented a Special Research Section to select candidates taking the NCLEX-RN exam. This section takes 30 minutes to complete and is not taken by everyone. This section does not count as part of the NCLEX score.

Management of Care

Advance Directives/Self-Determination/Life Planning

Advance directives, such as a living will or durable power of attorney, are forms that state a patient's choices for treatment, including refusal of treatments, life support, and stopping treatments when the patient chooses. **Do not resuscitate (DNR)** status, and its varying types, is also included in advance directives. The preoperative interview should include discussion of advance directives and DNR status. If the patient has advance directives, a copy should be placed in the medical record, and they should be reviewed by the nurse and physician. If the patient has a code status of anything other than full resuscitation, a conversation among the surgeon, anesthesiologist, and patient is necessary to discuss the patient's wishes in detail. Older schools of thinking suggest all patients, regardless of preoperative DNR status, are considered full code while in the operating room; however, this is not true. A patient with DNR status of no intubation and no CPR may proceed with the surgical procedure if the surgeon and anesthesiologist have a conversation with the patient and a plan is agreed upon among them. Consent must be obtained by the patient if there is a change in status or a suspension of the DNR order during surgery. However, if the patient wishes to keep DNR status of no intubation and no CPR during surgery, the surgeon and/or anesthesiologist may deem the patient a nonsurgical candidate. If a patient is entering surgery with a DNR order of anything other than full code, this must be communicated to the entire surgical team and documented in the medical record.

Advocacy

The American Nurses Association (ANA) provides this definition of **nursing practice**: "The protection, promotion, and optimization of health and abilities, prevention of illness and injury, alleviation of suffering through the diagnosis and treatment of human response, and advocacy in the care of individuals, families, communities, and populations." The ANA also addresses the importance of advocacy in its Code of Ethics, specifically in Provision 3: "The nurse promotes, advocates for, and protects the rights, health, and safety of the patient." The ANA Code of Ethics further states: nurses must advocate "with compassion and respect for the inherent dignity, worth, and uniqueness of every individual, unrestricted by considerations of social or economic status, personal attributes, or the nature of health problems."

Advocacy is a key component of nursing practice. An **advocate** is one who pleads the cause of another; and the nurse is an advocate for patient rights. Preserving human dignity, patient equality, and freedom from suffering are the basis of nursing advocacy. Nurses are in a unique position that allows them to integrate all aspects of patient care, ensuring that concerns are addressed, standards are upheld, and positive outcomes remain the goal. An experienced nurse helps patients navigate the unfamiliar system and communicate with their physicians. Nurses educate the patient about tests and procedures and are aware of how culture and ethnicity affect the patient's experience. Nurses strictly adhere to all privacy laws.

Advocacy is the promotion of the common good, especially as it applies to at-risk populations. It involves speaking out in support of policies and decisions that affect the lives of individuals who do not otherwise have a voice. Nurses meet this standard of practice by actively participating in the politics of healthcare accessibility and delivery because they are educationally and professionally prepared to evaluate and comment on the needs of patients at the local, state, and national level. This participation requires an understanding of the legislative process, the ability to negotiate with public officials, and a willingness to provide expert testimony in support of policy decisions. The advocacy role of nurses addresses the needs of the individual patient as well as the needs of all individuals in the society, and the members of the nursing profession.

In clinical practice, nurses represent the patient's interests by active participation in the development of the plan of care and subsequent care decisions. Advocacy, in this sense, is related to patient autonomy and the patient's right to informed consent and self-determination. Nurses provide the appropriate information, assess the patient's comprehension of the implications of the care decisions, and act as the patient advocates by supporting the patient's decisions. In the critical care environment, patient advocacy requires the nurse to represent the patient's decisions even though those decisions may be opposed to those of the healthcare providers and family members.

Professionally, nurses advocate for policies that support and promote the practice of all nurses with regard to access to education, role identity, workplace conditions, and compensation. The responsibility for professional advocacy requires nurses to provide leadership in the development of the professional nursing role in all practice settings that may include acute care facilities, colleges and universities, or community agencies. Leadership roles in acute care settings involve participation in professional practice and shared governance committees, providing support for basic nursing education by facilitating clinical and preceptorship experiences, and mentoring novice graduate nurses to the professional nursing role. In the academic setting, nurses work to ensure the diversity of the student population by participating in the governance structure of the institution, conducting and publishing research that supports the positive impact of professional nursing care on patient outcomes, and serving as an advocate to individual nursing students to promote their academic success. In the community, nurses assist other nurse-providers to collaborate with government officials to meet the needs that are specific to that location.

The nurse must function as a **moral agent**. This means that the nurse must be morally accountable and responsible for personal judgment and actions. Nurses who practice with moral integrity possess a strong sense of themselves and act in ways consistent with what they understand is the right thing to do. Moral agency is defined as the ability to identify right and wrong actions based on widely accepted moral criteria. The performance of nurses as moral agents is dependent on life experiences, advanced education, and clinical experience in healthcare agencies. Moral agency involves risk. It is an action that can be at odds with the traditional role of the nurse. As nurses assume more responsibility and accountability for client management and outcomes, it is essential to approach ethical dilemmas in a manner consistent with the caring component of nursing.

The role of moral agent requires nurses to have a strong sense of self and a clear understanding of the definition of right and wrong; however, nurses must also be aware that these perceptions of right and wrong will be challenged every day. In reality, nurses who act as the moral agents and are accountable for right and wrong decisions commonly encounter situations where the correct and moral action related to the patient's right to self-determination is opposed to the right and moral action with respect to competent patient care.

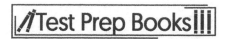

Assignment, Delegation, and Supervision

Assignment

Every day when the nurse reports to duty, a team of patients will be assigned to them. A caseload of patients will vary in size based on the acuity of the patients' illnesses and the unit policies that the nurse belongs to.

Acuity refers to the severity of the patient's illness. Some patients are high acuity, meaning a lot of time and resources are put into their daily routine due to the severity of their illness. Others are low acuity and do not require much oversight from the nurse to get through the day. High-acuity patients are a major sore point for many nurses because their care can often take away from the care of others. A team full of high-acuity patients, then, can be a great burden for a nurse to bear.

Dividing up teams of patients is often the task of the charge nurse. To fairly assign patient teams to nurses, the charge nurse must bear in mind each patient's acuity. Conflict arises when nurses feel that there is inequity in the assignment of patients and they are unduly burdened with an unfair patient load compared to other teams or units.

Nurse satisfaction directly correlates with patient care. If nurses do not feel their patient assignments are fair and the burden is too great, their performance suffers as well as their job satisfaction. Nursing performance can be linked to the following nurse-sensitive indicators: how well patient pain is managed; the presence and treatment of pressure ulcers, patient falls, and medication errors; patient satisfaction; and nosocomial or hospital-acquired infections.

When patient assignments become too burdensome for nurses, those nursing-sensitive indicators are the first signs that there is a problem. When the nurse is busy with a team of high-acuity patients, it is difficult to perform all the tasks of the day, let alone perform them carefully and thoughtfully. It is then in the best interest of those making team assignments for nurses to weigh carefully the patient load and ensure equitable and fair decisions are made.

Case Management

In the world of healthcare, one individual patient's case may look very different than the next patient's. Even if they have the same diagnosis, the same demographic and socioeconomic background, and live in the same geographical region, the fact that they are different people will cause their individual cases to vary.

Therefore, someone is needed to manage the patient's care and ensure that their needs are advocated for and the cost of care is kept to a minimum. This person is called a **case manager**. A case manager performs several roles while managing the care of the patient, including advocate, prescription manager, liaison with insurance companies and hospitals, and mediator between the patient and other health care providers.

Becoming a case manager requires special training in addition to the original nursing licensure and practice. The nurse must fulfill a prerequisite number of clinical hours and receive special case management training before testing for their case management certification. Once certified, the nurse is then ready to take on the role of case manager.

Some case managers work with a specific population, such as patients with cancer, HIV/AIDS, heart failure, kidney failure, and many more. Case managers are often needed for patients who have complicated conditions and require long-term care. Long, complex cases are best placed in the hands of a case manager to ensure the best possible outcome for the patient and to keep the cost of care down.

Anywhere there is a medical facility with patients, a team of case managers is likely to be found. Case managers work in offices where they manage patients' cases and call insurance representatives, physicians, and health care facility representatives. Case managers also spend time meeting with patients to discuss plans of care.

Periodically it is necessary to review a patient's plan of care. The purpose of a patient care review is to ensure that the patient's needs are being met, progress is being made toward the goal of recovery, and costs are being cut where necessary and possible. The case manager will be in on these reviews to give input from their perspective and ensure that the patient's voice and needs are being heard and met. The nurse has an insightful perspective on the patient due to their long-term relationship.

Often a case manager will be introduced to the patient at the beginning of an illness and stay with them throughout the experience, developing an intimate and caring relationship. This relationship both serves the care needs of the patient and is rewarding for the nurse. It is comforting to the patient to have this person with them for their whole journey, because other health care workers play important but often transient roles in the patient's care.

The case manager provides the patient with information regarding their plan of care. This may include educating them on their treatment options based on their particular illness, giving them access to helpful resources to guide their decision making, connecting them with community support groups, and advising them on decisions based on sound clinical judgment and experience. However, the case manager must be careful not to unduly pressure a patient to make a decision based on the case manager's own bias. The patient must be allowed the independence to make their own decisions according to their own belief system and worldview.

When the patient is allowed the independence to make their own decisions and assist with the plan of care, the plan of care is far more likely to be successful. This team model for health care planning is highly effective because it includes not only the input of the medical and nursing teams, but also the input of the most important member of the team, the patient.

To be a successful case manager, a nurse must be fluent in the language and policies of insurance providers. These include private and government-run programs such as Medicare and Medicaid. The nurse will often communicate with insurance providers to determine a patient's coverage for treatments and procedures, to advocate and appeal as necessary, and to look for cost-effective treatment plans.

The nurse organizing a patient's plan of care must be well organized. The nurse may oversee a large caseload of patients spanning the entire facility's population, and thus the nurse must keep all the details organized. Missing details could cost the patient time and money, and in the worst case, could delay their recovery.

The case manager must be, above all, a good communicator. The case manager is often called upon to translate the complicated jargon of medicine, insurance, and health care facility policies for the patient. Being able to turn complex messages into simple and digestible pieces for the patient is key to their comprehension of their plan of care. If the patient does not understand why they need to make it to their dialysis appointments or why insurance will not cover one treatment option but will cover another,

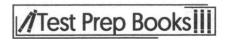

errors may occur. Miscommunications lead to frustration and inefficiencies, both of which the case manager strives to alleviate and correct.

The case manager must ensure that the medication included in the patient's plan of care is managed efficiently. The list of medications prescribed according to the patient's condition must be carefully considered, as to whether evidence-based practice backs up their use, whether the patient's condition will benefit from their use, and whether the patient is able to afford their medication plan. The case manager must consider affordability of the medications and whether the patient will comply with taking them. The case manager must determine the patient's understanding of their medication regime because misunderstandings regarding the treatment plan may lead to the patient's becoming non-compliant. If the patient understands their medications and their use, agrees with the plan, and can afford and access the prescriptions, then they are more likely to follow the prescribed medication regime. This success will hopefully translate to a better overall outcome with the patient's illness as well as a higher quality of life.

Client Rights

Each patient has certain rights that must be respected. When patients are admitted to a facility, they are put in a position of vulnerability. This special position of power held by the health care provider should never be abused to violate the rights of the patient. Caring for a patient is an honor, and certain rules of conduct should be followed. The following will be a discussion of patient's rights, violations, and consequences of violations, as well as appropriate avenues of reporting.

Patient Rights

The patient has the right to have health information kept private, and only shared with those who are given permission to view it. The **Health Insurance Portability and Accountability Act (HIPAA)** was passed by Congress in 1996 to protect health information. The term HIPAA is often used to reference patient privacy. There are many different ways a patient's personal health information can be shared: verbally, digitally, over the phone or fax, or through written messages.

The nurse plays an important role in keeping a patient's health information private. Sharing personal details—such as a patient's name, condition, and medical history—in an inappropriate way violates the person's right to privacy. For example, telling a friend who does not work in the facility that the nurse took care of the friend's aunt, without the aunt's consent or knowledge, is considered a violation of privacy. Another way a nurse could violate a patient's privacy is to access the medical record when they are not actually caring for that particular patient. For example, if a celebrity has been admitted to a different unit, and the nurse—curious to find out the details—accesses the celebrity's electronic health record, then they are in violation of HIPAA. Those who violate HIPAA and are caught could lose their jobs, among other punitive actions.

Along with protecting the patient's health information, the nurse must be respectful of the patient's privacy in general. Knocking on the patient's door before entering the room, keeping the door shut to the busy corridor outside the room, and not asking unnecessary personal questions are all ways the nurse can extend common courtesy to the patient. The nature of the nurse's relationship with the patient is already quite personal in nature (e.g., the nurse is giving the patient baths, helping him or her go to the bathroom, etc.), so there is no need to exploit that relationship.

The patient has the **right of self-determination**, which means that he or she has the right to make decisions regarding his or her own health care. Patients are members of the health care team along with the doctors, nurses, and nurses. What the nurse may think is the right course of action for a patient may not align with what the patient thinks is right, and that is to be respected. The health care team forms the plan of care and educates the patient as to what a plan entails, but it is the patient who makes the final decision to accept or reject a plan. If the patient is not capable of making his or her own decisions, the **power of attorney**—usually a close family member such as a wife, husband, or adult child—has the power to make health care decisions for the patient.

Along with self-determination, the patients also have the freedom to express themselves and their opinions. Simply being admitted to a facility does not take away their freedom of speech. Patients may have opinions about all aspects of their care, and they have every right to express these feelings. The nurse needs to be respectful, listen, and try to help when there is a problem that can be solved. Issues voiced by patients can always be escalated by the nurse, using the appropriate chain of command.

Each patient has the right to **fair treatment**. This means that no patient should be treated any better or worse than another patient for any reason, such as a racial bias or unfair prejudice based on the nurse's personal opinions and beliefs. Giving one patient preferential treatment over another is a violation of the patient's rights, and the nurse will be subject to disciplinary action if they are discovered to be treating patients poorly.

No patient should ever be abused or neglected. This should go without saying, but it is a patient right that is perhaps the most important. Abuse can be physical, emotional, sexual, mental, or financial. Neglect is when the patient's needs are being ignored, usually resulting in patient harm.

Responsibility for Recognizing and Reporting Violations

If the nurse suspects abuse or neglect, they are mandatorily required to report it to the appropriate entity. The charge nurse and/or nurse manager should be notified, so the appropriate action can be taken to right the situation. There are also hotlines that can be called, such as the National Center on Elder Abuse (1-800-677-1116).

Patient Abuse

There are different types of abuse. **Physical abuse** involves injuries to the body from punching, kicking, etc. If the nurse notes various bruises or cuts in various stages of healing without explanation, it may be a sign of physical abuse.

Sexual abuse is when sexual contact is made without the consent of one party, including rape, coercion into doing sexual acts, and fondling of genitalia. The nurse should look for unexplained bruising of or bleeding around the perineal area, new difficulty sitting or walking, or increased agitation/aggression as potential signs of sexual abuse.

Emotional or **mental abuses** are not quite as obvious as physical abuse as the damage inflicted is internal or hidden. Emotional and mental abuses are usually caused by verbal assaults. The abuser may belittle and criticize the victim to the point that the victim feels worthless, insecure, and afraid. If the nurse senses an uncomfortable relationship between an informal caregiver or family member and the patient, this should be monitored, investigated, and reported if abuse is suspected.

Financial abuse is a type of abuse in which the abuser limits the victim's access to money and financial information, sometimes stealing directly from the victim without the victim's knowledge. Being the caregiver of an older person grants a person special access to personal documents and financial resources; this privilege can be abused. If the nurse suspects that checks and other financial means

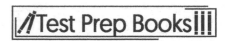

meant for the patient are being rerouted and misused by a caregiver, this abuse should be reported right away.

Diversity in the Workplace

Depending on the facility, a nurse will potentially work with a diverse group of fellow health care workers as well as a diverse patient demographic. People from all different cultural, racial, religious, sexual, and economic backgrounds converge in health care, and the nurse must know how to work within such an environment.

When working with a diverse population and with diverse peers, respectful behavior is the best strategy. The nurse will encounter belief systems different from their own, manifested in what people wear, what they eat, how they behave, and lifestyle choices they make. The nurse's initial reaction may be one of shock when they learn certain details about other cultures. It is healthy to be aware of these reactions and examine them and their origins. The best response is to educate oneself to cultivate a deeper appreciation for these different cultures, rather than making judgments or being dismissive.

A diverse workplace, serving a diverse population of patients, can be an enriching environment in which the individuals working together are greater than the sum of their parts. There is no reason why differences in beliefs, lifestyles, and cultures should hinder the work of caring for the sick. The nurse steps into this world, becomes a part of it, and can take away a better understanding and broader perspective of the people of this planet.

Grievance and Dispute Resolution Techniques

There may be times during a nurse's career where they have a grievance against the entity for which they are working or have a dispute with a peer or patient. This is another instance where the chain of command should be followed. Usually the nurse manager is the one to go to with issues that cannot be resolved by the charge nurses. The nurse manager can act as a mediator and meet with the two disputing parties and try to reach a resolution. It is in the best interest of the nurse and all involved to remain professional during times of conflict, avoid personal attacks, and keep the issue private so as to not disrupt patient care.

Patient Personal Property

Each facility will have specific policies protecting the property of patients. When patients enter the facility, they are entrusting the staff to take care of certain items, such as clothing, family photos, and other treasured objects. The nurse must follow facility policy regarding such items and take special care not to lose or damage them. Many patients will have designated spots in their rooms, such as closets and/or lock boxes, where items can be kept safe from theft and damage. Patients should be encouraged to keep valuables at home whenever possible.

Collaboration with Interdisciplinary Team

Interdisciplinary rounding can provide an opportunity for team collaboration after a patient's surgery. Much like a clear hand-off process, interdisciplinary rounds reduce patient care errors, decrease mortality rates, and improve patient outcomes. Interdisciplinary rounds are an excellent place to discuss social service needs, nutritional care services, and transportation needs with all teams coordinating care for the patient in a single setting.

The patient's service needs may vary in depth for the inpatient stay and at the time of discharge; however, there should be an evaluation of these needs and a coordination of care for those services in which there is a need. Nurses document the action plan as it relates to services and requirements for the patient and collaborate with members of the interdisciplinary team to see that next steps are executed in a timely fashion. In many instances, rounding may not be possible due to the rapid pace and turnover of the medical environment, and thus, clear documentation will be an absolute must to allow for synchronous care coordination.

Nurses, physicians, surgeons, nurse aids, physical and occupational therapists, mental health professionals, and medical assistants are just some of the members who may be collaborating on the care of one patient. Perception of power between these professionals can sometimes create a stressful environment that can also affect patient outcomes. The ability of each one to collaborate with the other is imperative so that patient safety does not become an issue. **Collaboration** involves joint decision-making activities between both disciplines rather than nurses only following physician orders. Although each role may have a particular focus throughout the assessment and plan of care activities, they must jointly come together to formulate the best possible treatment plan throughout the treatment period. Studies show that an attentive communication style between nurses and physicians has the most positive impact on patients.

Ongoing education of physicians and nurses may be a necessity to support a collaborative environment. In addition to continuing education and in-services, job shadowing, which exposes both the nurse and physician to each one's role, can assist in promoting understanding and teamwork.

Concepts of Management

Delegation
Nursing staff take on many responsibilities that can be delegated to other clinical and non-clinical colleagues. However, learning how to effectively and safely delegate tasks, while still making patients feel cared for, is a skill that can take time to develop. It requires knowing not only what the needs of the patient are, but also the strengths and weaknesses of assistive personnel and how to best communicate professional needs with them. It also requires personal development in becoming comfortable with outsourcing responsibilities, as the nurse who delegates still remains accountable for the patient.

Assistive personnel may be supervised by nurses, but clinical assistive staff can provide basic medical assistance such as monitoring patients' vital signs, assisting with caretaking duties, monitoring any abnormalities or changes in the patient, maintaining a sterile and safe environment, and any other request made directly by nursing staff. Non-clinical assistive personnel, such as front desk staff, can assist with patient communication (such as wait times), managing paperwork and ensuring it is complete, and performing any other administrative task that may support the nursing staff's cases.

When nursing staff choose to delegate tasks, they may feel worried about risking their own accountability or work ethic. However, relating with assistive personnel, understanding their strengths and weaknesses, understanding their interests, and remaining transparent about the needs that are present in the department can ensure that delegated tasks are a good fit for the person who is taking the responsibility. In this regard, nursing staff take on a leadership and managerial role that requires developing their problem-solving, time management, and interpersonal skills. Some effective tools for delegation can include standardized checklists that cover the procedure that is being delegated, formal and informal meetings about assistive personnel's comfort levels and interests in performing certain tasks, and matching professional needs with individual qualifications. When delegation is effective, it can help the entire department work in a more efficient manner. Additionally, both nursing staff and

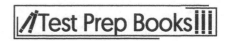

assistive personnel are more likely to feel like part of a cohesive team and less likely to feel overworked or undervalued.

Supervision

After the nurse has successfully and effectively delegated a task, the nurse then takes on the role of supervisor of the person to whom they delegated the task. Delegation requires supervision, to ensure the task is done appropriately and to protect the nurse's own licensure.

The key to supervision is the follow-up. After the task is delegated, the nurse must then make a note to investigate whether the task was done, whether it was done in a timely manner, and whether it was done correctly. Asking the person who was supposed to perform the task to report back is appropriate. All conversations and interactions must be performed professionally and with respect for both the inferior and superior party.

Many nurses were once **certified nursing assistants (CNAs)** and understand the role and responsibility of the person they now delegate to. If the two nurses were former co-workers and one has risen to the role of nurse from CNA, tensions may arise. Tensions that arise between nursing staff and those they delegate to may be resolved through careful interactions in which each party is respected and an effort made by both parties that shows they are both working hard together with the best interest of the patient at the forefront of their mind.

At times, it may be necessary for the nurse to coach and support the staff member, giving tips for better performance where appropriate. Again, this interaction must be done with professionalism and respect. It is important as an employee in any field to be receptive to constructive criticism, as well as being able to offer it when appropriate and allowing plenty of discussion on the point.

The nurse must ensure that the task delegated, such as taking vital signs or cleaning up an incontinent patient, has been appropriately documented. Documentation is necessary for legal reasons, to show that proper care was given to the patient. If the person to whom the task was delegated did not document the task, it is necessary for the nurse to confront them directly and confirm that it was done.

Confidentiality/Information Security

Patient privacy and confidentiality is a constant for all health care providers. Given the sensitivity of medical procedures, the health care team must maintain strict patient confidentiality. Under the Health Insurance Portability and Accountability Act (HIPAA), a patient's information is required to be protected and kept confidential regardless of the form, including electronic, written, and spoken communication. **Protected health information (PHI)** should be shared only on an as-needed and minimum necessary basis. When discussing patients or cases in settings where other personnel may overhear the conversation, the medical team should be careful not to include any PHI that may violate the patient's confidentiality. Additionally, when information is displayed electronically to families and visitors in waiting rooms, patient names should be avoided. HIPAA violations can have negative consequences for the providers and/or the facility.

The nurse plays an important role in keeping a patient's health information private. Sharing personal details—such as a patient's name, condition, and medical history—in an inappropriate way violates the person's right to privacy. For example, a nurse telling a friend who does not work in the facility that the nurse took care of the friend's aunt, without the aunt's consent or knowledge, is considered a violation of privacy. Another way a nurse could violate a resident's privacy is to access the medical record when they are not actually caring for that particular patient. For example, if a celebrity has been admitted to a different unit, and the nursing assistant—curious to find out the details—accesses the celebrity's electronic health record, then they are in violation of HIPAA. Those who violate HIPAA and are caught could lose their jobs, among other punitive actions. Nurses should also ensure that other staff members—such as nursing assistants—as well as patients understand the confidentiality requirements of the facility, state, and country.

Continuity of Care

If one imagines a patient's illness as a road, what would the ideal road look like? Smooth, no potholes, appropriate signage to guide and direct the patient from illness to wellness, right? In the real world of health care, the road the patient travels from illness to wellness often has bumps and miscommunications. Things do not go as planned, missteps are taken, unexpected events and miscalculations can and unfortunately do occur.

All members of the health care team should be striving to provide patients with a high quality of care over time, or continuity of care. This continuity is the metaphorical smooth road mentioned above. The patient begins their journey with an illness, at a doctor's office, convenient care clinic, or an emergency room. From there the road proceeds through various tests and procedures to diagnose and treat the illness. Management teams that include doctors and nurses provide input into this process, and resources also contribute.

The patient is at the center of the **continuity of care model**. The patient is the object of the health care processes at work, it is the patient's case that is being managed, and they use the health care resources to reach their goal of wellness. In continuity of care, the whole patient is treated, not just an organ or an illness. Ideally, the community surrounding the patient is also involved in promoting good health and high quality of life.

The roots of continuity of care lie in a meaningful, long-term relationship between the patient and the health care provider. This relationship ensures that the patient is known. Their needs are anticipated through regular check-ups and follow-ups after the illness has run its course. The ideal is to form a firm bond of trust between the health care provider and the patient. This trusting relationship and deep knowledge of the case allow the provider to better advocate for the patient.

The physician or nurse practitioner coordinating care for the patient will look for ways to make the plan of care cost-effective for the patient. Tests and procedures are carefully weighed for their usefulness in the patient's case, looking for ways to eliminate wasteful healthcare spending.

The main idea behind continuity of care is to avoid what happens all too often in health care: fragmentation of care. The responsibility of the patient's case is often shifted from one entity to another over the course of an illness. Initially, the patient's case is handled in a primary care setting or perhaps an emergent care setting, depending on the illness. Then the patient may become hospitalized, at which point the hospitalist and various specialists step in and take over. At discharge, the patient's case is then handed over to their primary care physician and community centers. Due to this shifting of care, it becomes ambiguous just who is overseeing the patient's care. The patient has a fragmented experience rather than continuity of care.

One issue faced by health care providers is not having the infrastructure to effectively coordinate patient care and avoid the problems associated with fragmented care. A case manager comes into play here because their role is perfect for coordinating the patients' care as they move through the system.

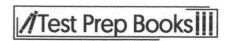

Primary care physicians face a hurdle when coordinating patient care because they have limited communication with the hospital team when their patient is admitted. Nowadays, there is a team of health care providers called "hospitalists," whose job it is to care for patients while they are in the hospital, but not pre- or post-admission. This is helpful because they know the ins and outs of the facility and have good communication with the hospital's specialists and surgeons. They can all work together to get the patient in and out of the hospital relatively quickly.

A **patient-centered medical home (PCMH)** comes into play pre-admission to prevent a costly hospital visit. The idea of a PCMH is to combat fragmentation of care and promote better continuity of care for the patient on their road to wellness. The PCMH is a model of care that is well-coordinated, proactive, and centered on the patient. In this model, a patient is paired with a personal physician to oversee their care. Their family and loved ones are recruited to assist in promoting a whole patient–focused wellness plan. The PCMH moves away from fee for service; instead, it focuses on fee for value, meaning the level of success in keeping the patient healthy determines how the health care team is reimbursed. The patient must regularly keep in touch with their primary care physician, a factor that has been associated with better patient outcomes.

Many communities are adopting the PCMH model of health care, attempting to promote a better continuity of care for patients on their road from illness to wellness.

Establishing Priorities

The ability to establish priorities is one of the nurse's most important skills. The nurse must be able to look at their patient load for the day, assess the needs of each patient, organize tasks in chronological order, and prioritize each task based on its importance and necessity.

When prioritizing the tasks for the day, the nurse must first employ their knowledge of the body, how it works, and what it needs to function. The nurse starts with **ABC:** airway, breathing, and circulation. Are any patients compromised in these respects? If so, they are immediately placed at the top of the list of priorities. If the patients cannot breathe, they are hemorrhaging, or their heart has stopped beating, they require the nurse's immediate assistance. The ABCs are considered the first priority of patient needs.

Emergency Trauma Assessment
- A: Airway
- B: Breathing
- C: Circulation
- D: Disability
- E: Examine
- F: Fahrenheit
- G: Get Vitals
- H: Head to Toe Assessment
- I: Intervention

After the ABC patient needs are taken care of, the nurse can move down the scale to the next priority. A helpful acronym to remember is **M-A-A-U-A-R**. These are considered second-priority needs.

- M is for mental status changes and alterations
- A is for acute pain

- A is for acute urinary elimination concerns
- U is for unaddressed and untreated problems requiring immediate attention
- A is for abnormal laboratory/diagnostic data outside of normal limits
- R is for risks that include those involving a healthcare problem such as safety, skin integrity, infection, and other medical conditions

Along with the ABC-MAAUAR methods of prioritization, the nurse may also utilize **Maslow's hierarchy of needs.** Maslow argues that physiological needs such as hunger, thirst, and breathing are among the first that have to be met. The same goes for patients. For example, a patient in pain needs to be addressed before a patient who needs education on a procedure that is to happen tomorrow.

After the basic physiological needs have been met, the nurse knows that on the next level of the pyramid are safety and psychological needs. Mental health fits on this tier of the hierarchy and is a crucial step toward wellness. Love and belonging follow; for this part of care the nurse can enlist the help of social services and family members. The next level of Maslow's hierarchy is "self-esteem and esteem by others." In nursing terms, this level represents the patient's need to feel they are a respected and esteemed member of the care team. The final level of Maslow's hierarchy is **self-actualization**, in which a person reaches their fullest potential and highest level of ability. The nurse does everything they can to help the client reach this level, pushing them to do their best and be their best at all points in the care journey.

Recognizing the patient's needs and establishing priorities based on Maslow's hierarchy, the nurse can then move on to the next step of the process: after goal-setting and client care delivery comes the evaluation stage. In fact, evaluation does not happen only at the end. The nurse must be continually evaluating the plan of care for each patient. The plan may need tweaking and revision throughout the day, based on how the patient responds to interventions. Quality evaluation of interventions ensures needs are being met and proper care is being delivered.

Sound nursing judgment will guide the nurse as they endeavor to prioritize and adequately meet the needs of their patients in a timely manner.

Time Management and Work Prioritization

One of the most important skills a nurse must master in the busy health care environment is that of time management and prioritization of tasks. The work day is filled with tasks, scheduled activities, unexpected time conflicts, and constant interruptions.

As best as the nurse can, they should have a way of planning the day. Some find it best to have some sort of written system to take notes and jot down vitals in between charting periods. Meal times can be the busiest times of day, so it should be accounted for in planning.

Countless interruptions will occur throughout the day, such as a call light going off when the nurse was planning to start a bath or a patient needing assistance to the bathroom when the nurse was planning on taking a break. It is vital that the nurse prioritizes tasks and make sure the most important tasks get done in a timely manner. It is easy to put off tasks for later that really should be done immediately, but that sort of procrastination can have adverse results. The day will be busy; that is a given. Developing one's time management and prioritization skills will help the day go a lot more smoothly.

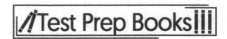

Ethical Practice

Healthcare providers routinely face situations with patients where they must analyze various moral and ethical considerations. In the emergency department, where quick judgment and action is necessary to care and where patients are often not fully sound in body or mind, ethical dilemmas can arise without much time to process resolutions.

Nurses are held to the **American Nurses Association's Code of Ethics**, which states moral and ethical guidelines that nurses should incorporate into their practice. Above all else, nurses have the responsibility to do no harm while advocating for, promoting good health outcomes for, minimizing injury to, and protecting the overall health and functioning of their patients. It is important to consider the patient holistically when applying these values, such as considering what the patient may view as a good quality of life, what family values the patient holds, other family members that may be affected (such as a spouse or children), legal considerations, and logistical considerations (such as how much time and medical resources are available). When patients are unable to make decisions autonomously, or even to indicate consent to treatment (as can be common in emergency cases), nurses should act from these responsibilities to make wise and compassionate decisions on the patients' behalf.

Dilemmas that can arise for nursing staff include situations where the patient may have cultural or personal beliefs that prevent lifesaving treatment. For example, a female emergency patient may not want to be treated by any male staff, or a patient that needs a blood transfusion may not accept this procedure due to religious beliefs. In cases where the patient is able to directly communicate their wishes, the nurse may need to defer to the patient's wishes in order to preserve the patient's autonomy. This may mean providing alternative means of care (such as finding available female medical providers to assist with the female patient that does not wanted to be treated by male staff). It may mean withholding treatment that the patient refuses. If the patient's life is in question and rapid medical action is necessary to save the patient's life, nursing staff may need to intervene even if it is against the patient's wishes. Ethical considerations like these will vary by case and patient, and will depend on the severity of the case, the medical and personal history of the patient, and the judgment of the nurse in question. In all cases, it is ideal if the nurse and patient are able to communicate openly with each other about the case and potential medical options, and hope that the resolution is able to be for the greatest good.

Informed Consent

Before a major medical procedure can be performed, the patient's consent must be obtained. Obtaining this consent requires educating the patient on what the procedure is, how it is performed, what types of outcomes are to be expected, and most importantly, why the procedure will be done. This process of educating the patient and getting their permission is called informed consent.

There are two key aspects of the term **informed consent**. The term "**informed**" implies that the patient has been given information pertaining to the procedure. This requires a conversation between the patient and their health care provider. Education must be provided to ensure that the patient has been given information about the procedure to be done as well as time to consider their options. If a patient signs a consent without having a proper understanding and comprehension of what's to be done, it is not a true informed consent.

The second part of the term is "**consent.**" This means that the patient agrees with the plan and gives their permission for what is going to be done. Without consent, it is illegal or improper to perform certain healthcare procedures.

Consent can be given through three different avenues: implied, verbal, and written. In **implied consent**, the patient has given the health care worker permission to perform interventions on them without writing it down or saying it. This can get into a gray area on some issues, but for the most part, it's agreed upon care that is needed. For example, let's say a patient drops to the floor in full cardiac arrest. They are unresponsive. A nurse witnesses the fall and begins cardiopulmonary resuscitation (CPR) and activates the emergency response system. The patient did not say they agreed to have CPR done on them nor did they sign a document agreeing to the procedure, but it is assumed that the patient is complicit. This is due to the patient's being in danger of death and in need of swift action. On a much smaller scale, a patient coming into a doctor's office does not sign a document of consent to have their vital signs taken, yet they willingly comply with having their blood pressure taken. All parties present assume and agree upon certain procedures and thus no formal consent is required.

Verbal consent is obtained by having the patient saying something along the lines of "Yes, it is okay to do this." This is the in-between consent, slightly more formal than implied consent and less formal than the signed legal document that is informed consent.

Written consent involves a formal conversation between the health care provider, the physician performing the procedure, and the patient. It is vital that the patient is adequately educated on the procedure and has a full understanding before consenting. Obtaining consent without proper patient education is fraudulent and poor practice. Not properly informing the patient may lead to legal trouble down the road for both the nurse and the physician, not to mention potential complications following the procedure. Above all, it is a violation of a patient's rights to not be properly informed before giving consent.

While the physician is legally responsible for satisfying all elements of informed consent, nurses are ethically responsible for assessing the patient's ability to process and understand the implications of informed consent. Nurses should ensure that the patient understands the purpose of a procedure and any possible risks, whether the physician or the nurse themselves explained the information to the patient. The nurse should also be sure the appropriate person to provide informed consent for the patient has been identified and understands the procedure. This may be the patient, his or her legal guardian, parent, etc. Nurses protect the patient's autonomy by raising these questions and concerns.

Information Technology

Information technology (IT) is a field of nursing that continues to evolve with the rest of health care. Nurses must not only understand the science that is associated with nursing, but they must also be able to navigate various forms of technology. While there are nurses still in the workplace who can recall what it was like to physically fill out forms and track vitals on paper, there are also nurses who have no concept of having documented their activities in these systems. All nurses must be able to function within today's technologically advanced world.

IT is important for many reasons including:

- Cost savings/reduction of costs
- Need to decrease or eliminate medication errors

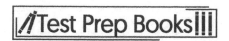

- Improving documentation efficiency by removing paper charting
- Enhancing accessibility to quality health care

Medical technology needs to be fully integrated with a larger system within an institution to support the continuum of patient care. This connection provides information sharing throughout each stage of the treatment period and eventually allows for the collection of statistical data at a later date.

Next, medical technology has to support the user's ability to navigate without difficulty. The goal here is to not slow down the pace of the medical environment but allow for increasing efficiency so that technology is seamless. These qualities then allow for real-time data and real-time decision-making capabilities while reducing the risk of errors or redundancy.

There are a few gaps that remain on the IT front of the medical environment that have their roots in the computerized physician order entry (CPOE) arena. In some instances, CPOE software is not able to meet the needs of various interdisciplinary roles in the OR. The reason for this is that it tends to favor the inpatient setting.

Health Care Information Technology

Health care IT, or HIT, has characteristics that are steeped in supporting broad processes or functions.

HIT is software that can perform operations associated with:

- Admissions
- Scheduling
- Clinical documentation
- Pharmacy
- Laboratory
- Clinical Information Technology

Clinical IT (CIT) concentrates on a particular set of clinical tasks, instruments, equipment, and imaging.

Radio Frequency Identification

Radio frequency identification (RFID) provides support for real-time surgery scheduling. This technology has been shown to drastically enhance the structure and functions within medical software. RFID functions on wireless networks and helps to "tag" items and track the movement of the items as they remain on or leave a particular unit. This may be especially important when tracking equipment or supplies that are used to care for the patient or during a surgical procedure.

Nurses will need to stay current with IT trends and engage in ongoing education and exposure to technology. Continuing education and training can be accomplished through independent reading, e-learning, and live classroom instruction.

Finally, nurses may encounter a broad range of technologies including:

- Robots
- Medication delivery devices
- Instruments
- Biotechnology and nanotechnology
- Digital tracking
- Mobile and wireless devices

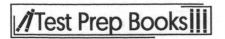

- Nurses and Informatics

Nurses may assist in the development of standards for **EHR (electronic health record)** or other clinically based IT systems that nurses utilize for their sphere of health care. In today's landscape, many nursing applications fall into a variety of categories including:

- Internet-based patient education systems
- EHR
- Telemedicine and telenursing

These systems have the capacity to exchange information and enable the decision-making process to progress along the continuum.

Some nurses possess a master's degree in informatics and also work in a variety of roles to assist with development of clinical systems designed to support nurse activities including:

- Business or clinical analyst
- Project management
- Software developer

These systems are designed to accommodate patient education resources, nursing procedures, and critical pathways, to name a few.

Nurses may also serve in the role of perioperative robotics nurse specialist. As robotic surgery utilization continues to evolve into standard practice, the robotics nurse specialist supports a variety of tasks ranging from scheduling maintenance to assisting during surgery.

Legal Rights and Responsibilities

The nurse must uphold and answer to certain legal rights and responsibilities within their profession. From simple things like managing a patient's property to more complicated issues such as reporting abuse and neglect, the nurse has a legal responsibility to act, or their license could be in danger.

Nurses need a knowledge of the common legal terminology in their practice. The following is a list of terms the nurse should know:

- **Common law:** Common law is based on legal precedents or previously decided cases in courts of law.

- **Statutory law:** These are laws based on a state's legislative actions or any other legislative body's actions.

- **Constitutional law:** Laws based on the content of the Constitution of the United States of America are referred to as constitutional law.

- **Administrative law:** For a nurse, this is a type of law passed down from a ruling body such as a state nursing association. For example, each state's nursing board passes down regulations on continuing education requirements for licensed nurses.

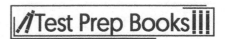

- **Criminal law:** This type of law involves the arrest, prosecution, and incarceration of those who have broken the law. Such offenses as felonies and misdemeanors are covered under criminal law.

- **Liability:** Nurses are liable for their actions while practicing. Thorough documentation and patient charting are important. If an act is not charted, it was not done, so to speak. Nurses must protect themselves legally to maintain their practice.

- **Tort:** In a nursing context, this legal term refers to nursing practice violations such as malpractice, negligence, and patient confidentiality violations.

- **Unintentional tort:** Negligence and malpractice may be unintentional forms of tort.

- **Intentional tort:** On the other hand, torts may be proven to be intentional, including such violations as false imprisonment, privacy breaches, slander, libel, battery, and assault. A nurse using a physical restraint without meeting protocol or getting a physician's order is guilty of false imprisonment. Slander is a form of defamation in which the person makes false statements that are verbal, and libel is written defamation.

A nurse is legally responsible for maintaining an active licensure according to their state's regulatory board's laws. Failure to maintain licensure requirements such as continuing education credits will result in disciplinary action. Nursing licenses may be revoked or suspended because of disciplinary actions.

Nurses must report abuse, neglect, gunshot wounds, dog bites, and communicable diseases. Nurses are also legally mandated to report other health care providers whom they suspect may be abusing drugs or alcohol while practicing, because they are putting patients and themselves at risk.

Nurses have a legal obligation to accept the patient assignments given to them, if they believe they are appropriate and it is within their scope of practice to perform duties related to these patients.

Laws at the national, state, and local level must be complied with by practicing nurses. Such laws include those in relation to the Centers for Medicare and Medicaid services. Another example would be adhering to local laws regarding the disposal of biohazardous waste.

Legal Reporting Obligations

Reporting patient information and work issues in a timely manner and using the correct route on the chain of command are a legal obligation of nurse. Not reporting important information could result in serious ramifications and punitive action for the nurse, up to loss of employment and/or revocation of certification. When important information goes unreported, it can result in patient harm or unresolved conflicts that turn into bigger problems to deal with later on. Addressing patient issues and resolving conflicts all start with accurate and timely reporting.

A basic definition of a **report** is the relaying of information that one has observed or heard. When this report is given to an authority figure who can intervene, it will contain different elements, such as patient name, situation, time of event, and circumstances surrounding the event.

As one shift ends and another begins, there is a **handoff report** that is given from the off-going team to the oncoming team. The nurse who has completed the shift will tell the nurse beginning the next shift all pertinent information related to each individual patient. Another type of reporting is the exchange of smaller pieces of information between members of the health care team that occurs throughout a shift.

In the handoff report, the nurse should strategically relay information in a simple, concise manner that is easily understood by the oncoming nurse. It can be easy to get carried away with reporting and include every little detail of the day, opinions about patients or other coworkers, and stories of particular conversations or interactions that occurred during the shift. These superfluous details should be limited, and the report should be kept to the essential items only.

Some organizations employ the **SBAR method** to help guide communication. SBAR is an acronym for situation, background, assessment, and recommendation. An SBAR report starts with the situation: why is this communication necessary? The background is a brief explanation of the circumstances leading up to the situation. The assessment is what the reporter thinks the issue is, and the recommendation is what the reporter needs in order to correct the situation.

In addition to reporting patient information, the documenting of patient information and interventions performed is also important. A patient's chart is a legal record of observations about the patient and any care given for the patient. Most facilities use an electronic health record, which the nurse will generally be trained to use as a part of new employee orientation. Documentation may include time of observation, time task was performed, what was done, how it was done, and reaction to intervention.

There are various charting systems used to document patient data by patient care facilities. Documentation requirements will be dictated by facility policy and regulatory guidelines. Two methods are used: charting by exception and comprehensive charting.

Charting by Exception

Charting by exception means that besides recording of vital signs, only abnormal findings are documented. This charting method is somewhat controversial as so much information about the patient is usually left out. It is sometimes argued that this is the safer way to chart, as only what is deviant from normal is noted, and thus, there is less room for documentation errors. The normal is assumed, unless otherwise noted. This method also saves time, as less information needs to be documented, leaving more time for patient care.

Comprehensive Charting

Some facilities prefer a **comprehensive method** of documentation, charting everything about the patient—normal and abnormal—in a very thorough manner. This way, when the patient's chart must be reviewed, especially in the case of a safety incident (e.g., a pressure sore develops or a patient falls), all details surrounding the event should be present in the medical record. This method works as long as everything is actually documented, although it can be quite time-consuming and take away from patient care time.

Documentation provides a defense for health care workers and patients in the case of patient incidents to show what was done for the patient. There is an adage that says, "If it wasn't charted, it didn't happen." The nurse needs to be mindful that the medical record is a legal document—a complete, thorough, and accurate documentation of care, according to facility policy.

Performance Improvement (Quality Improvement)

Performance improvement is a mechanism to continuously review and improve processes in a system to ensure that work is completed in the most cost-effective manner while producing the best possible outcomes. Healthcare facilities are constantly hoping to drive down cost and increase reimbursements while delivering the highest quality of healthcare and utilizing analytical methods to achieve this. These

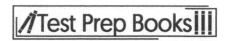

analyses and implementations may be done by top administrative employees at the organization and be executed across the healthcare system, or within a particular department. Leadership support is always crucial for positive change to occur and sustain itself.

All processes should be regularly monitored for opportunities for improvement. Common opportunities include areas of reported patient dissatisfaction; federal, state, or internal benchmarks that are not being met; areas of financial loss; and common complaints among staff. While multiple opportunities for improvement may exist, focusing on one at a time usually produces the greatest outcome. When choosing a process to improve, it is important to select a process that can actually be changed by the members involved (i.e., medical staff often do not have control over external funding sources). Processes where minimal resources are required for change, but that can produce positive end results, are also preferable to costlier improvements. Once the process has been selected, a group of stakeholders that are regularly involved in the process should map out each step of the process while noting areas of wasted resource or process variation. From here, stakeholders can develop a change to test.

The **PDCA cycle** provides a framework for implementing tests of change. Plan, the first step, involves planning the change. This will include accounting for all workflow changes, the staff members involved, and logistics of implementation. It should also include baseline data relating to the problem. Do, the second step, involves implementing the change. During this step, data collection is crucial. For example, if a department believes that implementing mobile work stations will decrease nurses' wait time between patients, the department should keep a detailed record of the time spent with and between each patient. Check, the third step, involves checking data relating to the change with the baseline data and determining if the change improved the process. Act, the final step, involves making the change permanent and monitoring it for sustainability.

Evidence-Based Practice

Evidence-based practice (EBP) is a research-driven and facts-based methodology that allows healthcare providers to make scientifically supported, reliable, and validated decisions in delivering care. EBP takes into account rigorously tested, peer-reviewed, and published research relating to the case, the knowledge and experience of the healthcare provider, and clinical guidelines established by reputable governing bodies. This framework allows healthcare providers to reach case resolutions that result in positive patient outcomes in the most efficient manner. This, in turn, allows the organization to provide the best care using the least resources.

There are seven steps to successfully utilizing EBP as a methodology in the nursing field. First, the work culture should be one of a "spirit of inquiry." This culture allows staff to ask questions to promote continuous improvement and positive process change to workflow, clinical routines, and non-clinical duties. Second, the **PICOT framework** should be utilized when searching for an effective intervention, or working with a specific interest, in a case. The PICOT framework encourages nurses to develop a specific, measurable, goal-oriented research question that accounts for the patient population and demographics (P) involved in the case, the proposed intervention or issue of interest (I), a relevant comparison (C) group in which a defined outcomes (O) has been positive, and the amount of time (T) needed to implement the intervention or address the issue. Once this question has been developed, staff can move onto the third step, which is to research. In this step, staff will explore reputable sources of literature (such as peer-reviewed scholarly journals, interviews with subject matter experts, or widely accepted textbooks) to find studies and narratives with evidence that supports a resolution for their question.

Once all research has been compiled, it must be thoroughly analyzed. This is the fourth step. This step ensures that the staff is using unbiased research with stringent methodology, statistically significant outcomes, reliable and valid research designs, and that all information collected is actually applicable to their patient. (For example, if a certain treatment worked with statistical significance in a longitudinal study of pediatric patients with a large sample size, and all other influencing variables were controlled for, this treatment may not necessarily work in a middle-aged adult. Therefore, though the research collected is scientifically backed and evidence-based for a pediatric population, it does not support EBP for an older population.) The fifth step is to integrate the evidence to create a treatment or intervention plan for the patient. The sixth step is to monitor the implementation of the treatment or intervention and evaluate whether it was associated with positive health outcomes in the patient. Finally, practitioners have a moral obligation to share the results with colleagues at the organization and across the field, so that it may be best utilized (or not) for other patients.

Evidence-Based Practice Flowchart

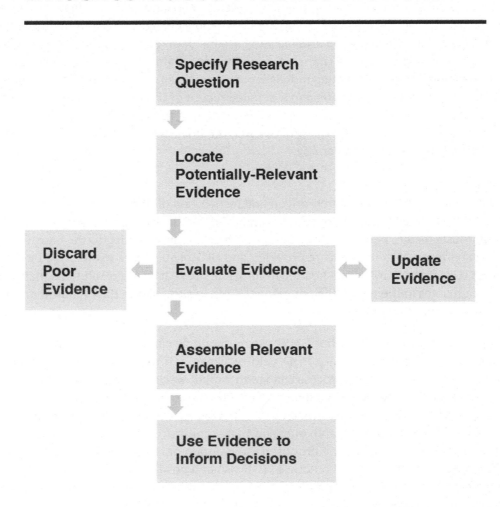

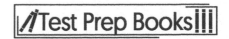

Referrals

As patient advocates, nurses should be knowledgeable about referring clients when a need arises. The nurse is aware of many different branches of the health care tree that are designed to assist with each patient's specific needs. A **referral** is a method by which the nurse contacts another member of the healthcare team to meet the patient's care needs in the most appropriate setting. This is part of care coordination and must happen throughout all stages of the client's continuum of care. Case managers play a key role in making appropriate referrals.

Referral occurs during the first stage of the nursing process: assessment. The nurse assesses the patient and identifies a need. For example, a school nurse may become aware of students who have learning or developmental disabilities. In these cases, the nurse may refer the child and their parents to a speech therapist, a language therapist, or a developmental therapist, depending on the case.

In the hospital environment, the nurse may recognize the need for an auxiliary team and refer the client to them. Such auxiliary teams include the palliative care and hospice team, respiratory therapy, physical and occupational therapy, and speech/language therapy. Community resources should be used when appropriate, such as extended-care therapy, social service support, and shelters for the homeless and disadvantaged. Patients may also need spiritual care, in which case clergy can be requested to make a bedside visit.

With any referral, the nurse must follow the appropriate protocols and remain within their scope of practice. Other members of the health care team such as physicians and nursing management should be consulted. Doctor's orders must be obtained where necessary.

After the referral has been made, it is vital that the nurse or case manager evaluates the patient for their response to care. Evaluation is a key component of the nursing process. Without evaluating for effectiveness, the process is incomplete. Only after evaluation has shown effectiveness and the patient is on their way to recovery can the plan of care be deemed successful.

Safety and Infection Control

Accident/Error/Injury Prevention

The majority of accidents that occur in the older population happen in their homes, with falls being the most common accident. **Accident prevention** involves maintaining a clean home and living area and recognizing potential hazards. In addition, individuals should be knowledgeable and aware of their level of health and their own body's capabilities and weaknesses. Keeping regular appointments at the physician's office and following any medication regime correctly will keep one's health in check. It is important for people to understand and be aware of potential side effects of any medications that they may be taking. Recognizing a side effect could be a way to prevent an accident, especially if it relates to mental status or mobility. For example, blood-pressure medications have the potential to lower blood pressure to the point of the person passing out, ultimately causing a fall. Informal caregivers such as family members should check on elderly family to ensure they are able to continue taking care of themselves and to survey the home for safety hazards.

If an older adult is still living in their home, the following measures should be addressed to avoid accidents related to poisoning, burns, hypothermia, and fires. The main causes of poisoning in adults aged sixty-five and older are medicines and gases. Gases would include carbon monoxide and pipeline gases, such as propane or natural gas for heating the home. Fuel-burning devices should be checked regularly for proper functioning. Chimneys and flues should be cleaned once a year.

Older adults are often on a complicated medication regime involving multiple pills, various dosages, and the different times of the day and week that they should be taken. Medicines should be taken exactly as prescribed, and an organized schedule should be in place to prevent mistakes. One example for organizing medications is a pillbox that has individual compartments for each day of the week.

Burns and scalding in the home can be prevented if water heaters are not set too high, and if the cold water is turned on first. Kettles should be avoided if possible. If necessary, spout-filling kettles, cordless kettles, or wall-mounted heaters can be used instead. Items in the kitchen and the flow of the kitchen should allow for the least amount of distance for carrying hot food or beverages. On the stove, rear burners should be used and handles should be kept away from the edges in order to avoid accidentally knocking a pan off the stove.

An additional accident not often thought of in the older population is **hypothermia**, which means the body's temperature drops below 95 °F. Strategies to prevent hypothermia in the elderly include making sure the home is heated properly in colder weather, providing several layers of clothing, encouraging movement and exercise around the home to increase body heat, and making enough food and drink available.

As previously discussed, falls are the most common accident in the older adult population. Whether the person lives in their home or in a care facility, there are preventative measures that should be put into place.

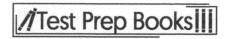

Fall-prevention interventions include:

- Identification of patients at high risk for falls
- Assessment of the patient's room or environment for hazards that can be removed, such as:
  - Rugs
  - Slippery floors
  - Clutter
  - Poor lighting
- Use of assistive devices, such as:
  - Canes, used for stability
  - Walkers, used for balance because of their wide base
  - Reachers or grabbers, used to pick up items off of the floor or reach items on a shelf
  - Gait belts, used with an aide or caregiver, placed around the patient's waist to assist in walking or when standing up from a sitting position
  - Railings in bathrooms, hallways, and tubs
- Proper footwear is worn, such as rubber-soled shoes
- Staff, family-member, and patient education on fall-prevention strategies
- Assistance for patients with daily activities and routines if necessary
- Stairways that are well lit, have railings, and are lined with nonslip flooring

Fall prevention for bed-ridden patients includes:

- Keep two side rails up at all times when a patient is in bed.
- Keep the call light and personal items on a table within reach of the patient's bed.
- Place bed alarms on the patient's bed to alert the staff of any attempt to get out of bed.
- Offer toileting at least every two hours to prevent patients from getting up without assistance.

Falling with a Patient

Sometimes it becomes necessary to assist a person to the ground safely if it becomes clear that they are about to fall. When standing in front or behind the falling person, spreading one's legs apart allows for a wide base of support. Try to keep an arm under their shoulders or under their arms and ease them to the floor. Always attempt to protect their head first, and try to direct them away from hard objects, such as furniture.

Healthcare facilities should identify which patients are at a higher risk for falls, as these patients will require special fall precautions. Some facilities have signs on patients' doors that say "Fall Risk," or a patient may wear a certain color bracelet as a reminder to staff and/or family. Keep in mind that all patients or patients are at risk for a fall, especially if they are elderly. Staff will be educated regarding how much assistance is needed for each patient. For example, patient A may be able to walk with assistance or walk with stand-by assistance. Patient B may need assistance x 2, or two staff persons, to help transfer.

Assistance for Ambulation

The types of assistance needed for ambulation are as follows:

- **Stand by assistance (SBA):** This patient does not require any assistance to move and can walk independently, though someone should be standing by to monitor. A gait belt is not required.

- **Contact-guard assistance (CGA):** This patient requires an assistant to be within reach in case of a fall. These patients can walk independently but have a high risk for falls.

- **Minimum assistance (MIN):** This patient needs a little support when moving about, and an example would be the use of a gait belt.

- **Maximum assistance (MAX):** This patient is unstable and may not be able to walk or stand without help. At least two staff persons are needed for assistance.

Patients who use assistive devices for ambulation need instruction on how to use them and may need reminders to ensure they are still using the device properly. It is important to stay with a patient who is learning to use an assistive device. A gait belt should be used while the patient is learning to use a walker.

Canes

The purpose of the cane is to help stabilize a leg that is weak. Steps for using a cane are listed below:

- Have the patient place the cane in their strong hand and move the cane out one step while stepping the weak leg out with the cane.
- With their weight on the cane, have them step out with their stronger leg.
- After each step, the patient can rest to ensure they feel balanced.

A Walker Without Wheels

A walker is used to give the patient extra stability when a patient is weak in both legs or has trouble with balance when walking. Steps for use are listed below:

- Instruct the patient to stand inside the walker while holding onto the walker with both hands.

- Have the patient lift and move the walker forward so that the back legs of the walker line up with their toes.

- With their weight on their stronger leg, have the patient take a step with their weaker leg while gripping the handrails of the walker. They should step into the center of the walker.

- Finally, their stronger leg steps up to evenly meet their other leg. They may rest in between steps if necessary.

Care must be taken to ensure that the flooring surface is flat when using a walker or a cane. Trips or falls can occur if rugs or thick carpet get caught in the walker or cane. Some walkers have wheels on the bottoms of the legs so that a patient can push the walker while walking. The wheels may be on all four legs or just the front two legs. The patient's weight is placed on the walker with their hands, and this helps with extra support as they lean forward. These types of walkers are not lifted during walking and allow for a bit faster pace. Make sure while walking that the walker does not move too far ahead of the patient.

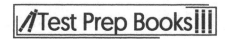

Here are steps for moving from a chair to standing with a walker:

- Place the walker in front of the patient and have the patient place their hands on the arms of the chair.
- Assist the patient with standing up.
- Encourage the patient to place one hand at a time onto the handgrips of the walker.
- Ensure the patient feels steady and is not dizzy before walking.

Use of Crutches

Crutches can be used on a short-term basis when a patient has limitations for weight bearing on a leg. An example would be a patient that has a cast or a splint on their ankle, foot, or leg. Putting weight on an injured leg may interfere with healing and may be painful. A physical therapist will be responsible for fitting the crutches. Ensure the crutches are the appropriate length for the patient. The armpit, or axilla, rests should fit into the patient's armpit without lifting the shoulders and without causing stooping. The pads should be one to one-and-a-half inches below the axilla. If the crutches are too tall, the patient could trip over the crutches and too much pressure will be placed in their armpits. If the crutches are too short, leaning over will put unnecessary strain on the patient's back. The handgrips should also be adjusted so that the arms are slightly bent at the elbow. The grip should be comfortable.

Crutch Gaits

The **three-point crutch gait** helps with an inability to bear weight on one leg, such as with fractures, pain, or amputation.

- Move both crutches and the weaker leg forward. Then place all weight down on the crutches and move the stronger or unaffected leg forward. Repeat this pattern.

- Good balance is required for this type of gait.

The **two-point crutch gait** is used for weakness in both legs and poor coordination.

- Move the left crutch and right foot together.
- Then move the right crutch and left foot together.
- Repeat the pattern.
- This is a faster gait but difficult to learn.

The **swing-through crutch gait** helps with an inability to bear full weight on both legs.

- Move both crutches forward then swing both legs forward at the same time. The legs must swing past the crutches.

- This is the fastest gait but requires a lot of arm strength and energy.

- It will not be used in the elderly.

The **swing-to crutch gait** is used for patients who have weakness in both legs.

- Move both crutches forward.

- Put weight on both crutches and swing both legs forward together to the crutches. The legs must not swing past the crutches.

- This requires good arm strength, so it most likely will not be used for the elderly.

Standing up with crutches:

- Have the patient hold both crutches on their injured side, and then lean forward off of the chair while pushing off with their arm from the chair.

- Once standing, place the crutches under the arms.

Sitting down with crutches:

- Have the patient place both crutches on their injured side.

- Holding the handgrips in one hand, they can use their other hand to brace on the chair as they sit.

Using crutches on stairs should not be attempted until the patient is confident on level ground. Until then, or at any time, the patient can also slide up or down the stairs on their bottom. Also, the railing of the stairs can be used with one hand while holding the crutches in the other arm.

- The crutches should stay on the step the patient is standing on.

- The good leg is brought up to the next step while letting the injured leg lag behind.

- As the patient straightens up to their good leg, they should bring the crutches and their injured leg up onto the step.

Going down steps:

- Have the patient place the crutches on the next step lower and bring their injured foot forward.

- Next, the good foot is moved down to meet the crutches on the lower step. The weight is on the crutches at this time.

Emergency Response Plan

In the case of an emergency, a nurse must be prepared to recommend certain clients for an immediate discharge, activate the emergency response plan, and participate in disaster drills. Each facility must have plans for emergency situations, and the nurse may be a part of such planning.

Disasters can be internal or external. Examples of internal disasters include fires; violence in the workplace; failure of utilities such as water or electricity; or electrical outage or flooding in the building caused by weather disasters such as tornadoes, hurricanes, or earthquakes. An external disaster can include a serious community event in which a population sustains many injuries. Such events can include mass shootings, train wrecks, and airplane crashes. Acts of terrorism or bioterrorism can affect a facility both internally and externally. Weather events can affect a health care facility both internally and externally, depending on the extent of damage that occurs.

A recent example of an act of terrorism that caused a massive influx of patients to local hospitals was the Route 91 shooting in Las Vegas. This was an external event that caused the activation of certain emergency response plans to deal with the influx of incoming patients. Such events must be discussed

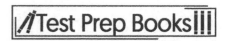

as a potential occurrence in each facility. Health care facilities must put plans in place to deal with such catastrophes in a smooth, coordinated manner to effectively care for the maximum number of patients.

The hurricanes Irma and Harvey that recently struck the Gulf states are an example of an external weather situation that directly affected those communities with electrical power losses, flooding, destruction of property, and injuries and illness related to the flooding and high winds. The health care system must be ready for these situations with an effective emergency response plan.

One of the first steps when activating an emergency response plan is to discharge patients who are medically stable enough, in order to clear beds for incoming patients. Facilities only have a set number of beds available for patients. When the influx of patients is greater than the number of beds available, a crisis arises. When a catastrophic event occurs, the nurse is part of a triaging process that determines whether certain patients can be relocated to open beds for incoming patients. Unstable clients will stay put; they are at the top of the rung of patients to stay. Stable patients may be discharged only if it is likely they will remain stable without ongoing nursing and medical care. On the bottom rung below unstable and stable clients are ambulatory and self-care clients. These are patients who are walking around and able to independently care for themselves outside a hospital facility. Ambulatory and self-care patients will be discharged to clear beds for incoming disaster patients.

The nurse plays a key role in disaster preparedness and knowing that role is key to a successful execution of each emergency response plan. During a fire, for example, the nurse must competently implement all four elements of the **RACE acronym**, as follows:

- **R** is for rescuing all those in danger, including patients, visitors, and staff.

- **A** is for activating the alarm after those in danger have been cleared.

- **C** is for containing the fire in the smallest possible area. This is accomplished by closing all windows and doors, preventing the fire from spreading.

- **E** is for extinguishing the fire if it is small enough and the nurse can do so safely.

Concurrent with knowledge of the RACE acronym during a fire is knowledge of how to use a fire extinguisher. There are five main types of fire extinguishers: Type A, Type B, Type C, Type AB, and Type ABC. **Type A extinguishers** are used for common solids such as paper, mattresses, and clothing. **Type B extinguishers** target oil, gasoline, and grease fires, common in kitchens. **Type C extinguishers** fight electrical fires. **Type AB** combines the roles of Type A and Type B, while Type ABC combines all three. **Type ABC** is the most commonly seen due to its ability to extinguish all types of fire sources. This is likely the type of extinguisher located within a hospital facility for that reason.

When attempting to use a fire extinguisher, the nurse must remember the acronym "**PASS**," which describes the following steps for effective use:

- **P** is for pull, pulling the pin to begin using the fire extinguisher.

- **A** is for aim, aiming directly at the bottom of the fire.

- **S** is for squeeze, squeezing the trigger to release the spray.

- **S** is for sweep, moving from side to side across the base of the fire. This will effectively extinguish the fire.

Along with knowing their role when fire threatens the safety of patients, the nurse must also know what to do when the hospital's utilities fail. Electricity powers many life-supporting machines for patients, such as oxygen delivery systems and mechanical ventilation machines. Most hospitals have back-up generators to keep these machines going when the power goes down. The nurse must alert maintenance and management immediately if the power goes off. Many hospitals have special red outlets into which important patient machinery should be plugged for just that reason.

There are times in the workplace when the nurse may encounter violence, harassment, or aggression. The source of these behavioral conflicts may be a visitor, fellow staff member, or patient. Causes of workplace violence may include delirium and disorientation, especially in hospitalized patients with illness and medication side effects in play. Visitors and family members may become disruptive for any number of reasons, including misunderstandings about care during high-stress and emotionally charged health care situations involving a loved one. Whatever the cause, the nurse must work to de-escalate the situation verbally as well as enlisting help from team members and hospital security staff.

Each health care facility will have explicit guidelines that must be followed in the case of a weather emergency, such as a hurricane, tornado, or earthquake. Closing windows, doors, and curtains as well as moving patients to the appropriate pre-determined safe place are all part of the nurse's role during these situations.

For all these emergencies, a chain of command needs to be established long before a catastrophic event occurs. This lays out in clear terms who is in charge during the disaster, who needs to know what, who takes on leadership roles, and so on. Clearly defining the roles of each team member and rehearsing what will happen by using emergency drills ensures that things are run smoothly and efficiently in the event of a disaster.

Ergonomics Principles

Ergonomics is the science of matching the physical requirements of a job to the physical abilities of the worker. Musculoskeletal injuries can occur if physical demands are greater than the employee's physical capabilities. Body mechanics refers to how the body moves during activities of daily living. Understanding and practicing the use of proper body mechanics is imperative to preventing associate injury. The physical requirements of a job are explained during the interview process, and the physical capabilities of the associate are assessed during the pre-employment physical examination. Education on the use of proper body mechanics begins in nursing school and continues during employment. New associate orientation should include validation of proper body mechanics.

Principles of Body Mechanics
One way the nurse can take care of themselves is to employ proper body mechanics. The job of the nurse is often highly physical in nature, with much time being spent on turning patients in bed, transferring them from the bed to the chair or bedside commode, and assisting with **ambulating** (walking) patients to the bathroom or around the unit. Moving another person, especially one with limited ability to assist, can be extremely difficult and taxing on the body.

Depending on the facility in which the nurse works, different equipment will be available to assist with moving patients. Becoming acquainted with how and when to use this equipment will be part of the nurse's training in that facility. The nurse should use this equipment whenever possible, even if it takes a little more time to do so.

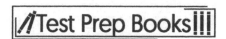

Basic **safe lifting techniques** include lifting with one's legs, not one's back, avoiding twisting and awkward positions when lifting and moving the patient, and keeping the back upright as much as possible to avoid straining. The individual should make sure to keep their feet as balanced as possible and not rush lifting or moving a patient. The nurse should ask for help from other nurses or nurses whenever needed to avoid injury.

The medical environment can present potential hazards that increase risk of injury to the nurse. Examples of these are transferring the patient from the cart to the operating room bed, positioning the patient, and standing for prolonged periods. Repetitive motions, such as turning the head to one side for visualization of monitoring equipment and holding a retractor for an extended time period, can also present ergonomic hazards. Proper body mechanics should be consistently followed to prevent injury. There are **three foundational principles of proper body mechanics** that should be followed by nurses. First, bending at the hips and knees instead of at the waist uses the large muscle groups of the legs instead of the back muscles, and helps to prevent back injury. Second, standing with feet at about shoulder-width apart helps to reduce risk of injury by providing foundational support. Finally, the nurse should keep the back, neck, pelvis, and feet aligned when turning or moving. Twisting and bending at the neck and waist can increase risk of associate injury.

As a standard of care, many healthcare institutions have mandated use of **safe patient mobilization (SPM)** equipment in an effort to reduce associate injuries, as well as to promote patient safety. SPM equipment in the medical environment can be used during patient transfers and positioning. Slide sheets are often used in patient transfers. These sheets are placed underneath the patient prior to lateral or vertical transfer. They decrease the surface tension, making transfers easier for the associates. However, since the slide sheets do decrease surface tension, they must be removed after use, so that the patient is not at risk of sliding off the operating room bed. Inflatable blankets can be placed under the patient to assist in lateral transfers, as well. When engaged, the forced air blanket helps to support the weight of the patient, making lateral transfers easier. The mattress should be deflated after completion of transfer. Another type of SPM equipment is lift equipment. Lift equipment works by placing a sling under the patient's limb or underneath the entire patient, connecting the sling to the lift machine, and programming the machine to lift the body to the desired height. The weight limits of these machines vary, so the nurse must ensure the patient's weight does not exceed the weight limit set by the manufacturer.

Injury Prevention

A member of the health care team who is not careful could easily become injured, potentially resulting in physical harm, missed days of work, lost wages, and medical bills. Nurses are at high risk for injury due to the amount of lifting they do during a shift. Using the appropriate lifting techniques can help prevent an injury to the back and strains or sprains to the joints of the body. The nurse should employ assistive devices such as gait belts and mechanical lifting devices whenever possible. It is important to ask for help whenever necessary to prevent injury. The following depicts eight steps to use when lifting a heavy object:

1. Plan for lift and test the load
2. Ask someone for help
3. Get a firm footing
4. Bend your knees
5. Tighten stomach muscles
6. Lift with legs
7. Keep the load close to you

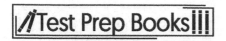

8. Keep your back straight

Self-Care

The job of a nurse is physically, mentally, and emotionally stressful. The strain of moving and lifting patients, along with going from room to room constantly answering the needs of the patients for a long shift, can be physically exhausting. One must organize one's time, prioritize tasks, answer questions, and have countless conversations with the health care team and patients and their families, all of which can take a mental toll. Dealing with patients who are sick, in pain, suffering, and, in some cases, facing death, can drain a nurse's emotional reserves, which can quickly lead to burnout if left unaddressed. Being aware of this potential for overall fatigue is the first step to managing stress and maintaining one's own health.

It is important that a nurse knows how to cope with the effects of stress positively. **Negative coping mechanisms** include unhealthy eating habits and binging behavior, abusing substances such as alcohol and drugs, acting recklessly with one's own safety, and becoming abusive in personal relationships.

Positive coping mechanisms include finding an activity to engage in to unwind and relieve stress in a healthy way. Activities such as daily exercise, spending quality time with friends and family, cooking, yoga, biking, and hiking are all ways to deal with the stress of a demanding job in a healthy way.

The nurse should be careful not to work too many hours as well. It can be tempting to take on extra shifts continually to earn extra money for gifts, vacations, or simply to pay the bills and support a family. These extra shifts and long hours can put a nurse in a danger zone if they are using up too much mental, physical, and/or emotional energy. It is better to be well rested and have adequate mental and physical energy for a shift than to put the patient and oneself at risk for harm.

Being properly nourished, getting adequate exercise, and maintaining healthy sleep habits will all positively contribute to a nurse's health. The nurse's health is vital to helping their patients regain or maintain their own health and, thus, should be made a high priority. If one needs help learning healthy eating habits, meal planning, how to get involved in an exercise program or routine, or other methods of managing stress, many facilities have programs to help guide employees toward better health. There are a plethora of available online resources aimed at improving one's health as well.

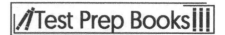

Handling Hazardous and Infectious Materials

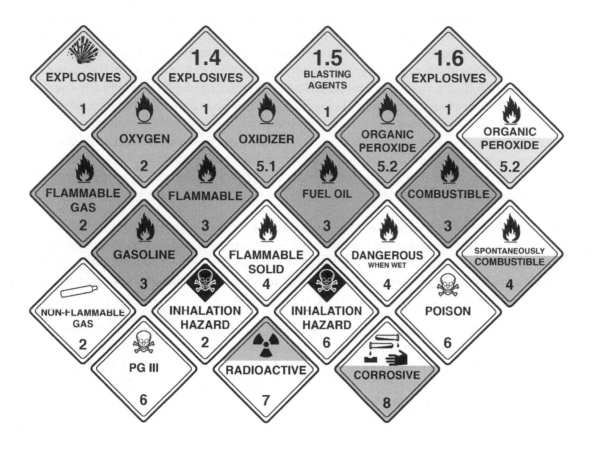

According to the Institute of Hazardous Materials Management (IHMM), a **hazardous material** is defined as "any item that has the potential to cause harm to humans, animals, or the environment, either by itself or through interaction with other factors." A hazardous item may be biological, chemical, radiological, and/or physical in nature. Agencies such as the United States Environmental Protection Agency (EPA) and the Occupational Safety and Health Administration (OSHA) provide regulation and guidelines as to how hazardous materials are handled.

Hazardous materials in the medical environment can include biological, chemical, radiological, and physical hazards. Biological hazardous materials are commonly referred to as **biohazards**. These are materials that present a threat to the health of living things, primarily humans. Biohazards are typically introduced into the medical environment in the form of patient body fluids and excreta. Examples of biohazardous materials are blood, body fluids, viruses, and bacteria. Items in the medical environment that have been exposed to biohazardous materials are considered to be biohazardous, as well, until the decontamination process is completed. For example, used surgical instruments are considered biohazardous until they have been cleaned of bioburden and sterilized.

Chemical hazardous materials in the medical environment include solid, liquid, or gas materials that pose a threat to health. Primarily, solid and liquid chemical hazards include materials used to clean, disinfect, and sanitize the medical environment. They may also include cytotoxic and chemotherapy medications. Gas chemicals are primarily anesthetic gases. Containers for chemical hazards are labeled with symbols representing the type of potential hazard, along with instructions for steps to take in the event of exposure.

Radiological hazards found in the medical environment are seen in the forms of thermal, radioactive isotopes, and electromagnetic radiation. The most common thermal radiological hazard is in the form of laser. The use of lasers exposes the patient and the health care team to risk of eye damage, as well as increasing the risk of fire in the operating room. Laser operators must be trained on the correct usage of the laser, along with indicated safety precautions. Radioactive isotopes are used in brachytherapy. **Brachytherapy** is a form of cancer treatment where radioactive beads are inserted near or inside a cancerous tumor in order to deliver a high dose of radiation to the tumor while sparing the surrounding healthy tissue. Electromagnetic radiation is seen in the form of x-ray and ultraviolet radiation. During a procedure where electromagnetic radiation is used, the patient is protected by shields and/or drapes specifically designed to minimize exposure to the radiation. The perioperative team utilizes shields, gowns, and eyewear to minimize radiation exposure.

Physical hazards also exist in the medical area. **Autoclaves** are used to steam sterilize surgical instruments, and this steam can potentially cause burns. Removing surgical instruments straight from the autoclave can cause burns to the hands if the proper gloves are not used. Liquid on the floor can cause someone to slip or fall, causing injury. Handling carbon dioxide tanks or cryogenic material can cause severe burns to the hands if gloves are not worn.

The types of hazards should be discussed at the beginning of employment in the medical environment. This should include identifying the potential hazards and known hazards, steps to minimize exposure to them, and discussing the necessary steps to take in case of exposure. Healthcare facilities are required to provide materials safety data sheets (MSDS) and keep them in a central area. For most healthcare facilities, education on hazardous materials management is done on an annual basis.

Home Safety

The nurse works to promote patient safety by ensuring their home environment is safe. The nurse will begin this process by first assessing the client's home for safety opportunities. This can be done by walking through the client's home taking mental and written notes as well as interviewing the patient and their caregiver.

The patient themselves must be assessed for their ability to live safely in their own home. Patients with dementia, Alzheimer's, and other cognitive dysfunctions present more of a risk to themselves than a patient whose cognitive faculties are well intact. The nurse may assess whether the patient is able to live independently, need constant supervision, or need assistance with only a few daily activities. An important consideration is how well the patient can follow their own medication regime. The nurse should consider whether the use of divided days-of-the-week pill boxes would be appropriate, for example. Once the client's cognitive function is assessed and addressed, the nurse can then move on to ensuring the external environment is safe.

The external environment of the patient's home poses many potential safety hazards. The patient may live in a multiple-story house, in which case the stairs present a fall risk for elderly and deconditioned patients. A hand rail may be helpful if it is not already present, as well as safety treads on the staircase. Some patients with chronic conditions that restrict them from climbing up and down stairs may require a chair elevator. The nurse can connect the patient and their family to community resources for such items.

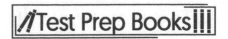

The lighting in the home is as important as the lighting in a hospital room. One of the classic fall prevention tips in the hospital is to ensure the patient's room is adequately lit both in the daytime and at night. The same goes for the client's home. The nurse needs to ensure nightlights are available in rooms that the client may need to ambulate across during the night, such as the bedroom. Visits to the bathroom should be unencumbered and easily navigated, without fall risks in the way. Due to medication and chronic illnesses such as heart failure, visits to the bathroom often increase in the elderly patient, thus increasing fall risk.

The nurse should discourage the use of throw rugs in the homes of patients at risk for a fall. This type of rug can easily catch the client's foot, throwing them off balance and potentially causing a fall.

The house should be well kept, clean, and sanitary. If the client is not able to keep up with their normal housekeeping duties, assistance should be sought. The nurse can, again, connect the client to community resources in this case. Perhaps a church friend, community volunteer, or local housekeeping service if affordable for the client may be used. A cluttered home may present a fall risk, and it also negatively affects the mental health of the client, causing anxiety and depressive symptoms.

Some clients, such as those with diabetes, may have syringes to administer insulin that will need proper disposal. The nurse may provide the client with a sharps container for syringe disposal as well as educating the patient on proper syringe hygiene and disposal. The nurse should ensure that the client understands these concepts to prevent at-home injuries.

Food hygiene is an important topic to address with the client if they are still preparing their own food. Hand hygiene before, after, and during food preparation is vital to preventing the spread of food-borne illnesses. The client should be educated on the proper handling of meats, ensuring that they not only perform frequent hand hygiene, but that they properly sanitize surfaces that raw meat touches, such as cutting boards.

The nurse needs to assess household alarms such as fire, smoke, and carbon monoxide alarms and ensure that they have fresh batteries and are in working order. The client should be educated to monitor these alarms as needed so they are ready to go in the case of a fire or carbon monoxide leak.

Patients receiving oxygen therapy should be educated on proper oxygen use and maintenance of their oxygen tank. They will be taught not to smoke while receiving oxygen, because this is a fire hazard. They will also need to monitor the tank's gauges to make sure they know when they are running low on oxygen and need a replacement tank.

Reporting of Incident/Event/Irregular Occurrence/Variance

If there is an unanticipated or adverse event, the nurse should follow the facility's policies and procedure for reporting and documentation. One of the first activities, of course, after the patient is stable, should be to inform the respective manager or charge nurse of the event. The facility may have internal processes to follow as well to ensure they are protected as best as possible from medicolegal action.

One of the more common reportable events that the nurse will be involved in is an incorrect count. In the event of an incorrect count, the circulator should make attempts to recover the missing item. The circulator should also follow the facility's policies and procedures; at some facilities, x-ray may not be required for needles smaller than a certain size because they are typically not visible on x-ray. If an intraoperative x-ray is required for a potentially retained object, the team should ensure that the integrity of the sterile field is maintained because the x-ray may be performed prior to full closure of the incision.

Following reasonable attempts to recover the potentially retained object, the circulator should complete the necessary documentation in the patient's chart, such as which count is incorrect, what actions were taken to recover the object, and who was notified. In addition to the documentation in the patient record, the facility's policies may require reporting of the incident in an internal system. This allows the facility to gather additional data that may not be appropriate for the patient record. In the event of a retained foreign object, the facility can use this information to determine if all appropriate actions were taken.

Safe Use of Equipment

The use of medical devices, including equipment used in the operating room, is regulated by the United States Food and Drug Administration (FDA). The Joint Commission (TJC) and the Centers for Medicare and Medicaid Services (CMS) also provide oversight on the proper use of surgical equipment. Both TJC and CMS require the presence of manufacturer's **instructions for use (IFU)** to be present in areas where the equipment is used. Prior to surgical equipment being used on patients, the IFU are established by the device manufacturer. It is important for care providers to use the equipment only per manufacturer guidelines, since these guidelines are the ones tested and approved as safe for patient use by the FDA. If a safety concern regarding the equipment arises, the FDA recalls the product until the safety issue is resolved. For example, if a specific type of surgical guidewire breaks off at the tip and causes patient harm, the product may be recalled and pulled from circulation until further investigation.

The product manufacturer's IFU indicates if the equipment poses a fire, electrical, laser, or radiation hazard. If the product does pose one of these hazards, the IFU indicates the type(s) of hazard and the recommendations for protecting the patient and equipment users from the hazard. For instance, if the product poses a fire hazard, the IFU contains information stating which type of fire extinguisher should be available. Also, the IFU states whether to have liquid (sterile water or sterile saline) on the surgical field as a precautionary measure.

TJC and CMS observe infection control practices such as chemical disinfection and sterilization of surgical instruments during site visits to ensure healthcare facility compliance. If disinfection and sterilization are not performed according to manufacturer guidelines, the cleanliness/sterility of the surgical equipment cannot be verified. Manufacturer instructions for use should be available in each area where surgical equipment is used. Many healthcare facilities utilize **OneSOURCE**, an online database of manufacturer instructions for use. Since OneSOURCE is an electronic database, the contents are updated automatically, eliminating the need to update unit-based binders.

Security Plan

Within the healthcare facility, maintaining a strong security system is vital for patient and staff safety. The nurse will likely be trained in and involved with the hospital's security team, playing an active role in promoting a safe environment.

There are many ways a hospital can be threatened. A baby may be abducted from the hospital nursery, a hacker may breach the hospital's firewall and access private patient data, a violent person may enter the hospital and begin shooting people, a patient may run away, or a person may make a bomb threat.

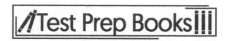

Whatever the threat, the facility will likely have a plan in place to quickly deal with the threat and neutralize it.

The nurse may be involved with a hospital security planning team. These types of teams meet to discuss potential threats and draw up a plan. The nurse can voice their opinion and contribute helpful ideas to effectively deal with the situation. The security team can share key tips with the rest of the staff based on their training and experience. These tips benefit the overall security of the facility. Planning, training, and drills all ensure that if a threat were to happen, the team is ready to respond.

Within the hospital, there are various methods of alerting the staff to a security breach. There may be alarm systems, announcements made over a PA system, or a text alert system on the staff's phones that notifies everyone of the situation. Many hospitals have closed circuit television security monitoring systems that employ cameras and video screens to monitor high-risk areas such as entrances and isolation rooms for violent patients. Certain security doors may be used to keep areas of the hospital off-limits to visitors or can close off areas of the hospital as needed.

Many hospitals use identification badges and bands to identify who is who and ensure only authorized persons and personnel are in certain areas. For example, the mother and father of a baby often get a special ID band identifying them as such, ensuring that no one else is permitted access to a baby, in case they might attempt an abduction.

If the nurse receives a bomb threat over the phone, they should attempt to stay on the line with the person making the threat as long as possible. The nurse may alert other staff of the bomb threat to get the security team in action, while trying to collect as much data on the perpetrator as possible. This information can include sound of their voice, whether they are male or female, and any other information the nurse can get out of them such as their location, the bomb location, and their motive. The nurse may even be able to de-escalate the situation over the phone if they remain calm and collected, but the situation should be handed over to the experts on the security team as soon as possible.

Standard Precautions/Transmission-Based Precautions/Surgical Asepsis

Infection prevention is an important theme in health care, particularly in the surgical patient population. A main focus of nurses is protecting patients and health care associates from transmission of infectious organisms. **Standard precautions** are applied during direct patient contact and the patient's environmental contact. Standard precautions are followed universally by health care providers, and they are the foundation for preventing disease transmission in all health care settings. Included in standard precautions are hand hygiene, **personal protective equipment (PPE)**, environmental control, and sharps safety. Hand hygiene is the gold standard for preventing disease transmission. In compliance with standard precautions, the nurse performs hand hygiene before and after patient contact, before and after applying exam gloves, after touching anything in the patient's environment, before eating, and after using the restroom. PPE protects the nurse from coming into contact with the patient's bodily fluids and other potentially infectious material. Examples of PPE are gloves, masks, gowns, shoe covers, and eye shields. Surfaces in the patient environment are laden with bacteria and other infectious agents. Environmental contamination is directly linked to pathogen transmission and hospital-acquired infections (HAIs). Reusable laundry and textiles should be changed and laundered between each patient and in a health care–accredited laundry facility. Syringes and needles should be limited to single-patient use in compliance with evidence-based care related to infection control. Sharps should include safety devices, when possible. Angiocaths (IV needles) and surgical blades are available with built-in safety features that cover the sharp when not in use, decreasing the change of needle-stick exposure to patient body fluids. Transmission-based precautions are to be used with patients with known or suspected infection with highly transmissible pathogens. These are to be used along with standard precautions.

Transmission-based precautions are classified in three ways: contact, droplet, and airborne. **Contact precautions** are used with patients infected or colonized with microorganisms transmitted by direct or indirect contact. These include *Clostridium difficile (C. diff),* methicillin-resistant *Staphylococcus aureus* (MRSA), and vancomycin-resistant *Enterococcus* (VRE). When caring for these patients, the nurse dons a gown and gloves prior to entering the patient room. The PPE is discarded immediately prior to leaving the patient room, and hand hygiene is performed immediately. **Droplet precautions**, in addition to standard precautions, are used if a patient has a confirmed or suspected infection transmissible through respiratory droplets. PPE associated with droplet precautions are gloves, gown, and mask. The patient is also placed in a single-patient room. Influenza and respiratory syncytial virus (RSV) are indications for droplet precautions. **Airborne precautions** are taken when providing care to a patient with known or suspected infection transmissible via airborne route. The patient's respiratory particles are airborne for prolonged time periods and are carried by normal air currents. PPE for these patients includes gloves, gown, and surgical mask with respirator level of N95 or higher. The most common airborne-transmissible infections are tuberculosis, measles, and varicella.

Spread of Disease-Causing Organisms

Microorganisms that cause infection can be spread by touching surfaces, equipment, people, and bodily fluids, as well as by breathing in **airborne droplets**, such as those that exit the nostril when a person sneezes. Touching infectious microorganisms followed by contact on the hands, face, mouth, eyes, or with food can spread the germs. A clean environment and good handwashing not only protect healthcare workers from infectious germs, but protect the patients as well. Infections can spread from patient to patient, from caregiver to patient and vice versa.

There are three types of infections: viral, bacterial and fungal. **Fungal Infections** are caused by spores of fungus that usually affect the skin but also can be inhaled and cause respiratory infections. Examples of fungal skin infections include Athlete's foot, ringworm, and yeast infections. Fungal infections can be spread by touching the lesion or skin area that is infected.

Bacteria and **viruses** are caused by microbes, or microscopic organisms. Both of these types of infection can produce similar symptoms, including:

- Coughing and/or sneezing
- Inflammation (swelling)
- Fever
- Vomiting
- Diarrhea
- Fatigue

Bacteria and viruses are both too small to see without a microscope, but they differ in how they infect the body. Bacteria are complex and can reproduce or multiply on their own. They can live in extreme environments, such as heat and cold, and can infect both the bodies of animals and humans. Bacterial infections are usually localized or found in contained areas of the body, such as the sinuses (sinus infection). Most bacteria are harmless and actually necessary to the body. One example is the bacteria

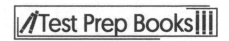

in our gut, which is important for digesting food. Bacterial infections are treated with antibiotics, which will either kill the bacteria or stop the growth of the bacteria that has entered the body.

There are many different types of bacterial infections. Some common bacterial skin infections include cellulitis, folliculitis, impetigo, and boils. Foodborne bacterial infections usually cause vomiting, diarrhea, fever, chills, and abdominal pain. Harmful bacteria may be in raw meat, fish, eggs, and poultry, and in unpasteurized dairy products. The bacterial growth can be caused by unsanitary food preparation and handling.

Sexually-transmitted bacterial infections include chlamydia, gonorrhea, syphilis, and bacterial vaginosis. There are many additional types of infections, such as otitis media (ear infection), urinary tract infections, and respiratory tract infections. Infections in the respiratory tract can be from bacteria or a virus, and they can cause a sore throat, bronchitis, sinus infections, tuberculosis, or pneumonia.

Viruses are different from bacteria in that they need another cell in order to reproduce, or multiply. They attach to a cell in the body and change the cell to make more of the virus. Eventually, the original body cell dies. Viral infections do not respond to antibiotics and are more difficult to treat. Unlike bacteria, most viruses cause infection. The common cold is most often caused by a virus in the rhinovirus family and is an example of a mild virus. An example of life-threatening viruses is the human immunodeficiency virus (HIV). Vaccines do a good job of protecting against viruses such as polio, chicken pox, influenza, and measles. There are antiviral drugs available to treat certain viruses.

Common types of respiratory viruses include influenza-causing viruses, respiratory syncytial virus, and **rhinoviruses,** which is most often the cause of the common cold. Viral skin infections can include **Molluscum contagiosum** (small, harmless bumps on the skin), herpes simplex virus-1 (cold sores), and **varicella zoster virus**, which is similar to the chickenpox. Foodborne viral infections are the most common cause of food poisoning and can include the hepatitis A virus, norovirus, and rotavirus. Viruses that are transmitted sexually include human papilloma virus, hepatitis B, genital herpes (herpes simplex-2), and HIV. Other types of viruses include Epstein-Barr, West Nile, and viral meningitis.

Bacteria and viruses can be spread by:

- Droplet contact from coughing and sneezing
- Contact with infected people
- Contact with infected animals, like livestock, pets, fleas, and ticks
- Contact with infected surfaces, like tabletops or railings
- Contact with contaminated food or water

Microbes can cause acute infections, chronic infections, or latent infections. **Acute infections** last for a short period of time and chronic infections can last for weeks, months, or years. **Latent infections** may not show any symptoms at first and then may reappear, or show up after months or years.

Handwashing with soap and water is the number one way to prevent the spread of germs. The soap removes the visible dirt and invisible germs from the hands, and the water rinses them off.

Handwashing steps:

- Remove any jewelry or watches and pull long sleeves up past the wrists.

- Turn on the water and use warm water.

- Place soap in one hand and rub for at least twenty seconds.

- Make sure to rub the top and palms of the hands. Rub between the fingers and around the nails.

- Wash above the wrists.

- If there was contact with bodily fluids, wash for at least one minute.

- Be sure not to touch the sides of the sink during the process (the washing process would then need to be repeated).

- Rinse hands with fingers facing down so that the soap and germs run off, rather than back up the arms.

- Dry hands with a paper towel, or clean hand towel.

- Use the towel to turn off the faucet.

When to perform handwashing:

- After using the bathroom
- After sneezing or handling tissues
- Before and after eating
- Before entering a patient's room
- Before and after feeding a patient
- Before and after performing a procedure on a patient
- Before and after coming in contact with a wound
- After coming in contact with dirty linens or clothes
- After coming in contact with bodily fluids of any kind (blood, urine, vomit, mucus, or stool)
- After leaving a patient's room

Cleansing the hands with an alcohol-based hand sanitizer is also available in healthcare facilities, but it is best to wash with soap and water. Hand sanitizers can get rid of many, but not all, microbes. For example, **clostridium difficile,** commonly referred to as "**c-diff**," is a microbe that is not killed by alcohol-based sanitizers. A c-diff infection causes a patient to have copious amounts of watery diarrhea. In addition to standard infection-prevention precautions, the nurse must wash hands with soap and water before and after caring for a patient with c-diff.

Hand sanitizer should not be used when the hands are visibly soiled, or if bodily fluids have been touched. After several uses of hand sanitizer, oils build up on the hands and should be removed by washing with soap.

Educating patients about cleanliness and proper handwashing will also help prevent the spread of disease. Make sure to assist patients with washing their hands, or use a soapy washcloth on their hands throughout the day, especially after toileting and prior to eating. Proper handwashing in the community reduces the number of people who get sick with diarrheic illnesses and respiratory illnesses, such as colds.

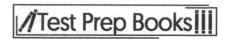

Use of Restraints/Safety Devices

Restraints can be defined as any device, material, or equipment that is attached to the body and intentionally limits a person's ability to move freely. Restraints, when applied properly, cannot be easily removed or controlled by the person. In addition to physical form, restraints can also be emotional, chemical, or environmental. Use of restraints is very controversial due to the ethical issue of personal freedom. These are a temporary solution to a problem and must always be used as a last resort. Restraints are used to limit a patient's movement to prevent injury to themselves or others, and they always require a physician's order.

Types of restraints include:

- Physical: vests, wrist restraints, straps, or anything that confines the body
- Emotional: verbal cues or emotions used to coerce the patient to act a certain way
- Environmental: side rails, locked doors, closed windows, locked beds
- Chemical: any medication used to change a patient's behavior

The medical doctor or practitioner is responsible for ordering the use of restraints. Nurses and caregivers are responsible for applying restraints safely and for the management of a patient with a restraint. After an order is given and a restraint is applied, the physician must visit the patient within twenty-four hours of placing the order to assess its further necessity.

Alternatives to Restraints

Other methods must be tried before restraints. They include:

- Talking with the patient about being cooperative
- Using distractions such as television, music, knitting, and folding towels or cloths
- Placing the patient within view of a caregiver, such as near the main desk
- Having someone sit with the patient
- Moving the patient to a quiet area
- Ensuring that the patient's bathroom needs are being met
- Ensuring personal items are within reach

When to Use Restraints

Each facility will have a specific protocol that must be followed for restraint use. Circumstances under which restraints are used include:

- Signs of patient aggression toward self, staff, or other patients
- Interference with important medical devices, such as an IV or a catheter
- Patient movements that are potentially harmful to their health, or may cause further injury
- Potential for a patient to interfere with a procedure

Applying Restraints

- Always follow the facility's restraint policy.

- Obtain an order from a physician or medical practitioner unless it is an emergency situation.

- Obtain consent from the patient or from next of kin if the patient is not capable of understanding.

- Explain to the patient what is going to happen, even if the patient is unable to understand due to confusion or dementia.

- Always monitor the patient per facility policy—check the positioning of the restraint every thirty minutes and remove every two hours for range of motion. Remember to reposition the patient and offer toileting every two hours.

- Explain the need for restraints and how long the restraints will be used.

Applying Physical Restraints

Vests have holes for the arms and the opening crosses in the back. The straps will be secured on either side of the bed or chair, depending on the patient's location. Tie it in a quick-release knot to a lower part of the bed that does not move. Make sure that two fingers fit underneath the vest on the patient's chest, so that it is not too tight.

Wrist or ankle restraints are cloths that wrap around each wrist or ankle. They have a strap that is tied to a lower, immovable part of the bed or chair. Tie it in a quick-release knot. Ensure the restraints aren't too tight and that the patient's arms or legs aren't in an awkward position. Usually a pillow will be placed under the arms and/or the knees and heels.

Legal Implications in the Use of Restraints

If restraints aren't used correctly or are used for the wrong reasons, the patient's family can take legal action against the facility. A patient in restraints becomes completely vulnerable and may feel helpless. They are at a greater risk of sexual abuse, elder abuse, psychological abuse, or violence from other patients/patients.

Possible injuries from restraints can include:

- Broken bones
- Bruises
- Falls
- Skin tears or pressure sores
- Depression or fear due to lack of freedom
- Death from strangulation

Health Promotion and Maintenance

Aging Process

Across the lifespan, from conception to birth, infancy to school-age, adolescence to adulthood, and middle age to death, the human experience is not unique. Like most other mammals, humans are said to be sentient beings, in possession of all of the five senses and self-awareness. With self-awareness, comes the realization of one's own mortality. The aging process is linear, beginning at the moment of birth. Distinctly, the **aged population** is generally said to include those over the age of sixty-five. Although many expect to see a marked decline in physiological and neurological functioning, this is not necessarily the case. Depending on individual lifestyle choices, high-risk behaviors, and adherence to annually recommended health screenings, the aging process can be uneventful.

For all patient populations, one of the most important topics to discuss is their diet. Especially for older adults, proper nutrition is critical. Income fluctuations due to retirement or lost income from a deceased or divorced spouse may affect the grocery budget. Vitamin deficiencies can quickly become problematic, resulting in a brief or prolonged hospitalization. Neurological concerns may also affect memory, and patients may simply forget to eat. Simple questions regarding favorite meals, restaurants, or eating preferences can yield answers. It is important to note that missing meals can also become commonplace if a depression diagnosis exists. Inserting a brief depression inventory early in the visit may reveal the major reason for the patient's current health status and uncover areas of concern regarding daily nutrition.

Exercise is also a crucial piece of the assessment puzzle when discussing healthy lifestyle choices. Chronological age is not synonymous with physical decline, and patients should be encouraged to continue with exercise as tolerated. Simply walking daily for 30 minutes, broken into segments if necessary, is a great starting point. Weight-bearing exercise, isometrics, swimming, yoga, pilates, or Tai-Chi all provide patients with the opportunity for gentle movement if some mobility issues exist. If needed, physical or occupational therapies can aide in the restoration of mobility and should be suggested after injury or with sedentary patients. Older patients must be reminded that retirement is not a signal to simply age, but the opportunity to age well.

Apart from the maintenance of diet and exercise is the importance of socialization and hobbies. Aging can be an isolating experience, especially as adult children move away and manage separate families. Less time may be spent with extended family and, once retired, the older adult may see less need for meeting new people in general. It is important for the nurse to assess the patient's perceived need for companionship. What do they do for fun? How do they unwind? Do they have a bucket list and what's on it? These types of open-ended questions not only create dialogue but can quickly become a goal-setting session.

When discussing high-risk behaviors with members of the aged population, it is imperative that the nurse include sexual activity. Although thought to be less sexually active than younger patients, this age group has seen a dramatic increase in sexually transmitted disease (STD) in recent years. Many have lost a spouse or life partner to death or divorce, and experience bouts of profound loneliness and sexual frustration. Although some may be seeking to remarry, most are interested in companionship and may not consider STDs to be a major concern. It is not as necessary to discuss birth control with a postmenopausal woman or elderly man as it is to discuss chlamydia, gonorrhea, herpes, and HIV. A simple question regarding intimate partners or social life will likely yield more information that the nurse can use to gently introduce the subject.

Nurses must carefully assess the likelihood of the progression of both medical and mental health concerns. Historically, the longer an individual manages chronic disease, the more complicated the illness becomes. More biological systems are impacted, leading to further physiological compromise. For example, diabetes mellitus, if managed well over a number of years, may still result in renal, visual, and cardiovascular complications in later years. The nurse must discuss basic diabetic care with the patient at every encounter. Annual eye exams, podiatric care, consultation with a diabetic nutritionist or dietician, and adhering closely to the diet plan, are all essential.

An additional, distinctive aspect of the aged population is neurological decline. Alzheimer's disease and dementia are said to contribute to a majority of hospitalizations and nursing home placements. Nurses must be familiar with a brief **neurological assessment**, also referred to as a **mental status exam**, in order to provide appropriate care. It is also necessary to assess the patient frequently for abrupt decline in functioning. Patients have a tendency to be forgetful, combative, and/or behave in a childlike manner. Neurological compromise can affect balance and gait, often resulting in falls and injury. Careful consideration to the safety of the patient's home environment is critical. Caregivers must be educated, trained, and prepared regarding the signs and symptoms of neurological impairment, along with appropriate interventions. It will also be necessary to discuss or review end of life care plans.

One final integral piece to the assessment of the older adult is preparation for the treatment and care of the patient and the family at the end of life. Some patients may have previously determined their preferences for end-of-life and palliative care. Obtain a copy of all advance directives and review for accuracy with the patient or caregiver. Does the patient possess the ability or desire to make changes to the documents? Are the primary and secondary proxy agents present or readily available if needed for consultation? The nurse must approach the discussion of comfort care with an awareness of the appropriate parties to include from the patient's preferred circle of confidants. If the nurse is unfamiliar with these topics, enlisting the assistance of a chaplain, social worker, or hospice care professional is vital. Respite care, bereavement counseling, and support-group referrals also are essential for the patient and family to ease their transition through the dying process.

Ante/Intra/Postpartum and Newborn Care

Excellent nursing care prior to, during, and immediately following childbirth is essential. Pregnancy as a medical state comprises several distinct stages: antepartum, intrapartum, postpartum, and newborn care. **Antepartum care** can be defined as care during pregnancy. During this period, the pregnant patient must be assessed periodically for appropriate fetal growth, responsiveness in-utero, and the mother's overall health status. Any fluctuations in these areas signal the potential for maternal or fetal distress. It is necessary to obtain a complete medical, gynecological, and obstetrical history. The nurse must be aware of any sexually transmitted diseases, previous abortions or full-term pregnancies (gravida), any complications, and the number of vaginal and cesarean births (para), as well as estimated date of delivery (EDD) and current birth plan.

The term **intrapartum care** refers to care provided during childbirth. Pregnancy is a progressive medical state; nursing care during the intrapartum period is based on all information gathered during the antepartum period. The mother and fetus are monitored simultaneously for signs of distress. Although continuous fetal monitoring is the standard of care, intermittent auscultation is acceptable if performed hourly. On average, fetal heart tones range from 120 to 160 beats per minute (bpm), with periodic

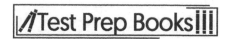

accelerations over 160 bpm denoting a positively responding fetus. The nurse must be equipped to discuss preferred treatment for uterine contractions and provide emotional support during delivery. Once cervical dilation reaches 10cm, the nurse must contact the provider and begin preparations for delivery of the infant. Once delivered, the mother and infant enter the postpartum stage.

The **postpartum phase** is considered to begin immediately after childbirth and ends after six weeks. Once the infant is delivered, it becomes a second patient and must be cared for separately from the mother. The nurse must assess both patients every 15 minutes for 2 hours to confirm that both mother and infant are adjusting well. Continued hospitalization is generally no longer than one day for a vaginal birth and two to three days for a cesarean section. Upon discharge—with infant care manual, feeding plan, and patient education completed—the couplet and other caregivers return to the home environment. Within weeks, the couplet will visit the physician, for well checks. This nursing assessment includes a depression inventory and discussions of progress with infant feeding.

Infants born prior to thirty-seven weeks gestation are considered to be **preterm** and at a high risk for complications at birth and throughout infancy. Specialized care of preterm infants and those born with twice-repeated APGAR scores below 7 must occur in the neonatal intensive care unit. Well infants are roomed in with their mothers, as a couplet. The postpartum nurse must be prepared to teach the parent(s) on feeding, changing, and general care of the infant. Umbilical cord care, as well as proper cleaning of a circumcised penis, is also vital in preparation for the discharge home. Within the first 24-to-48 hours after birth, careful assessment must be performed to ascertain if the infant is not adjusting to his or her new environment.

Developmental Stages and Transitions

Erikson's Psychosocial Stages of Development

As discussed in the first section under "Models of Human Behavior in the Social Environment," Erikson proposed a lifespan theory of psychosocial development as an alternative to Freud's psychosexual stages. According to Erikson's epigenetic principle of maturation, human beings pass through eight developmental stages, each of which build upon the preceding stages and set the groundwork for the stages that follow.

All eight stages are present at birth but remain latent until both an innate schedule and an individual's cultural upbringing cause a stage to begin to unfold.

An individual does not have to "master" a stage in order to proceed to the next stage, and the outcome of a particular stage may later be changed by an individual's life experiences.

As with Freud's theory, Erikson proposed that each stage of development is characterized by a crisis; however, for Erikson, the crisis involves a conflict between the needs of the developing individual and the needs of society.

Successfully mastering a stage and its psychosocial crisis leads to the development of a healthy personality and possession of basic virtues.

Erikson's theory centers on the development of ego identity, or a sense of self that is acquired by interacting with the social environment.

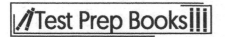

Self-Image Throughout the Life Cycle

Self-image has to do with how people view themselves. This concept includes **self-esteem**, whether a person has feelings of high or low worth. The concept of self evolves throughout the life span, but it always plays a significant role in a how a person functions in life.

Infancy: The ego is in charge. The baby thinks primarily of basic needs, such as food or warmth.

Childhood: In early to middle childhood, children tend to rate themselves higher than peers in terms of talents and intellect. As middle school approaches, there is a decline in self-evaluations. This could be related to feeling unattractive due to physical changes or being teased or bullied by peers in that age group.

Adolescence: In the early stage of adolescence (ages nine to thirteen), another drop in self-esteem occurs. This is thought to be related to the need to let go of childish pleasures, such as a beloved toy or previous interests, and step up to the plate of becoming a more responsible person. This can be a painful sacrifice for some youth. The next drop in self-worth occurs at the end of adolescence and beginning of young adulthood (ages eighteen to twenty-three). It is during this period that the young adults realize that they truly are responsible for their own lives, yet they have not yet achieved a sense of mastery in the academic or vocational world. They are fearful and full of doubt about the ability to be successful as an independent adult.

Adulthood: Studies indicate a small but steady increase in self-image by mid-twenties. In general, during this period, men tend to have higher self-esteem than women. Persons who live in poor socioeconomic conditions tend to have lower self-esteem than their more financially stable peers. As later adulthood nears (the seventies), women tend to catch up with men in terms of how they evaluate themselves. Women in their eighties tend to have a more positive self-image than male counterparts. As a general rule, for both genders, there is a gradual increase in one's sense of self-worth throughout the life span until late middle age. Research shows that most adults' self-image peaks at around age sixty.

Influence of Age on Behaviors and Attitudes

There are various, and sometimes conflicting, hypotheses with regard to how and whether attitudes change with age.

- **Impressionable-years hypothesis:** The environment and socialization that people experience when they are young shape their worldviews and have a profound effect on their attitudes for the remainder of the lifespan.

- **Increasing persistence hypothesis:** People exhibit flexible and impressionable thinking when they are younger but become increasingly inflexible with age.

- **Life-long openness hypothesis:** People exhibit flexible and impressionable thinking throughout the lifespan, and their attitudes are dependent upon evolving life circumstances.

Some changes in behavior and thinking may be related to the changes that older adults often experience as they navigate their later years. For example, they may experience a loss of independence due to impaired health or a loss of identity and confidence as they cope with retirement. People who have always had difficulty with change are particularly likely to experience negative effects of change during older adulthood.

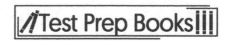

Examples may include somatic complaints, denial that change has occurred, feelings of powerlessness, rigid thinking, isolation, anger, depression, grief, or regression to earlier behavior.

Health Promotion/Disease Prevention

Two of the most important aspects of providing exceptional nursing care are health promotion and disease prevention. Both are integral to ensuring the physical and psychological well-being of individuals, groups, and the community at large.

Health promotion can be loosely defined as the direct or indirect presentation of information, specifically designed to influence behaviors that are expected to result in positive health outcomes. When presented directly, the instruction may be in written form such as brochures, books, or articles in magazines or newspapers. Historically, these publications were typically available in physician's offices, clinics, and hospitals. For nurses, health promotion is no longer relegated to easily discarded brochures or pamphlets. With the introduction of the Internet, information targeting healthy activities can be found instantly after several keystrokes. Nursing interventions can be provided via webinars, face-to-face coaching sessions, telephonic care, and social media sites. These mediums allow the nurse to contact thousands of individuals at once and increase exposure.

Indirect presentation of healthy lifestyle choices often occurs through billboards, signage, or posters in physicians' offices, as well as strategic mention or product placement in movies and television shows. Increasing numbers of "reality TV" stars can be seen holding bottles of a specific brand of vitamins or diet pills, or leaving a restaurant noted for healthy dishes. Albeit not as successful as the direct-to-consumer approach, this allows for health promotion to sneak in the back doors of viewers' minds, slowly affecting their daily habits. Traditionally, nurses are not involved in this type of health promotion, but nurses can use this type of behavior when interacting with patients. Ensuring that hand washing posters are present in restrooms, display cases of vitamins and supplements in the office waiting area, and sponsorship or participation in local health fairs all support higher awareness.

In an effort to actively guide the prevention of disease, community health nurses employ numerous tactics. Each strategy is specific to a particular population to intervene at several stages of the disease process.

Primary prevention consists of the nursing strategies implemented to prevent the onset of a particular disease process. One well-known example of primary disease prevention is the "say no to drugs" movement. Nurses in this campaign can specifically target young children and teens to prevent their initial use of drugs with the use of buttons, posters, commercials, and rallies. Secondary prevention focuses on the early detection of disease and prevention of considerable damage from the disease process. Using the same example, "pill checks" at rave parties would represent secondary prevention. Nurses and often paraprofessionals attend parties with teens to test the pills of party goers. This is done onsite, in the presence of the user, explaining what is found in the pill and offering to discard it. Finally, tertiary prevention efforts with this same patient population would be nursing interventions implemented in drug treatment centers, clinics, and detox units in the hospital. These nurses work with the patients actively addicted to substances and collaborate to manage their disease.

Health Screening

Historically, nurses have been primarily responsible for conducting health screenings. Every biological system within the human body should be screened periodically to ensure that it is operating at optimal levels. At the start of every developmental stage, it is recommended that patients be screened and, if found deficient, treated and monitored for progress. Health screenings are suggested based on chronological age to guide both individual treatment and trends for developing community outreach. Armed with the data, nurses collaborate with patients, providers, and caregivers to formulate an effective treatment plan.

Nurses working within the community health sector also utilize health screenings to guide disease-prevention efforts on a larger scale. Nurse researchers can use the data to aide in the creation of medications and advertisement campaigns to target those individuals on the borderlines of a particular disease process. Further, community-health nurses can conduct health screenings to identify gaps in access to healthcare, barriers to care, and disease maintenance. Once the information is disseminated to surrounding healthcare providers, clinics, and local government officials, the community-health nurse can begin the dialogue to effect policy changes. More engagement with health fairs, educational seminars, and print and social media campaigns may also result from health screenings.

Overall, health screenings are an integral piece of the healthcare puzzle. As nurses, it is often necessary to discuss the importance of annual health-screening recommendations upon each patient encounter. If patients reject or accept the recommended testing, they become aware of any present risk factors. Nurses can probe for information as to their ambivalence. For example, while completing a depression screening, a nurse can determine if an individual is at risk for depression. A patient who scores higher on the questionnaire can reveal if the answers are an accurate representation of daily high-risk behavior, or situational in nature.

Cancer Screening

Cancer screening tests relevant to several organ systems have effectively decreased the incidence and mortality of cancer in those systems. Common screening tests include the PAP test for cervical cancer, colonoscopy for colon cancer, and mammography for breast cancer. Recently, screening for lung cancer with advanced computed tomography (CT) technology in patients with a history of smoking has been proposed, in an effort to identify lung cancers at an earlier stage that may be treated more successfully. Conversely, the research indicates that there is insufficient evidence to support any relationship between decreased disease incidence and morbidity and the prostate-specific antigen test (PSA) measurements for prostate cancer, or the annual full-body skin assessments by a dermatologist. In addition, there are no screening tests available for ovarian cancer.

Osteoporosis Screening/Bone-Density Scan

Osteoporosis is the "thinning" of the bone, which most commonly affects postmenopausal women. The degree and progression of the changes associated with osteoporosis can be measured by the bone-density exam, which compares a patient's test results with the results of younger patients who are disease free.

Domestic Violence Screening and Detection

The efficiency of domestic violence screening and detection is often hampered by the reluctance of the abused individual to report the abuse. Institutions and insurance companies have included routine assessment questions related to a patient's perceptions of personal safety; however, the widespread acceptance and effectiveness of these measures are not known.

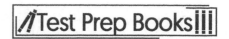

High Risk Behaviors

High-risk behaviors can be defined as actions that have a high probability of yielding a negative consequence. Nurses must develop a rapport with patients in an effort to create open communication so the patient will be more likely to reveal conduct that could have detrimental health outcomes. This technique can also encourage patients to ask questions about their risky behaviors. The nurse can then use the established rapport to discern if the patient's level of comfort and commitment to the behaviors is amenable to change.

One of the most effective methods of encouraging open communication with patients is motivational interviewing. Nurses use motivational interviewing to assess, collaborate, plan, and implement treatment with patients. There are five major components of motivational interviewing: express empathy, illustrate incongruity, manage resistance, encourage self-validation, and promote independence. The nurse can employ these steps when combatting ambivalence to change. For example, when working with a patient who is considering smoking cessation, begin with simple statements regarding the difficulties involved with quitting. This often results in the patient remarking about the number of attempts to quit, along with reasons why his or her prior attempts did not end in success. Next, draw from earlier statements concerning lifestyle choices, the patient's own reasons for quitting, and the potential for negative outcomes. In the next step, the nurse can tie the elements together, choosing carefully which area of resistance to target. What might the patient gain from quitting? What are the potential barriers to success from the patient's viewpoint? Asking these open-ended questions will help patients draw their own conclusions, validating the ability to self-navigate through possible obstacles. Once able to verbalize how the desired outcome could be achieved, the patient has managed to break through his or her own resistance, and the groundwork has been set for more internal dialogue.

Lifestyle Choices

Traditionally, nursing interventions are designed to target the lifestyle choices that affect disease processes. During every patient encounter, the nurse must ask open-ended questions in order to determine which interventions should be implemented. The acronym **SMART** (specific, measurable, attainable, relevant, and timely) is a concise reference for patients. When it is clearly what the main objective is, the likelihood of achieving that goal is increased.

When addressing multiple issues, chose one area with the highest likelihood of success to build momentum and patient confidence in the process. For example, when discussing diet, it is important for the nurse to first establish what the patient's current diet and exercise plan includes. This dialogue will open the door to likes, dislikes, preferred cooking methods, and diet history. As the discussion expands, inquire about budgetary constraints and actual access to healthy food options. Once eating habits are known, define daily scheduling conflicts that may become barriers to success. Create a contingency plan, with multiple options. Another major area of importance for lifestyle choices is exercise. Upon reviewing current diagnoses, medications, and any mobility or chronic pain concerns, the nurse can partner with the patient to formulate a reasonable plan. Set a specific goal on the type and duration of exercise; measure steps or activity as accurately as possible with a pedometer. Can they commit to exercise daily? What is an appropriate form of exercise? Maintain the stance of advocate and collaborator to preserve patients' autonomy and validate their experiences whenever possible.

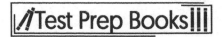

Techniques of Physical Assessment

One of the most important skills that a nurse can possess is that of the physical assessment. Practically every area of nursing practice requires that a nurse have an accurate recall of normal physical functioning and be capable of observing areas of compromise. The nurse's awareness of baseline functioning for a patient within the specific age group and associated health concerns is essential. Physicians, nurse practitioners, and other healthcare providers routinely depend on the nurse's initial assessment of patients to guide their overall treatment of patients.

The **initial assessment** of a patient does not begin in the face-to-face interaction. As an expert, the nurse must start with any available historical data. Review prior history and physical records, diagnoses, medications, and treatment plans. Certain medications and disease processes can impact daily functioning and the nurse must consider this prior to patient interaction. Immediately upon introduction, the nurse must observe: gait, posture, and balance, skin tone, voice intonation, responsiveness, eye contact, hand grip with handshake, and general stature. While taking vital signs, assess mood, level of consciousness (LOC), orientation, short-term and long-term memory, bowel and urinary habits, and medication list. The aforementioned portions of the assessment can aide in the formulation of the rest of the clinical picture. It is also necessary to discuss daily habits, work schedule, social interactions, and physical activity. Those factors can influence adherence to suggested treatment plans. Once a full clinical picture falls into place, the nurse can utilize the findings to discuss interventions that would be helpful to the patient.

Psychosocial Integrity

Abuse/Neglect

Abuse and neglect can take many forms and affect people of various demographics. Children, women, and the elderly tend to be the vulnerable victim populations. Abuse and neglect cases can often put the victim in the emergency room, so nurses and other medical personnel should be aware that they likely will come across these unfortunate situations, and intervention may be necessary. It is important to know how to spot abuse and neglect cases for legal and ethical reasons.

In children, abuse and neglect can come from a biological or adoptive parent, guardian, close adult in the child's life, or stranger. Younger children are the most vulnerable individuals in this demographic. This is because they may not be able to speak, defend themselves, or understand that they are being abused, or they may be fearful of reporting a caregiver.

Child abuse can be **emotional** (such as refusal to provide affection or emotional comfort, criticizing the child in a cruel or unusual manner, or administering humiliation or shame tactics) and may be hard to detect or penalize legally. **Physical abuse** of a child involves intentional acts of physical violence that could result in injury. **Sexual abuse** of a child includes sexual acts or interactions by an adult; even if the child provides consent, it is considered abuse, due to the emotional and mental immaturity of the child. In the United States, legal age of consent varies by state. Signs of abuse in children can include physical indicators, such as cuts, bruises, genital pain or bleeding, and persistent yeast infections. There can also be behavioral indicators, such as slow development, aggression, anxiety, suicidal tendencies, fearful natures, antisocial or awkward behavioral habits, statements describing inappropriate physical or sexual interactions, visibly unusual relationships or interactions with a parent or caregiver, and a lack of desire (or even refusal) to go home.

Child neglect refers to a parent, guardian, or other caretaker's inaction to provide basic care such as food, water, education, medical and dental treatments, safe supervision, and clean and safe living accommodations. Signs of neglect in children can include chronic illness, malnutrition, lack of personal hygiene, above-average school absenteeism, anxiety and depression, and substance abuse.

A single sign may not mean that abuse or neglect is present, but it should be taken seriously by asking further questions and potentially seeking resources, such as legal and social support agencies, to prevent further abuse. Most states require that knowledge of potential abuse or neglect be reported to legal and child protective services. The process of reporting varies by state, and practitioners should familiarize themselves with abuse and neglect reporting practices of the state in which their nursing services will be provided.

Domestic violence between adult partners, also known as **intimate partner violence and abuse**, is also a common form of abuse that can require emergency department visits. While this type of abuse can be experienced by partners of either gender or orientation, it is most commonly inflicted by male partners on female victims. Physical indicators of abuse from a partner include marks such as bruises, black eyes, genital or anal damage, scratches, and welts. Behavioral indicators include a fearful nature, low self-esteem, isolation, anxiety, depression, constant excuses for the abusing partner's dangerous actions, and suicidal tendencies. Again, the presence of one sign may not indicate that abuse is occurring, but it can be a call to action to provide resources for the victim's safety.

Elder abuse and neglect may occur by family members or other caregivers. Elderly people are vulnerable, as they may be physically weak or have other physical and mental limitations, handicaps, or disabilities. Signs of abuse in elders are similar to those seen in children but can also include the occurrence of adult-minded activities that happen without the elder's consent, such as mishandled financial transactions or health care fraud. Physical indicators of abuse in the elderly include bruises, broken bones, and signs of physical restraint. Behavioral indicators include poor relationships with caregivers, anxiety, depression, and a fearful nature. Indicators of neglect in the elderly include missed or improper medication administration, signs of poor hygiene, genital or anal rashes, and malnutrition. Unfortunately, many signs of elder abuse and neglect are similar to signs of dementia, a natural reaction to ailing health, and other behaviors commonly exhibited by this age demographic. Therefore, due diligence by nurses and medical personnel is necessary. All states have elder abuse prevention laws, though procedures for reporting may vary by state, so it is important to know the process for the state in which nursing services will be administered.

Behavioral Interventions

The overall theme of any effective nursing intervention is the implementation of behavioral change to produce healthy outcomes. Nursing interventions combine medical and psychosocial interventions to guide patients to live healthier lives. The most successful nursing interventions to promote disease prevention also incorporate the utilization of the patient's support network, stress-management techniques, building effective coping skills, and encouraging healthy lifestyle choices. The best illustration of how all of these components can produce the greatest impact is depicted in the following example.

Consider a nurse providing intensive case management to a morbidly obese patient seeking bariatric surgery. The incidence and prevalence of morbid obesity is rapidly increasing as the number-one cause of adverse health conditions in the United States. Despite primary, secondary, and tertiary health promotion efforts, the waistlines of Americans are continuing to grow at exponential rates. Disordered eating, sedentary lifestyle, poor impulse control, and inaccurate perceptions about how to maintain a healthy diet are commonplace. It is essential that the nurse providing case management services to patients seeking morbid-obesity surgery create a specialized treatment plan to help ensure the patient's success.

After conducting the history and physical interview, it is determined that the patient recently received a dual diagnosis of type II diabetes and hypercholesterolemia. With a family history of both parents diagnosed with diabetes and hypertension, there is some concern that the disease will progress rapidly. Newly diagnosed, the patient has not yet been prescribed daily oral medications. Instead, the attending physician has ordered a case management consultation for the patient to discuss morbid-obesity surgery. In this instance, the nurse will assume the role of case manager with the final result being to recommend or deny the request to approve the patient as a candidate for bariatric surgery.

Although the primary mechanism remains under investigation, bariatric surgery has been said to resolve myriad obesity-related comorbidities. As the body mass index of Americans has grown, physicians have observed an inverse relationship with healthy lifestyle choices. Studies have shown that both type II diabetes and hypercholesterolemia are among the main diseases that significantly contribute to the development of cardiovascular disease. These conditions often require extensive, ongoing treatment. Many patients reach a state where traditional medical treatment becomes ineffective in the daily management of their symptoms. As the disease state progresses, dietary interventions also become ineffective. Surgeons who regularly perform bariatric procedures have found that it is the combination

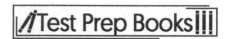

of substantial dietary restriction and increased physical activity that can lead to an almost complete resolution of disease. For these reasons, thousands of patients make the decision to pursue bariatric surgery.

Once the initial assessment is completed, the next task for the nurse is to verify the eligibility requirements dictated by the patient's insurance carrier. The nurse will contact the patient's health insurance provider and obtain an explanation of benefits. This information will help the nurse prepare the patient to complete any required criteria. This is an integral step to ensuring that surgery can be approved. Without clear direction, the treatment plan is incomplete. It is customary for the patient to be required to receive diagnostic testing, meet with a dietician, and complete a psychological evaluation to confirm his or her readiness to succeed after surgery. The nurse will then discuss the benefit criteria with the patient to assess the patient's commitment to the process. The final step in this preliminary phase is to obtain both written and verbal agreement from the patient to receive and actively participate in medical case management.

During the engagement phase of treatment planning, the nurse will begin to utilize the SMART goal-setting process. This type of behavioral intervention focuses on the presentation of the problem, developing a solution to the problem, and outlining the necessary steps to resolve the problem. Additionally, this technique encourages patients to brainstorm ways to meet their own needs. For this scenario, the nurse will describe the criteria that must be completed in order for the patient to be approved for bariatric surgery, along with any associated time frames within which those criteria must be met. In most cases, patients must complete a physician-supervised lifestyle modification program, for a specific number of weeks. The nurse will ask the patient what steps can be taken to adjust his or her lifestyle in order to satisfy that requirement. Patients can work with a nutritionist, dietician, or their primary care physician. How will those appointments be scheduled, and with whom? What specific lifestyle modifications will the patient need to make and why? What will it look like when the changes have been made? Does the patient believe that they can make the necessary lifestyle modifications? Do the changes seem appropriate, based on the patient's previously stated goals and needs? How long will it take? These questions lead to the development of SMART goals.

SMART goal setting requires a series of question-and-answer sessions. This technique will continue for each objective, in an effort to guide the patient to lead the treatment-planning process. If goals are ambiguous, the patient will not understand what to do. Goals are not measurable if there is no way to track progress. Goals must also be practical in their application. The goal must make sense to the patient and contribute to the overall completion of the desired outcome. The patient must be able to see the big picture and have a clear understanding of how and why all of the tasks are interdependent. It is also necessary for the nurse to periodically check in with the patient to determine if each task is being completed according to the timeline. Creating a plan in this way will affect how the patient thinks about goal setting in general. It is important for the nurse to allow the patient to take responsibility for completing each task. The patient will monitor his or her own progress and troubleshoot with the nurse as needed. This technique is self-empowering for the patient and reinforces the self-determination necessary for goal setting in the future.

Coping Mechanisms

Unpack coping mechanisms, and you will find at their core a whole-hearted but poorly defined resistance to change. Effective stress management combined with adaptive coping skills are directly related to the execution of a treatment plan. It is the acquisition and application of adaptive coping skills that promotes overall well-being. If coping skills are maladaptive, no matter how applicable the treatment plan is, there will be no effect if the patient is ill-equipped to navigate the stages of change. It is essential that the nurse work collaboratively with the patient and other members of the healthcare team to formulate a treatment plan that is based on patient-centered care.

Consider how a nurse working in an inpatient mental health unit would respond during the assessment of a teenage girl admitted for observation after a suicide attempt. The initial physical assessment uncovers evidence of what appear to be a series of self-inflicted cuts, in various stages of healing, on the patient's inner thighs. A thorough interview with the teen reveals that the patient has been cutting herself in response to bullying from fellow residents in her boarding school. The teen also reported that the bullying has occurred for several years and had escalated to threats of physical harm. School officials were notified, and the students were expelled. Despite the fact that the offending students no longer attend the school, the patient has been unable to relinquish cutting herself. Self-injurious behaviors have increased in the last 48 hours, after the teen ended a long-term romantic relationship. According to the patient, the break-up created feelings of hopelessness and overwhelming depression. In a deep state of depression, the student swallowed a bottle of Tylenol, hoping to end the pain. The admitting diagnosis of the attending physician is depression, with a rule-out diagnosis of bipolar disorder.

On an inpatient unit, there is often an interdisciplinary team assembled to develop a collaborative treatment plan. Although the therapist and social worker will conduct additional interviews with the patient, it will be necessary for the nurse to formulate nursing diagnoses and interventions that complement the overall plan of care. In this case, the most appropriate nursing diagnosis would be: risk for harm associated with feelings of hopelessness secondary to the diagnosis of depression. Suitable interventions would be centered around the application of the adaptive coping skills learned through ongoing individual and group therapies while admitted to the inpatient unit. The nurse will dispense antidepressant medications prescribed by the attending physician, reinforce the techniques demonstrated in therapy, and guide the patient to begin safety planning.

Types of Coping Skills

- **Self-Soothing:** Comforting the self through the five senses

- **Distraction:** Taking mind off the problem for a while

- **Opposite Action:** Doing the opposite of the initial impulse that's consistent with a more positive emotion

- **Emotional Awareness:** Tools for identifying and expressing one's feelings

- **Mindfulness:** Tools for centering and grounding the self in the present moment

- **Crisis Plan:** Supports and resource information for when coping skills are not enough, such as therapist, family, friends, or a crisis team

The nurse must also remain aware that the stress of managing emotional turmoil can create feelings of powerlessness and depression. The patient may have grown accustomed to denying intense feelings and instincts in an effort to be insulated from the source of pain. The goal is to focus on rebuilding the patient's coping skills from the inside out, in order to promote a sense of hope and self-determination. Discuss the difference between adaptive and maladaptive coping skills. Encourage the patient to define which behaviors they engage in that they would place into each category. What the patient perceives to be most effective is not necessarily the healthiest response. Educate the patient on how healthier choices lead to healthier outcomes. Discuss how the self-inflicted wounds could become infected or

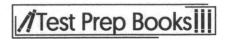

disfiguring. Offer information on the benefits of aerobic exercise to release endorphins known to naturally elevate the patient's mood. Encourage the patient to consider journaling, writing, or creating art to express suppressed emotions. Pet therapies have also been effective in the treatment of depression, providing much-needed emotional support. Finally, encourage the patient to consider attending local support groups for depressed teens. The communal aspect of a support group is helpful, as other teens battling depression can validate the patient's experience.

The customary discharge plan for depressed patients at risk for suicide includes several components. First, the patient must agree that they will no longer make any attempts to harm themselves in any way. Instead, the patient will create a detailed list of at least two alternatives to self-harm. The nurse must also highlight patients' current coping skills and encourage his or her ability to support themselves and to utilize their stress management skills. Which alternatives to self-harm that could produce similar feelings of release will the patient practice? Second, the patient must verbalize understanding that any episodes of self-harm will result in immediate hospitalization. What steps will the patient take when feeling overwhelmed? Does the patient have an accountability partner? Finally, the patient will be equipped with a personalized list of contacts to utilize when stress-relieving techniques are ineffective. This list will include a 24-hour suicide hotline, as well as the contact information for the local therapist assigned prior to the patient's discharge.

Crisis Intervention

Crisis-intervention skills are an essential component of providing exceptional patient care. Crises strike unexpectedly and, by definition, necessitate immediate intervention. Nurses in particular must have robust crisis-intervention skills in order to address the myriad issues that patients and their caregivers face. Why is crisis intervention so important? Why do nurses need to acquire this dexterity? It is because proper nursing care involves the astute assessment of the patient's overall well-being. At some point during the provision of care to patients and families, the nurse will encounter a situation in which they will have no other choice but to intervene. This is primarily because the nurse is often on the front lines of healthcare and the first to interact with the patient. The integration of nursing care, stress-management techniques, and assisting the patient navigate through the stages of grief are of paramount importance. Not unlike every other nursing technique, crisis-intervention skills will be enhanced with repeated use and more progressive problem solving.

Consider the importance of the nurse's adaptability to crises with reference to assisting patients and families impacted by natural disasters. Upon deployment to an area destroyed by torrential rains and subsequent flooding, a nurse could encounter families in need of not only immediate medical care, but ongoing crisis intervention. In conditions such as these, patients are often overwhelmed by their physical pain as well as concerns for how to meet their basic needs for food, shelter, and clean water. Disaster relief relies on medical triage to determine the appropriate level of care needed by patients and is typically assessed based on a four-tier model. Black/blue is reserved for the deceased; red for immediate care such as chest wounds or gunshots; yellow for those with stable wounds or head injuries; green for minor injuries such as fractures or burns. In this situation, the nurse must be prepared to rapidly assess the patient's level of injury, the most expedient treatment needed for stabilization, and move on to the next case within minutes. Does the patient or anyone in the family maintain a specific medication regimen to manage chronic illnesses? Have any doses of required medications been missed? Are any assistive devices such as hearing aids or canes needed? It is important to note that the nurse will need to focus on the medical stabilization of patients in this stage rather than delving into psychosocial and emotional trauma.

During disaster-relief efforts, nurses are normally dispatched to both acute care and follow-up care zones. Once immediate medical needs are addressed, patients are transferred to a safe holding area. This space is set aside for psychosocial triage, where patients' basic emotional and physical needs are met. Social workers and chaplains are readily available to debrief survivors. Consider the example of a nurse working with a family impacted by the previous illustration. Having lost their home and belongings and facing recovery from minor injuries, they have been transferred to the holding area for processing. The nurse in this example would receive a brief synopsis from triage, but only regarding injuries and treatment. In this stage, the nurse would obtain a brief social history, information on chronic disease, and feasible relocation options. Then, the nurse will need to begin guiding the patients through processing the emotional trauma of the incident. Are all family members accounted for? Does anyone in the family unit manage any mental health conditions that have been triggered? What, if any, legal or illegal substances are used or abused by anyone in the family unit? These questions are to help determine if the survivors' emotional responses are directly related to the recent trauma.

Responses to acute traumatic events often mirror the typical response of those who have experienced chronic trauma. The nurse must also assess patients for underlying mental health conditions that may have been exacerbated. In this instance, the most appropriate nursing diagnosis would include ineffective coping. Typical nursing interventions would require the nurse to work with the patient to access previous successful navigation through other traumatic events. Present viable options for next steps and allow the patient the time to process the best response to the traumatic event.

Cultural Awareness/Cultural Influences on Health

Patients will come from all backgrounds and cultures, and medical providers should be aware of the different cultural needs that may present themselves in the emergency department. **Culture** can encompass anything from a person's geographical location, race, ethnicity, age, socioeconomic status, and religious beliefs that influence the behaviors, traditions, and rituals that he or she chooses to engage in each day. It is important to note that cultural considerations will present themselves daily. Some patients may be unable to speak English and will need interpretive services. Some patients may request that only same-sex providers treat them. Some patients may need to keep culturally valuable adornments in place that could interfere with treatment (i.e., a metal symbol on a patient that needs magnetic resonance imaging, a procedure where metal poses an extreme danger). Respecting and attending to different cultural needs will provide the patient with a better healthcare experience, lead to increased patient satisfaction, and impact overall health outcomes (as patients will be more likely to seek out care if they feel comfortable doing so).

Medical providers can show that they consider cultural differences by kindly and compassionately asking patients to share cultural viewpoints, to share aspects of the medical system and services that make them comfortable or uncomfortable, and to continuously create rapport that allows the patient to feel comfortable in voicing their concerns. Medical providers should be mindful of any preconceived notions that they hold of certain cultures, and if possible, actively work to dispel these. Medical providers should also be mindful to not make presumptions, even if those presumptions come from an intention to be empathetic. For example, a patient who looks to be of Asian descent may have been born and raised in the United States and not identify well with any part of Asian culture. Finally, many healthcare organizations offer internal trainings that cover cultural considerations and cultural diversity. For staff that feel their knowledge and experience is limited in this aspect, these trainings can provide an avenue for personal and professional growth.

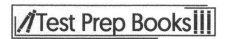

Having a diverse emergency department staff can be extremely beneficial when servicing a patient demographic that encompasses many cultures. Having a medical provider who is able to relate directly with a patient's culture can make the patient feel more comfortable and open. Additionally, a diverse emergency department staff can overcome common obstacles such as language barriers or lack of patient education. In this regard, healthcare organizations and nursing leadership should work to actively recruit a diverse workforce.

End-of-Life Care

At least once during their career, it is inevitable that a nurse will care for a patient near the end of life. Caring for patients near the end of life can occur in numerous settings. Whether on an inpatient hospice unit or in an outpatient setting, the patient's home, or a skilled nursing facility, the primary objective is to ensure that the nurse provides patient-centered palliative care. There is a stark difference between hospice and palliative care. Both of these, however, fall under the umbrella of end of life care. Specifically, **end of life care** includes the care that is received at the end of a patient's illness. While **palliative care** is considered to be basic comfort care, **hospice** is the more familiar term, and usually begins once all curative treatments have been stopped.

Hospice, or end of life care, can be loosely defined as: primarily palliative and, secondarily, medical care provided to patients deemed by at least two physicians to be terminally ill, with a projected life expectancy of six months or less. This means that the primary objective of hospice care is to provide comfort care to patients. This comfort care is provided under the primary diagnosis. The secondary medical care is typically provided whenever necessary to maintain the patient's comfort. For example, consider a patient who has been receiving hospice care for a primary diagnosis of dementia for four months. Upon admission to the inpatient unit for a weekend of respite, the patient is diagnosed with a kidney infection. The elevated fever, flank pain, nausea, vomiting, and rapid heart rate detract from the patient's overall comfort. The kidney infection is considered to be secondary to the diagnosis of dementia and will be treated. Conditions that are not considered to be comfort care are curative in nature, with the primary objective to prolong life.

It is essential for the nurse to remember that when providing care to a patient who has been placed on hospice, there is always more than one patient to be considered. The spouse or significant other, as well as whomever the patient perceives to be a member of the familial unit, will also be impacted by the patient's diagnosis and subsequent death. The family dynamics will be especially important in these cases, as they must also receive extensive treatment. The nurse can expect to see caregiver burnout, family members struggling with feelings of loss, and anticipatory grief. Most notable is the prospect of funeral planning while the patient is still alive. Although it is not uncommon for the patient or family members to reach end of life without preparing for the funeral, the finality of the task must be worked through. Both the patient and the family may need the intervention of the social worker and/or chaplain in order to facilitate this discussion. It may be necessary to obtain the patient's final wishes separately from the caregiver or family, to be shared upon the patient's demise, if the stress and grief of preparing for death becomes too overwhelming.

Although the patient is still considered to be terminally ill, they will continue to have desires, hopes, and may even want to create a plan for the future. It will be necessary to coordinate the patient's care with the interdisciplinary team (social worker, chaplain, physician, and nurse). All involved will have the opportunity to review the patient's electronic medical records, as well as current diagnosis, medications, and treatment plan. It is usually the nurse who initially notices the beginning of the patient's decompensation. As it is uncommon to accurately predict the precise date of the patient's death, the patient must be guided to prepare advance directives if not completed when enrolled into hospice. The nurse must review these documents carefully, looking for information from the patient's history for evidence of being an organ donor, specific religious affiliations, or stipulations against certain visitors.

A final word regarding the compassionate care of individuals receiving end of life care: If the nurse is managing a patient who has specific details in the care plan, or religious beliefs that heavily impact healthcare decisions, additional consultation may be required. For example, for a patient who identifies as Jewish, he or she may prefer to assign an additional family member to sit with the patient once deceased. As this is the religious custom, the nurse must respect this as much as possible. It is imperative that the nurse seek a consultation with the available social worker, chaplain, or member of the hospital/facility ethics board for guidance if any request is questionable. If an internal or professional conflict of interest might prevent the nurse from effectively delivering care to the patient according to his or her religious beliefs, the nurse would be best served to recuse herself in the best interests of the patient.

Family Dynamics

The term "family" holds a different level of significance to different people. No matter how the nurse chooses to define family, it is imperative that a neutral stance be maintained regarding the patient's familial network. If the nurse cannot maintain a sense of compassionate objectivity, it may cloud the nurse's responsiveness to cultural issues that affect patient care. Whenever possible, the nurse must consider that the family dynamic remains as the unseen influence on the patient. Stress-management techniques, as well as the cultural and familial roles assigned in the family, may have an undue influence on the patient's healthcare decisions and adherence to treatment.

A visual assessment of this dynamic can occur within several minutes. Observe how the family members interact; choices of conversation topics and responses can often reveal a great deal about who is the leader in the household. For example, upon the initial assessment of an obese teen and a morbidly obese parent, it can quickly become apparent that the dietary choices made by the teen are a mirror of those made by the primary caregiver. Both may lead a relatively sedentary lifestyle, punctuated by frequent visits to the local fast-food restaurant. As the nurse, it would be necessary to simply ask about their daily vegetable and water consumption, hobbies, or even the teen's favorite meal. During the discussion, the nurse will be better able to discuss SMART goals: specific, measurable, achievable, relevant, and timely. This type of goal setting allows for the patient to set realistic goals, with the opportunity to self-check for progress along the way.

When one member of the family is not performing at peak capacity, the dynamic shifts, causing all others to adopt different roles. If the family dynamic is cooperative, all parties will seek to reach a reasonable state of homeostasis. This means that if there is a recognized deficiency in one member of the family, each member will want to contribute to activities that will restore his or her health. This informal agreement is one of the ultimate goals of the nursing intervention. If the family dynamic is conflictual, then the parties will seek to satisfy their own needs, rather than help the ill family member achieve better health outcomes. As the nurse, it is important to utilize the familial bond, no matter the type, to influence the best result for the patient.

For the aforementioned example, the nurse would attempt to co-op the conflictual family members and align their needs with those of the patient. Offering healthier alternatives to staple meals, cheaper recipes, and suggestions for more physical activity would likely appeal to all parties. Alternatively, the nurse could propose that the teen prepare healthier meals themselves, allowing a busy parent much-

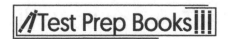

needed respite from cooking daily. During the average professional nursing career, it will become clear that family members' personal health selections can derail patients' lifestyle choices. It is incumbent upon the nurse to incorporate all aspects of the patient's life in order to create the most effective treatment plan.

Grief and Loss

Grief Process

Everyone grieves differently after the death of a loved one. Grief, and how it manifests itself, is different in each individual and depends on the relationship with the deceased. For some, grief will be brief, and for others, it will be prolonged. There is a general guideline for the grieving process, but it is descriptive, not prescriptive. Individuals may experience all stages in order, some stages, but not all, or switch between stages out of order at various points in time.

The **Kubler-Ross grieving model** includes five stages: denial, bargaining, depression, anger, and acceptance. For example, when a terminal diagnosis for a loved one is received, the family members may deny what is happening and not acknowledge reality. After this stage of **denial**, they may begin to **bargain**, or try to make deals with whoever they believe has the power to change the circumstances for their loved one. This could include long arguments with the health care team over care or praying to a higher power for a healing miracle. After bargaining, they may fall into a **depression,** with feelings of helplessness or powerlessness against the forces of the disease. This may be followed by a stage of **anger** in which they act outwardly or express frustration that they cannot change the circumstances. The last stage of grief is **acceptance**, and this is considered the stage in which the grieved person is finally at peace with the circumstances and can begin healing.

As mentioned before, these categories of grief are a rough guideline of what a person may experience. Grief varies in intensity from person to person and depends a great deal on the nature of the relationship with the deceased. The nurse need only be familiar with the stages in order to recognize them in family members and/or the dying person, who may go through these stages as well. If one recognizes the grief process is occurring, one is more sensitive to the needs of the grieving.

Emotional Needs of the Patient, Family, and Caregivers

Grief is a highly emotional process. The range of emotions experienced by those grieving the loss of a loved one is vast. The initial reaction of shock and disbelief may morph quickly into anger, then sadness, and even fear. Sometimes the patient or family may feel such intense emotional pain that physical symptoms such as chest pain, gastrointestinal issues, and shortness of breath may occur. The stress of losing a loved one is both physical and emotional. The nurse can recognize this and be of assistance.

The best way to help those who are grieving—whether it is the anticipatory grieving the dying patient may feel or the grief that occurs after the patient passes on—is to be there to support the family. It's incorrect to assume that one can imagine or alleviate what the grieving are feeling or thinking.

The role of the nurse is to help in any way possible, but not to offer empty optimistic statements or promises, such as "It'll be okay soon," or "You'll move on before you know it." These statements are not helpful and may aggravate the recipient. Instead, focusing on what can be done in the present to assist them is the best approach.

Grief cannot be avoided; it is a process that is different for each individual and is necessary for healing. The nurse can offer a listening ear, a hug, or a hand to hold if welcomed and appropriate, and can inquire how the patient or the family are doing. Simply asking how they are doing shows that the nurse cares and would like to be of assistance in any way possible.

Providing for the physical comfort of the grieving by offering a cup of coffee, a warm blanket, or a snack is a way to support them. The emotional pain they are going through may have caused them to ignore their own basic physical needs, such as eating and resting. Helping them focus on something besides their emotional pain can be helpful.

The nurse, doctor, and social worker will offer social services, grief counseling, and other resources that will connect the grieving to other forms of support.

Responses to Grief

Not only will each individual respond differently to grief based on personality and relationship with the deceased, but also the response will differ based on their own spiritual beliefs and cultural influences. These beliefs and influences affect how a person thinks they should act during the mourning period, what to wear, what rituals need to be performed, and what happens after a person dies.

Each individual culture will not be gone over in this discussion, as there are a multitude of variations of the death and grieving process. It is not necessary for the nurse to know each and every one, but rather have a general knowledge of differences and be respectful towards them.

Some cultures believe an outward show of emotion is appropriate and necessary. Sometimes, this entails an outward expression of weeping and wailing. Other cultures may be more conservative and think it is appropriate to be stoic, serious, and somber, without crying and losing one's composure. Some have specific rituals before and after the death, involving holy men, priests, or other clergy who prepare the person and/or the body for an afterlife. Some may not have any religious affiliation and may not believe in a life after this one.

Regardless of what cultural and spiritual beliefs are present, the role of the health care team is to respect those wishes as much as possible. It is imperative that the team explore the patient and family's wishes in this respect, rather than overlooking or refusing to allow them. It is always appropriate to politely ask how best to respect the patient and family's wishes when performing tasks for the dying or deceased patient. For example, some family members may prefer to clean the body themselves after death, an important ritual to express grief and ensure proper care in their view.

Each member of the health care team, including the nurse, needs to assess their own beliefs about death and dying. Self-knowledge on the subject is valuable as it may not be something one has consciously acknowledged. This self-assessment also helps reveal any unfair biases and prejudices towards cultures and people whose worldview is different than one's own. Discovering what one's own beliefs and others' beliefs are leads to a better understanding between groups. These groups can then begin to find ways to work together during the difficult end-of-life period.

Physical Changes and Needs as Death Approaches

As the patient approaches death, the nurse will play an important role in ensuring physical comfort. The patient may have increased pain, skin irritability, decreased control over bowel and bladder, decreased mobility, and decreased consciousness. There are concrete steps that the nurse can take to ensure the patient is as comfortable as possible during the last stage of life.

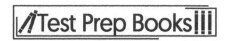

Monitoring the patient's level of pain is important. Pain medicine as necessary will be used to provide adequate comfort. The nurse should watch for nonverbal signs of pain, such as body tension, moaning, and facial grimacing.

Elimination may become difficult if the patient loses consciousness and mobility. The nurse can make elimination easier for the patient by assisting the patient to a bedside commode or bed pan, and/or checking for incontinence in order to perform perineal care to keep the patient clean and dry.

The patient's skin may become dry and brittle. Mouth breathing can cause the oral cavity to dry out quickly, sometimes called **cotton mouth**. Applying lotions, balms, and moisturizers to skin and lips, as well as making sure the oral cavity is well moisturized, are all steps that can relieve skin discomfort. Mouth sponges or swabs can be dipped in water to wet the mouth. Some patients find these sponges comforting to chew on or take a few drops of water from.

Preventing pressure ulcers or preventing existing pressure ulcers from worsening at the end of life is a consideration for nurses to keep in mind. These can cause additional pain and discomfort that might be avoided. Using pillows to prop and position at-risk areas, such as heels, buttocks, elbows, and the back of the head will help minimize pressure.

The patient will likely have difficulty regulating body temperature, and may experience periods of feeling hot, cold, or both. The patient may not be able to verbalize these needs, but the nurse can watch for nonverbal cues such as shivering or sweating. It is important to keep the patient comfortably warm or cool, using blankets and fans. Electric blankets should not be used, as the patient may not be able to verbalize if it is too hot, risking burn injuries.

Breathing may become difficult for the patient. They will likely develop increased secretions in the airway. The patient will likely be too weak to clear these secretions, resulting in a rattling or gurgling sound. Turning the patient's head to the side, providing a cool-mist humidifier (if available), and using suction equipment are all interventions that can alleviate the patient of these secretions. Depending on the facility, the nurse may or may not be able to perform the task of suctioning. The patient may be given supplemental oxygen via nasal cannula for comfort. Monitoring to make sure the prongs of the nasal cannula are in place and not causing discomfort to the patient is important.

The patient may not appear to be awake, but still may be able to hear and perceive what is going on around them. Because of this, it is always important for the nurse to identify oneself to the patient when entering the room and tell the patient what they are doing in the room. This courtesy may comfort a patient who is otherwise alone. The nurse aid should talk to the patient, provide quiet music, and keep the lighting low and/or natural. These environmental changes can all soothe the patient and should be guided by the patient and the family's wishes. Some patients may prefer a room full of visitors and others may be more private, preferring only a few close relatives and friends.

The nurse needs to be mindful of the family's needs as well. Again, their grief and emotional response in the moment may cause them to forget their own basic needs, such as eating and getting proper rest. It is important to remind them to rest when they need to, offer them drinks and snacks as appropriate, warm blankets, and any other offering available to comfort them during this difficult time.

The end of life need not be a lonely, miserable experience, lacking warmth, thoughtfulness, and care. The nurse can assist the health care team in providing comfort for the patient's physical needs as well as creating a soothing environment around the patient as they approach death.

Post-Mortem Care Procedures

After the patient has passed, the first step the nurse can take is to determine the family's needs. This is a time when spiritual and cultural considerations need to be respected. Some families may linger and talk over the body for hours before leaving the room, while others may say a brief goodbye and leave. The health care team should determine if there are any specific burial preparations that need to be done. Funeral and/or burial arrangements, such as cremation or embalmment, will be determined.

Once these considerations are determined, the health care team can prepare the body. Generally, the body will need to be cleaned, as bowel and bladder incontinence happens after death. Having an assistant, usually the nurse, is necessary, as the body will be difficult to move by a single person. Any excess tubes or IVs will need to be removed by the nurse, depending on facility policy. The body may need to be placed in a body bag, if in a facility with a morgue. This can be done using the same turning and repositioning techniques used to perform bath care.

The nurse should be aware that there are sights and sounds that one might see in a dead body that might be alarming and unexpected. For example, there may be a release of air from the lungs of the body as the nurse is cleaning or turning that may sound like a gasp or cry. The body may also have muscle twitches and slight movements as the neurological and muscular systems shut down. Both of these are normal. If the nurse and/or doctor have confirmed official death, post-mortem care can proceed.

After the body has been bathed and placed in a body bag, the body will be transferred to a gurney or some sort of transport stretcher. The body is then transported to the morgue. A **morgue** refers to the refrigerated room where deceased bodies are held pending funeral and burial arrangements. The cold temperature drastically slows down the decomposition process in the bodies, preserving them for the funeral presentation.

Some nurses may find post-mortem care to be uncomfortable, disturbing, and even depressing. This is an initial reaction, and many adjust to it with time and experience. Dealing with dead bodies is not something that the general public is used to experiencing. The nurse must keep in mind that post-mortem care is a continuation of respecting and caring for the patient. Everyone dies, and their bodies must be taken care of afterwards. Thinking of it as an act of respect and courtesy is perhaps the best perspective. The deceased must be treated with dignity, even in death. The nurse is in the unique position to provide such dignified care to the individual.

The reason that one enters the health care field should stem from an earnest desire to help others and care for them in their time of need. This extends beyond their life to their death by taking care of their remains appropriately and respectfully.

Mental Health Concepts

The mental status of a patient has the potential to impact every area of his or her life, resulting in an inability to respond to any nursing intervention. Compromised mental health has been known to affect a patient's coping mechanisms, lifestyle choices, and ability to manage stress effectively. Nurses who work with patients impacted by mental illness need to maintain awareness of numerous concepts. Chief among them is the nurse's effectiveness in conducting the initial interview. It is essential to assess the patient's mood, affect, body language, and tone. Asking open-ended questions about daily living, employment and relationship status, hobbies, and habits can help the nurse determine if any

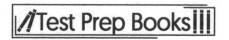

socialization deficits are present. Once the patient begins to respond, this will create an atmosphere of trust, which is necessary when conducting an assessment for depression.

One of the most frequently diagnosed mental illnesses is clinical depression. Although the vast majority of those diagnosed are women, many men are now seeking support. Once the nurse has completed the depression inventory and determines that some risk for clinical depression does exist, the next step will be to discuss how the patient's symptoms affect daily life. Within the last two weeks, has the patient felt increasingly depressed, hopeless, or helpless? Has the patient struggled to fall asleep, woken up early, or slept longer than expected? Are meal times less or more frequent? Has anyone that knows the patient remarked about a change in his or her mood? Have there been sudden bouts of tearfulness, sadness, or feelings of worthlessness? Is the patient engaging in self-harm or high-risk behaviors? Has the patient considered hurting themselves? If so, is there a plan? Does the patient have access to weapons or medications, and have there been suicide attempts in the past? This line of questioning will help the nurse to determine if the patient's depression is mild and situational, which is often transient, or if the depressive state is moderate to severe, requiring more immediate intervention.

Once it is determined that the patient is not in imminent danger or planning to commit suicide, the nurse can begin discussing nursing interventions to alleviate the patient's symptoms. If suicidal ideation does exist, safety planning and hospitalization may be necessary. Utilizing motivational interviewing to reveal the patient's readiness for change, the nurse can open the discussion from where the patient sits on the continuum. This type of nursing style is often necessary to confirm the feasibility of proposed nursing interventions.

If the patient is in **pre-contemplation**, the earliest stage of change, they may have an awareness of the symptoms but not know that those are symptoms of depression. At this stage, information is key. The nurse can explain the symptoms of depression and should be watchful of worsening symptoms. During the second stage, contemplation, the patient is aware that the symptoms are indicative of depression but remain ambivalent about change. The nurse will continue to provide feedback regarding the patient's own words, reflecting back his or her statements. The patient may wish for change but is not yet sure if it is possible.

Once the patient reaches **perception**, the ambivalence has turned into acceptance and the patient feels ready to take the first step. The nurse must have resources readily available regarding how to schedule an appointment with a counselor for talk therapy or to obtain a prescription for antidepressant medications. Be prepared to answer questions about untoward side-effects and how quickly the medications become effective. During the **action phase**, the patient may actually schedule the appointment or fill the prescription, with significant intent to continue. In this instance, the nurse must reinforce the patient's courage and utilize the SMART goal-setting technique to establish a timeline within which to act. Maintenance occurs once the patient actually takes the medication regularly, attends counseling, and is able to verbalize that change has occurred. The nurse should be able to validate the patient's improvement and continue to offer encouragement regarding the patient's own goals. Finally, during the **relapse stage**, something has occurred; a substantial stressor or an unexpected disruption creates imbalance. The patient will begin to miss numerous appointments, forget to refill prescriptions, and symptoms will resurface. At this stage, the nurse must realize that the patient may have returned to the preparation phase. They may believe that the counseling or medications were ineffective and be unsure which steps to take next. Outreach is often necessary, as the patient may be hesitant to return; depressive symptoms may also impact his or her decision making.

It is important to note that the stages of change are not linear. Patients can move along the continuum; moving between one stage and another frequently or skipping certain stages entirely is not uncommon. It is important for the nurse to remain neutral, mirroring the patient's ambivalence to allow for self-determined action.

Mood Disorders, Depression, Anxiety

A **mood disorder** is a mental health class that broadly describe all types of depression and bipolar disorders. The following are the most common types of mood disorders:

1. **Major depression:** having less interest in usual activities, feeling sad or hopeless, and other symptoms for at least 2 weeks.

2. **Dysthymia:** a chronic, low-grade, depressed, or irritable mood that lasts for at least 2 years.

3. **Bipolar disorder:** a condition in which a person has periods of depression alternating with periods of mania or elevated mood.

4. **Mood disorder related to another health condition:** having an acute or chronic medical illnesses can trigger symptoms of depression.

5. **Substance-induced mood disorder:** symptoms of depression that are due to the effects of medicine, drug abuse, alcoholism, exposure to toxins, or other forms of treatment.

Mood disorders may be caused by an imbalance of brain chemicals. Life events, abrupt changes in routine, and stress may also contribute to a depressed mood. Mood disorders also tend to run in families and are more intense and harder to manage than normal feelings of sadness. Children, teens, or adults who have a parent with a mood disorder have a greater chance of also having a mood disorder. Rates of depression are nearly twice as high as in women as they are in men. Once a person in the family has this diagnosis, their brothers, sisters, or children have a higher chance of the same diagnosis. Depending on age and the type of mood disorder, a person may have different symptoms of depression. The following are the most common symptoms of a mood disorder:

- Ongoing sad, anxious, or empty affect
- Feeling hopeless or helpless
- Having low self-esteem
- Feeling inadequate or worthless
- Excessive guilt
- Repeating thoughts of death or suicide
- Loss of interest in usual activities or activities that were once enjoyed, including sex
- Relationship problems
- Trouble sleeping or sleeping too much
- Changes in appetite and/or weight
- Decreased energy
- Trouble concentrating
- A decrease in the ability to make decisions
- Frequent physical complaints that don't get better with treatment
- Very sensitive to failure or rejection
- Irritability, hostility, or aggression

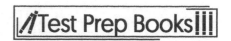

With a mood disorders, these feelings are more intense than what a person may feel occasionally. If these feelings continue over time, interfere with interest in family, friends, community, or work, or if there are thoughts of suicide, medical intervention is needed.

Antidepressant and mood stabilizing medicines, especially when combined with psychotherapy, have been shown to work very well in the treatment of depression. Treatment of bipolar disorder may include mood stabilizers such as lithium and carbamazepine, along with second-generation antipsychotics such as aripiprazole and risperidone. Psychotherapy is focused on changing the person's distorted views of self and the environment. It also helps to improve interpersonal relationship skills, identify stressors in the environment, and assist with avoiding them. Family therapy, electroconvulsive therapy, and transcranial stimulation may also be therapeutic.

Post-Traumatic Stress Disorder (PTSD)

PTSD is a disorder that develops in some people who have experienced a shocking, scary, or dangerous event. People who have PTSD may feel stressed or frightened even when they are not in danger. Fear triggers many split-second changes in the body to help defend against danger or to avoid it. This fight-or-flight response is a typical reaction meant to protect a person from harm. Most people recover from initial symptoms naturally but those who continue to be diagnosed with PTSD.

Symptoms usually begin within 3 months of the traumatic incident, but may occur later. Symptoms must last more than a month and be severe enough to interfere with relationships or work to be considered PTSD. The course of the illness varies, and it may become chronic. Some people recover within 6 months, while others have symptoms that last much longer. Re-experiencing symptoms may cause problems in a person's everyday routine. The symptoms can start from the person's own thoughts and feelings. Words, objects, or situations that are reminders of the event can also trigger re-experiencing symptoms.

To be diagnosed with PTSD, an adult must have all of the following for at least 1 month:

- At least one re-experiencing symptom
- At least one avoidance symptom
- At least two arousal and reactivity symptoms
- At least two cognition and mood symptoms
- Re-experiencing symptoms include:

  o **Flashbacks**—reliving the trauma over and over, including physical symptoms like a racing heart or sweating

  o Bad dreams

  o Frightening thoughts

Avoidance symptoms include staying away from places, events, or objects that are reminders of the traumatic experience and avoiding thoughts or feelings related to the traumatic event. Things that remind a person of the traumatic event can trigger avoidance symptoms. These symptoms may cause a person to change his or her personal routine. For example, after a bad car accident, a person who usually drives may avoid driving or riding in a car.

Arousal and reactivity symptoms include: being easily startled, feeling tense, having difficulty sleeping, and having angry outbursts. Arousal symptoms are usually constant, instead of being triggered by things that remind one of the traumatic events. These symptoms can make the person feel stressed and angry. They may make it hard to do daily tasks, such as sleeping, eating, or concentrating.

Cognition and mood symptoms include: trouble remembering key features of the traumatic event, negative thoughts about self or the world, distorted feelings like guilt or blame, and loss of interest in enjoyable activities. Cognition and mood symptoms can begin or worsen after the traumatic event, but are not due to injury or substance use. These symptoms can make the person feel alienated or detached from friends or family members.

Anyone can develop PTSD at any age. This includes war veterans, children, and people who have been through a physical or sexual assault, abuse, accident, disaster, or many other serious events. According to the National Center for PTSD, about 7 or 8 out of every 100 people will experience PTSD at some point in their lives. Women are more likely to develop PTSD than men, and genes may make some people more likely to develop PTSD than others.

The main treatments for people with PTSD are medications, psychotherapy, or both. Everyone is different, and PTSD affects people differently so a treatment that works for one person may not work for another. It is important for anyone with PTSD to be treated by a mental health provider who is experienced with PTSD. Some people with PTSD need to try different treatments to find what works for their symptoms. As genetic research and brain imaging technologies continue to improve, scientists are more likely to be able to pinpoint when and where in the brain PTSD begins. This understanding may then lead to better targeted treatments to suit each person's own needs or even prevent the disorder before it causes harm.

A 2012 study of 395 military veterans with PTSD found a link between risk-taking behavior and the disorder. In addition to the above forms of riskiness, vets with PTSD have a propensity for firearms play, potentially endangering their lives. People with PTSD have already survived dangerous situations and risk-taking behavior may give such individuals the feeling that they have more control over their present circumstances than those that led to them developing PTSD. Recognizing this propensity in their personality may help patients with risk-taking behavior, thus being the first step in remediating the problem. Behavioral and cognitive therapy, as well as psychological drugs such as antidepressants, may also aid in the treatment of this behavior.

Suicidal Ideation and/or Behaviors

It is important to take people seriously when they express having suicidal thoughts. Research has shown that about one-fifth of people who die by suicide had talked to their doctor or other healthcare professional about their decision. These types of thoughts may arise in people who feel completely hopeless or believe they can no longer cope with their life situation. Suicidal ideation can vary greatly from fleeting thoughts to preoccupation to detailed planning.

According to the CDC, for every 25 attempts, there is one suicide death, Suicide is the tenth leading cause of death for all ages in the United States, and the third leading cause of death among 15 to 24 year-olds. Patients with borderline personality disorder face an extraordinarily high risk of suicidal ideation and suicide attempts. One study showed that 73% of patients with borderline personality disorder have attempted suicide, with the average patient having 3.4 attempts.

Warning signs may include hopelessness, racing thoughts, insomnia or oversleeping, mania, loss of appetite or overeating, loneliness, alcohol abuse, excessive fatigue or low self-esteem. Research has found a variety of risk factors for suicidal ideation including the following:

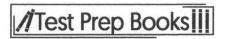

- Mood and mental disorders
- Adverse life or family events (divorce, death of a loved one, job loss)
- Chronic illness or pain
- Previous suicide attempt
- Military experience
- Witnessing trauma
- Family violence
- Owning a gun
- Being the victim of abuse or bullying
- Unplanned pregnancy
- Drug or alcohol abuse

An act that is intended to cause injury but not death is called a non-suicidal self-injury. An example of this type of behavior is when patients cut themselves. It is a method of relieving psychological pain through physical pain. Men are more likely than women to commit suicide, as well as more likely to abuse alcohol and drugs concurrently. Men are less likely to seek help when they are depressed. Veterans have seen an increase in suicides in recent years. It is important to note that despite these risk factors for suicide, it can occur across a wide span of age groups, genders, and life circumstances.

Some patients who are more vocal about their suicidal ideation may be crying out for help and must be taken very seriously. Treatment should include psychotherapy and antidepressants. It should be noted, however, that antidepressants sometimes have the adverse side effect of worsened suicidal behavior. Caregivers should be instructed to be watchful for deepening of depression and thus an increased risk for suicide. Suicide hotlines are available to help suicidal patients in moments of crisis.

Religious and Spiritual Influences on Health

Religious and spiritual beliefs can heavily influence a patient's decision to receive care. It is important for the nurse to determine if any specific religious or spiritual beliefs exist for the patient, and how those beliefs inform his or her decisions. Many people value certain dietary customs in accordance with their religion and strictly adhere to them. For example, for those who identify as Jewish, adherence to a strict Kosher diet is non-negotiable. Any attempts by the nurse to suggest any changes to this diet would be viewed as insensitive. It is for this same reason that religious and spiritual beliefs of any kind must be respected.

Congregants of the Church of Scientology have received significant media attention for what some perceive to be controversial beliefs. Formed by L. Ron Hubbard in the mid 1950s, this religious group focuses on the effectiveness of prayer over traditional Western medicine. Some who self-identify as a part of this group have also expressed particular mistrust of mental health practitioners in general. Although they do not forego all medical treatments, a nurse attending to patients following this religion must consider those beliefs when developing interventions and treatment plans. It may be more advantageous to encourage the patient to consult a church advisor and incorporate the tenants of Scientology into direct practice, if permitted.

Another religious group well known for their healthcare choices is Jehovah's Witnesses. Founded by Charles Taze Russell in the late 1800s, this group does not believe in accepting blood transfusions under any circumstances. A nurse caring for a patient who holds this belief must be prepared to discuss any viable options with the patient and church elders. Not all instances of receiving blood products are prohibited, so it will be important to confirm if the patient would consider using plasma, volume expanders, or artificial blood.

Additionally, ethical considerations regarding how to provide sensitive and compassionate care are important to highlight. It is the nurse's responsibility to seek a consultation with the unit chaplain, social worker, or facility ethics board to discuss any areas where there is a potential conflict of interest.

Sensory/Perceptual Alterations

Nursing interventions include a variety of holistic treatments. Among the most essential elements of nursing techniques that any nurse can employ are those associated with managing sensory and perceptual alterations. During the initial assessment or admission, the nurse must be diligent to perform a complete review of the patient's electronic medical record. Take note of medications that mask or augment neurological deficits. Observe the patient interacting with family members, caregivers, and other medical staff. Once the nurse has been able to gather the information necessary to form an initial impression, the next step is to evaluate the patient clinically.

It is customary to perform a basic screening neurological exam at every patient encounter. Diagnoses such as Alzheimer's disease and dementia are of special note, and the nurse is to follow facility protocols for treatment of these patients. If neurological decline is detected during the initial screening, it will be necessary to assess the patient periodically and, if not specifically ordered, according to the nurse's clinical judgement.

Once the initial chart review and assessment are completed, the nurse must develop a treatment plan and nursing interventions. All have as their primary objective to maintain patient safety. Some of the most common nursing diagnoses for these patients include basic recognition of the typical safety precautions that these patients often need. Bed alarms, keeping the call light within reach, slip-resistant socks, a writing pad and pen or dry-erase board for communicating, hearing and walking aides within reach, lifting one rail of the bed to allow only one route of access, and rooming the patient closer to the nurse's station are frequently instituted. All interventions are to be provided in a calming manner, being careful not to startle the patient. It will also be necessary to be aware of distractions to the patient like ambient noise or other patients in the immediate area. Additionally, the nurse must be prepared to teach all caregivers basic diversion tactics to de-escalate and soothe the patient's anxieties. Finally, take care to periodically evaluate the effectiveness of all interventions and be prepared to adjust as needed.

Stress Management

Stress management is a crucial piece of overall patient well-being. Poorly managed stress has the potential to cause significant health decline. When conducting an assessment, the nurse must carefully approach the topic of stress management. Since many of life's stressors cannot be completely changed, the nurse will be best served to listen actively, remarking about how certain activities or situations can worsen health conditions. Odd work hours, late night shifts, or working multiple jobs can negatively impact sleep patterns. Without restorative sleep, the patient will have difficulties focusing on treatment-plan adherence. As the lack of sleep continues, the patient can begin to lose focus on a previous goal of maintaining healthy lifestyle choices and return to easier high-risk behaviors.

Once the topic of known sources of stress has been initiated, the nurses can go one step further to inquire what steps have been taken to ameliorate those stressors. Next, the patient can be encouraged to state how they have worked to manage the stressors and what has been least effective. It is during

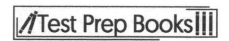

this exchange that the patient is more likely to accept recommendations and institute them in daily life. Notably, it is also necessary to uncover sources of stress that are not readily apparent. Ask probing questions about preferred forms of stress relief and relaxation techniques. Encourage patients to seek out trusted members of their support network to communicate their needs and ask for help. Overall, a patient's ability to institute the checks and balances required to alleviate stress is crucial.

Substance Use and Other Disorders and Dependencies

Substance abuse is defined, most simply, as extreme use of a drug. Abuse occurs for many reasons, such as mental health instability, inability to cope with everyday life stressors, the loss of a loved one, or enjoyment of the euphoric state that the overindulgence in a substance causes. Abused substances create some type of intoxication that alters decision-making, awareness, attentiveness, or physical impulses.

Substance abuse results in tolerance, withdrawal, and compulsive drug-taking behavior. **Tolerance** occurs when increased amounts of the substance are needed to achieve the desired effects. **Withdrawal** manifests as physiological and substance-specific cognitive symptoms (e.g., cold sweats, shivering, nausea, vomiting, paranoia, hallucinations). Withdrawal does not only happen when an individual stops abusing the substance, but also occurs when he or she attempts to reduce the amount taken in an effort to stop using altogether.

Some of the most commonly abused substances include the following:

Tobacco
People abuse tobacco either in cigarette, cigar, pipe, or snuff form. People report many reasons for tobacco use, including a calming effect, suppression of appetite, and relief of depression. The primary addictive component in tobacco is nicotine, and tobacco smoke also contains about seven hundred carcinogens (cancer-causing agents) that may result in lung and throat cancers, as well as heart disease, emphysema, peptic ulcer disease, and stroke. Withdrawal indicators include insomnia, irritability, overwhelming nicotine craving, anxiety, and depression.

Alcohol
Some individuals need a drink to "smooth out the edges," as it is a CNS depressant, which tends to calm and soothe and lower inhibitions. However, it also slurs speech and impairs muscle control, coordination, and reflex time. Alcohol abuse can cause cirrhosis of the liver; liver, esophagus, and stomach cancers; heart enlargement; chronic inflammation of the pancreas; vitamin deficiencies; certain anemias; and brain damage. Physical dependence is a biological need for alcohol to avoid physical withdrawal symptoms, which include anxiety, erratic pulse rate, tremors, seizures, and hallucinations. In its most serious form, withdrawal combined with malnourishment can lead to a potentially fatal condition known as **delirium tremens (DTs),** which is a psychotic disorder that involves tremors, disorientation, and hallucinations.

Other Prescriptions
Prescription medications, such as anti-anxiety, sleep, and pain medications.

Marijuana
Marijuana is considered the most frequently abused illicit drug in the United States. General effects of marijuana use include pleasure, relaxation, and weakened dexterity and memory. The active addictive ingredient in marijuana is tetrahydrocannabinol (THC). It is normally smoked (but can be eaten), and its

smoke has more carcinogens than that of tobacco. The individual withdrawing from marijuana will experience increased irritability and anxiety.

Cocaine

Cocaine is a stimulant that is also known as **coke, snow**, or **rock**. It can be smoked, injected, snorted, or swallowed. Reported effects include pleasure, enhanced alertness, and increased energy. Both temporary and prolonged use have been known to contribute to damage to the brain, heart, lungs, and kidneys. Withdrawal symptoms include severe depression and reduced energy.

Heroin

Also known as **smack** and **horse**, heroin use continues to increase. Effects of heroin abuse include pleasure, slower respirations, and drowsiness. Overdose and/or overuse of heroin can cause respiratory depression, resulting in death. Use of heroin as an injectable substance can lead to other complications such as heart valve damage, tetanus, botulism, hepatitis B, or human immunodeficiency virus (HIV)/AIDS infection from sharing dirty needles. Withdrawal is usually intense and will demonstrate as vomiting, abdominal cramps, diarrhea, confusion, body aches, and diaphoresis.

Methamphetamines

Also known as **meth, crank**, and **crystal**, methamphetamine use also continues to increase, especially in the West and Midwest regions of the United States. A methamphetamine is categorized as a stimulant that produces such effects as pleasure, increased alertness, and decreased appetite. Similar to cocaine, it can be snorted, smoked, or injected and eaten as well. Like cocaine, it shares many of the same detrimental effects, such as myocardial infarction, hypertension, and stroke. Other prolonged usage effects include paranoia, hallucinations, damage to and loss of dentition, and heart damage. Withdrawal symptoms involve depression, abdominal cramps, and increased appetite.

Nursing interventions for the individual addicted to tobacco, alcohol, and other drugs centers around the prevention of relapse, and treatment depends on the individual and the substance that is abused. Behavioral treatment assists with recognition of abuse triggers, habits, and drug cravings, as well as providing the tactics to help one cope with these issues. A physician may prescribe nicotine patches for the tobacco abuser and methadone or Suboxone to manage withdrawal symptoms and certain drug yearnings.

Non-Substance-Related Dependencies

Even some behaviors—such as exercise and work—are recognized as positive behaviors, but when taken to extremes, unpleasant consequences develop. For example, exercise addiction, in its least damaging form, may create anxiety when physical or weather conditions prevent participation. In more extreme cases, certain athletes will continue to train in spite of illness or injury, exacerbating the physical problem and sometimes causing permanent disabilities.

Overworking—sometimes referred to as "**workaholism**"—may also be viewed as positive by some standards. In the end, however, those working many hours of overtime may result in a life out of balance. They may also be using work as a means to avoid other responsibilities, such as family life. It can create stress and low energy, and it can lead to physical and emotional problems.

Sexual addiction, also known as **hypersexuality**, involves a preoccupation with sexual pleasures that can manifest itself in a multitude of ways. These behaviors prove harmful to themselves and potentially other people. One example is pornography. Those addicted to pornography find that having close and intimate contact with their long-term partner is less exciting than viewing stimulating films or pictures.

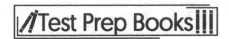

This creates intimacy problems and difficulty in one's primary relationship. The Internet has made it easier for people to access these materials, sometimes at no cost, creating a greater number of persons who view it addictively.

Gambling addiction may involve a desire for the adrenaline rush of making bets or a cycle of losing money via gambling and then gambling more to try to make up for previously lost money.

Overeating, based upon the number of obese and overweight persons in our culture, is on the rise. Some people use food much in the same way that others use alcohol or drugs—to feel a sense of pleasure or to numb feelings of depression or anxiety. The consequences of obesity are numerous from a social and physical standpoint, with the most severe of these being at higher risk for heart disease or stroke.

Some individuals are addicted to **self-harm** in the form of cutting, scratching, or mutilating themselves. This is often described as a means to bring relief from emotional pain as one focuses on the physical sensation of pain to distract from the emotional sensation. It may also be a type of self-punishment. Some people have horrendous scars from this compulsion. Others may contract infections. It is theorized that persons who self-mutilate are at higher risk of suicide than those who do not, making it a possible precursor to suicidal ideations.

Support Systems

Another contributing factor for overall patient well-being is a well-functioning support system. Even if there is no disease process present, a support system, as defined by the patient, is vital to healthy stress and disease management. During the assessment, the nurse must ask open-ended questions about patients' support systems: What hobbies do they enjoy? How do they spend the holidays, and with whom? Are they married or single? Do they have children? Answers to these few questions will help quickly decide if there are any gaps in socialization and open the discussion on how to fill them.

Whether it's family members, friends, or coworkers, some sort of support network usually exists for most patients. The nurse must make sure to encourage discussion about who the patient confides in and trusts. Those individuals can either add to or subtract from the patient's progression through and whole-hearted commitment to treatment. For those patients who report having no supportive network, the nurse can guide the patient toward viable options. One of the most effective and influential options would be to match the patient to a support group according to any comorbidities that they currently manage. Thousands of independent groups exist to provide a much-needed communal experience. Often run by health professionals or counselors, members of these groups can gain knowledge about their condition, daily symptom management, and possibly gain new supportive friends. Overall, the presence of a network of trusted friends and advisors is an invaluable facet of the therapeutic environment.

Therapeutic Communication

Overcoming barriers to communication requires practicing therapeutic communication. **Therapeutic communication** is a type of communication that assists the patient in the healing process rather than hindering it. There are a number of useful communication techniques the nurse can employ to aid in therapeutic communication.

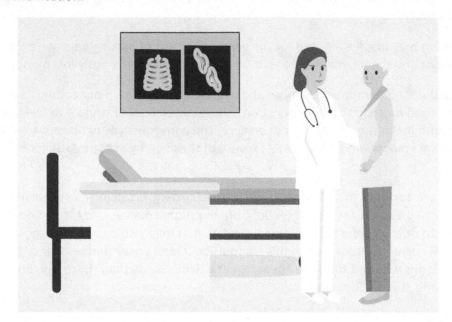

Sometimes, silence is the best way to get clarification from a patient, or simply asking them to clarify when one does not understand. Nurses may offer themselves to support the patient without providing personal details, by sympathizing and saying, "Yes, I have been through something similar." The nurse may ask the patient to summarize their thoughts or identify a theme when stories go on at length. This helps redirect communication in a positive direction.

Asking the patient how certain events made them feel is a way to investigate the patient's emotional status. The nurse may give information about their role and make observations, such as "I noticed you seem tense," to open the door to more fluent conversation. Giving the patient praise and recognition without overt flattery is a way to show support, such as complimenting a noticeable effort during a physical therapy session. The nurse may want to determine the chronological order of events, which can be helpful for reporting information.

Employing therapeutic communication aids smooth collaboration and cooperation between members of the health care team. Incorporating smart, simple, therapeutic communication techniques and overcoming barriers to communication are important parts of achieving this goal.

Therapeutic Environment

Within every milieu, the nurse must maintain awareness of the effectiveness of the therapeutic environment of the patient. The nurse must enter into each patient encounter with a plan to develop a rapport as quickly as possible. A warm greeting, using Mr. or Mrs., rather than using a first name, honey, or sweetie, will imply an equal and respectful relationship. The ability to work collaboratively with the patient is the foundation of cooperative treatment planning.

Although the nurse is generally much more comfortable during the assessment, it is important for the nurse to consider that the patient may be hesitant to disclose personal information. If the patient does not trust the nurse or feels unseen, unheard, or hurried through the interaction, the environment may

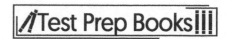

not feel safe. More important, when a patient does not feel safe enough to disclose, they will not share important health information, which could hinder treatment planning and adherence.

Another important aspect of the therapeutic environment for the nurse to be aware of is the treatment setting. For example, a patient in a correctional-facility hospital may be less likely to reveal sensitive information for fear of reprisal from inmates or staff. Alternatively, patients in a mental health or substance abuse treatment center may freely divulge information, as they often seek treatment of their own accord. In either instance, the nurse must utilize critical thinking to determine if the therapeutic environment is negatively impacted by the setting and seek ways to address any barriers to resolution.

Basic Care and Comfort

Assistive Devices

The nurse may discover during assessment that the client needs an assistive device. There are many such devices available for a variety of different client needs. **Assistive devices** may generally fall into the categories of assisting with sensorial deficits or mobility deficits.

Clients with sensorial deficits may first need a referral to the appropriate party. A client with difficulties seeing may need a referral to an ophthalmologist for evaluation and the prescription of appropriate lenses.

There are four main vision problems that can be treated with corrective eyewear in mild to moderate cases: myopia, presbyopia, hyperopia, and astigmatism. More severe cases may require surgical intervention.

For the client who requires eyeglasses, the nurse must take care to protect the glasses from damage. While in the hospital room, the glasses should be kept in a safe place, such as in their case on the bedside table. Most bedside tables in hospital rooms have pullout drawers underneath that can store items such as glasses, dentures, hearing aids, and other personal effects.

Patients with blindness, who are legally blind, or who have some form of low vision, will need assistive devices to help them navigate their environment. They may also need assistance with written communications such as discharge instructions and other patient education materials. Depending on the facility, the nurse may be able to give the patient access to devices that use Braille for written communication, software for a PC or smartphone that reads aloud written instructions, and magnifiers for computer screens, phone screens, or other devices. The patient with blindness or very low vision may require a special cane, a therapy animal, or a personal assistant to help them ambulate about their room and the facility. The nurse will assess for these needs and ensure the patient has everything they need for clear communication and a safe environment during their stay.

Patients who have difficulty hearing may require a referral to an audiologist who may then fit them with a hearing aid. Hearing aids, along with glasses, should be kept in a safe place when not in use. Small assistive devices such as hearing aids, dentures, and eyeglasses can easily be lost in the linens when they are changed or carried away with the food tray if they are left on top. The nurse and nurse's aid should work with the patient and family to ensure that these items are stored properly to avoid losing them. These items can be very difficult to track down if lost in the linens, in a bedside waste basket, or on the food tray. They are often very expensive to replace for the patient.

The nurse will further assess the patient with hearing loss for any other needed interventions that might assist with communication and ease of stay. Closed captioning is available on most TV sets for most programs so the patient can fully enjoy what they are watching. The patient may be a lip-reader, in which case the nurse needs to ensure they stand directly in front of the patient, face them, and make solid eye contact when communicating important messages. The patient will need to see the nurse, specifically their lips, to interpret the message. If the nurse's face is turned away or looking down, the patient will have difficulty understanding what is being spoken to them.

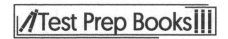

The nurse needs to ensure the patient understands the message by asking questions about comprehension. Some patients with chronic, severe hearing loss may have developed a coping mechanism of pretending they understood what was said by nodding or giving a short verbal reply. They may do this because they feel embarrassed or ashamed about their hearing loss. They may also not want the further hassle of admitting they did not hear or understand what was said and needing to have the message repeated. Without further embarrassing the patient, the nurse should gently inquire about comprehension of the medications they are taking, procedures they are to go through, and if they need anything to make their stay better. Patience and thoroughness are key to ensuring the message gets delivered.

A patient with a speech-language deficit may have difficulty forming meaningful communication as well as fully comprehending the messages that are spoken to them. The nurse who assesses such a need can refer the patient to a speech-language pathologist or therapist; most hospitals have a team of these specialists. They will evaluate the patient's speech-language capabilities and recommend assistive devices as needed.

Some such assistive devices include word boards in which the patient can point to a word or picture that helps them communicate a need. The speech-therapy team will work with the patient through exercises aimed at enhancing their abilities to their greatest potential. Patients who have experienced a cerebrovascular accident or stroke often experience speech and language deficits because of the cerebral tissue damage that occurs. Not all function may be restored, depending on the patient and the extent of the stroke.

Patients with difficulties walking may require assistive devices such as a walker, cane, or wheelchair. If the nurse assesses the patient and finds that such a need is there, they may contact the physical and occupational therapy (PT and OT) teams for assistance. PT and OT work to help the patient become mobile to their greatest functioning capability as well as assisting them in performing activities of daily living (ADLs). Common ADLs that PT/OT works with the patient to perform include getting dressed, tying their shoes, and bathing and feeding themselves.

The nurse will work with the patient and encourage them to use their assistive devices as needed. The nurse ensures the patient that they, along with the nursing assistant team, are always a call button away to assist the patient in getting out of bed, walking with the use of a cane or walker, or getting them into a wheelchair. Mobility in patients is always encouraged, as it helps them heal and achieve their fullest sense of wellness, but it must always be done with safety measures in place to prevent falls and injury.

The nurse may advise the patient using a wheelchair to avoid tipping themselves out of the chair by leaning forward. Their feet should be firmly planted in the foot rests to prevent getting caught in the wheels or dragging on the ground. The brakes should be locked at all times that the wheelchair is stopped or not actively rolling to avoid slippage. The patient in the wheelchair should avoid overreaching for objects, as this may also cause them to fall out. The patient's buttocks should be positioned as far back in the seat as possible to avoid falling out.

The nurse may have a patient with a prosthetic limb. Usually these patients arrive at the hospital with their own prosthetic limb that they have been properly fitted for, educated on, and actively use. If the patient is a new amputee, they will need a referral to the proper prosthetics expert for fitting. Patients with prosthetics should use the proper footwear for their prosthetic as well as adequate support to prevent falls. The patient will be aware that they should not allow their prosthetic limb to become wet. Thus, they will take the limb off when washing or taking a shower. The metal components of the prosthetic will rust if exposed to water. The patient should let the nurse know if their prosthetic device feels uncomfortable, as this may be a sign of misalignment and need adjustment. If the patient is hearing unusual noises from their prosthetic such as squeaks or crunches, this may be a sign of mechanical impairment and that the prosthetic needs repair.

Patients using crutches should start walking by putting all their weight on their good leg. With the crutches firmly situated in the armpits, the patient can then lift the crutches and set them down 6 to 12 inches in front of them, lean their weight into their hands, and then step forward with the good leg. This avoids putting weight on the injured leg, transferring all weight to the hands and the good leg, alternatively.

Elimination

There are many situations in a facility in which the patient is unable to **eliminate**—i.e., defecate and/or urinate—independently. Elimination is a basic and highly personal need for all people, and the nurse needs to be able to assist with this task appropriately and respectfully. Common issues in elimination are incontinence, constipation, and diarrhea. Some patients may have devices to assist with elimination, such as a colostomy, rectal tube, or urinary catheter.

Incontinence is a term meaning the patient cannot control their bladder and/or bowels. Some patients may be said to be incontinent of bowel, incontinent of bladder, or both. This can be for various reasons, including neurological impairment, such as paralysis or a physical impairment, such as a broken hip. In any scenario of incontinence, it is important to monitor the patient's elimination throughout a shift and assist when possible. If the patient is oriented enough to request help before having a bowel or bladder movement, the nurse should be as available as possible to assist. This may entail assisting the patient to the bathroom or providing a bedside commode or a bedpan.

If the patient is incontinent in bed, a partial bath will be needed along with a linen change. Checking for incontinence frequently is important, as a timely cleanup of a patient who has been incontinent is crucial to preventing skin breakdown. Proper hand hygiene needs to be performed before and after any perineal care to prevent spread of disease.

Constipation refers to a condition in which the bowels have slowed down their movement, preventing normal defecation and potentially causing discomfort to the patient. Immobility and medications may cause constipation as a side effect.

Monitoring of output is one way to discover constipation, along with the patient and/or family report of bowel patterns. If constipation is suspected, the health care provider may prescribe a stool softener, a laxative, or—in severe cases—an enema. Soap suds and fleets enemas are commonly used types.

Each institution has individual policies on who can perform enemas on patients. Other interventions used to alleviate constipation include encouraging mobility, encouraging intake of fluids when possible, and increasing fiber intake.

When the bowels are overly active and amounts of liquid stool are passed frequently, it is called **diarrhea.** Causes of diarrhea include food intolerance or allergy, infection, a medication side effect, or a reaction to a surgical procedure. A major complication of diarrhea is dehydration. Dehydration can occur rapidly in a patient with diarrhea due to loss of fluids. Intake and output need to be vigilantly monitored along with encouragement of fluid intake, if appropriate.

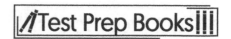

A **colostomy** is a surgically placed opening from the large or small intestines to the abdominal wall as a result of a bowel condition, such as colon cancer. A colostomy bag is attached to the skin around the colostomy to collect stool. Depending on how long the colostomy has been in place and how well developed the colostomy is, the patient may be able to care for their colostomy bag independently or may need varying levels of assistance from the health care team. Most colostomy bags are fairly easy to remove, drain, and replace when necessary.

Another assistive device for elimination of the bowels is called a **rectal tube**. A rectal tube is a tube that is inserted into the rectum to collect stool or relieve gas. At the end of the tube is a balloon that can be inflated to anchor it in place as it collects stool. The rectal tube is used in patients who are incontinent, at risk for or have skin breakdown, and/or have diarrhea. Each facility will have specific policies outlining when a rectal tube is needed. Complications, such as atony of the rectum and internal tissue breakdown, may arise when rectal tubes are in place for extended periods. The rectal tube drains into a bag that the nurse can empty and record as output in the medical record. Perineal care may be required around the site of the rectal tube if any leakage occurs.

The patient may have a **urinary catheter** for various reasons including immobility and monitoring of output. The catheter has an inflatable balloon at the end filled with normal saline that anchors the catheter in place as it drains urine from the urinary bladder to a collection bag. The nurse can then empty this bag and record the output in the medical record.

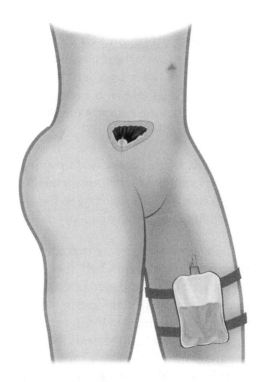

During the patient's daily bath or whenever perineal care is necessary, proper technique must be used to prevent a urinary tract infection (UTI). The nurse must follow the facility's policy regarding proper catheter care, including using warm water around the site to cleanse the urethra and always using a circular motion around the tube moving away from the patient. The nurse should never use a back and forth motion as this could introduce bacteria into the urethra, resulting in a UTI. Signs and symptoms of a UTI include fever, chills, cloudy urine, blood in the urine (**hematuria**), or a change in mental status. If any of these occur, the nurse should be alerted immediately.

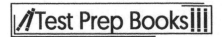

Mobility

Promoting Mobility and Proper Positioning

Proper positioning is important for a patient's comfort and safety. Some of the common patient positions are:

- **High Fowler's Position:** The head of the patient's bed is raised sixty to ninety degrees and the knees are either flexed or extended out straight.

- **Fowler's Position:** The head of the patient's bed is raised forty-five to sixty degrees.

- **Semi-Fowler's Position:** The head of the patient's bed is raised thirty to forty-five degrees.

- **Supine:** The patient is lying on their back.

- **Lateral:** The patient is lying on their side.

- **Prone:** The patient is lying on their stomach, with their head turned to the side.

When positioning a patient in bed, always raise the entire bed high enough to avoid bending over while assisting the patient. Be sure to lower the head of the bed to its lowest position before leaving the patient.

Promoting Function, Including Prosthetic and Orthotic Devices

A nurse should encourage patients to be as mobile as possible and help them correctly use assistive devices such as canes and walkers. Patients with prosthetic limbs should be given assistance with, and access to, these devices. When assisting a patient with a prosthetic limb, always note any redness or irritation that occurs where the prosthetic limb contacts the skin.

Safe Transfer Techniques

When transferring a patient, the safety of the patient and the nurse are of the greatest importance. Incorrectly performed transfers can cause injury to both. Be mindful of proper transfer techniques and body mechanics, such as keeping a straight back, bending at the knees, avoiding twisting at the waist, and, most importantly, asking for additional help if needed.

When assisting a patient out of bed, always make sure that the bed is in the lowest position. Then, assist the patient to sit upright on the side of the bed with both feet on the floor. While the patient remains in this seated position, make sure they aren't lightheaded or dizzy from the position change. If the patient needs significant physical assistance other than stabilization, an assistive device should be considered. To assist the patient in standing, the nurse should stand in front of the patient, place their knees in front of the patient's knees, and hug the patient under the arms for lifting. Then instruct the patient to help as much as possible. If transferring the patient to a chair after assisting them to stand, both the nurse and the patient should take small steps, pivoting around to the chair. Make sure the backs of the patient's knees are touching the front of the seat before lowering them into the chair.

When transferring a patient, make sure that all wheels are locked on the bed and/or chair before moving the patient.

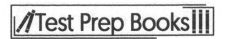

Devices that Promote Mobility

A nurse should encourage patients to use available assistive devices, such as canes, walkers, and wheelchairs. Before leaving a patient's room, make sure any assistive device that the patient uses independently is within their reach. Patients with lower-body immobility who still have upper-body strength might have a bed equipped with a trapeze. A **trapeze** is an assistive bar that hangs above the patient's bed and enables self-repositioning. Patients who are able should be encouraged to use the trapeze.

The use of assistive devices such as **gait belts** (also known as **transfer belts**) benefits both the nurse and the patient. When transferring or walking with a patient who needs assistance, it's advised to use a gait belt to prevent falls. When using a gait belt to assist a patient to walk, fasten the belt around their waist and hold it with both hands while standing to the side and slightly behind the patient. If the patient loses their balance and begins to fall, never attempt to catch them. Instead, continue holding the gait belt, bend at the knees, and slowly lower the patient to the floor.

Range of Motion Techniques

Range of motion exercises involve moving the body's limbs in particular ways to keep the joints healthy and flexible. **Active range of motion exercises** are performed by the patient independently. **Passive range of motion exercises** are done for patients who are unable to perform active ones. When performing passive range of motion exercises, gently guide the patient's limbs through their range of motion. Never force the limbs, as this can harm the patient.

With the patient resting in the supine position, take each joint through its range of motion. **Adduction** is the movement of a limb toward the midline of the body. **Abduction**, the opposite of adduction, is the movement of a limb away from the midline of the body.

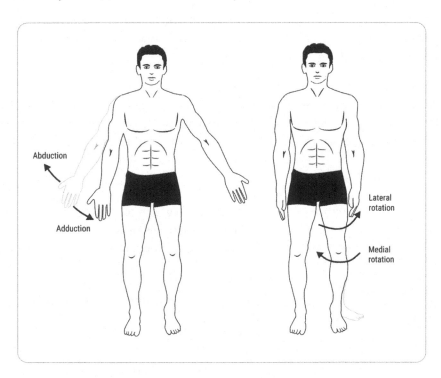

Flexion is the bending of a limb at the joint, while **extension** is the straightening of a limb at the joint.

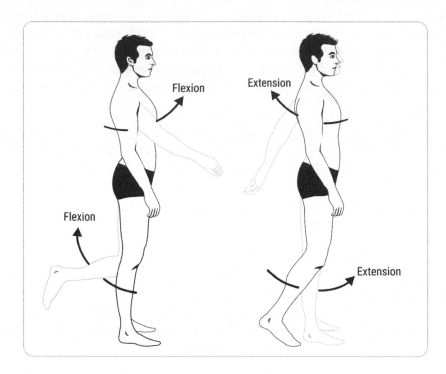

Effects of Immobility

Circulation and Skin Integrity

Patients with limited mobility are at risk for compromised circulation and/or skin breakdown. A nurse helps patients reposition themselves frequently (at least once every two hours), which prevents pressure sores and promotes adequate circulation.

Pressure sores (also called **bedsores** or **pressure ulcers**) are areas of skin breakdown that manifest when pressure on the skin minimizes circulation in that area. These usually occur over bony prominences such as the heel, ankle, coccyx, elbow, knee, or hip. Patients with pressure sores generally have some degree of immobility and are unable to reposition themselves frequently. Pressure sores are categorized by the following four stages:

Stage I

The skin of the affected area is unbroken, generally red, and warm to the touch. Skin discoloration remains even after the patient is repositioned and the pressure is relieved from the site. Patients may have associated pain. Stage I pressure sores can be difficult to recognize in patients with dark skin.

Stage II

Damage or loss of skin through several layers (partial thickness) with shallow ulceration of the skin, abrasion, or blistering.

Stage III

Full thickness skin loss (epidermal and dermal layers) with ulceration that can be deep enough to expose fatty tissue; however, muscle, bone, and tendon are NOT visible. Tunneling might also be seen in patients with Stage III pressure sores.

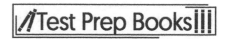

Stage IV

Full thickness tissue loss (epidermis, dermis, and underlying tissue damage) with deep ulceration and possible tunneling. Muscle, bone, and/or tendon are visible and palpable with Stage IV pressure sores.

To help prevent pressure sores, keep the patient's skin clean and dry, and reposition the patient at least every two hours. Whenever available, use assistive positioning devices such as pillows and wedges to help relieve pressure on bony prominences. These bony areas should not be massaged in patients who have, or are at risk of having, pressure sores. Clothing and bed linens should be straightened often to avoid wrinkles that can quickly lead to pressure sores in at-risk patients. Report any indication of skin breakdown to the nurse.

Deep vein thrombosis (DVT) refers to a blood clot in the body's deep veins, most commonly in the legs. Redness, swelling, and sometimes pain in an extremity can be signs of DVT. Patients with DVT are at risk for a **pulmonary embolism (PE)**, which occurs when a blood clot in the deep vein breaks off, travels to the lungs, and cuts off blood flow. Do not massage red or swollen areas in the extremities, as this can result in a clot breaking off and causing a pulmonary embolism.

Patients who are immobile are at an increased risk for developing DVT. If possible, patients should be encouraged to ambulate to avoid DVT. If a patient is unable to ambulate, assistance with range of motion exercises should be provided. **Anti-embolism stockings** (also called **TED hose**) and **sequential compression devices (SCDs)** are commonly used for patients who are confined to their beds. Both of these help to promote circulation in the lower legs and prevent blood pooling.

Elimination (Bowel and Bladder)

Immobility can lead to problems with elimination. Patients who are unable to care for their own toileting needs are at risk for incontinence. Be attentive to a patient's toileting needs and attempt to establish a routine with the patient. Immobility can also lead to constipation. If not contraindicated, a patient who is at risk for constipation should be encouraged to increase fluid intake. Patients can be reluctant to increase fluid intake because of their inability to self-toilet, so encourage the patient to increase their intake and be available for their toileting needs.

Sleep and Rest Patterns/Needs

Patients with immobility can have altered sleep patterns because of their limited ability to be physically active. Pain, discomfort, anxiety, stress, and certain medications are also common issues that can disrupt sleep. Older patients, as well as patients who are healing from illness or injury, require frequent rest and sleep periods. However, they should be encouraged to be active when they're able. Assist patients in establishing daily routines and encourage them to participate in daily living activities as much as possible. For instance, if a patient can sit in a chair for a meal rather than remaining in bed, encourage and assist them to do so. As another example, if a patient is able (with assistance) to transfer from using a bedpan to using a bedside toilet, encourage and assist them to do so. Any activities a patient can participate in will benefit their sleep, rest, and overall well-being. However, be attentive and careful not to overtire the patient. Any patient complaints of sleeplessness should be reported to the nurse.

Self-Image

When patients lose mobility, they can experience a sense of loss of independence. They can become isolated, depressed, and/or withdrawn and might begin to develop a negative self-image. Encourage these patients to participate in activities of daily living and give them as many opportunities as possible for autonomy.

Strength and Endurance

Patients who experience immobility can begin to lose muscle strength and endurance. If the immobile patient isn't cared for properly and their muscles aren't used, the muscles can begin to atrophy (weaken), the joints can begin to stiffen, and **contractures** (muscle shortenings) can develop. To prevent this from occurring, a nurse performs passive range of motion exercises with immobile patients during times of care, such as bathing and/or dressing. Patients who are able to perform active range of motion exercises are encouraged to do so.

Activity Tolerance

While patients should be encouraged to participate in activities of daily living as much as possible, be careful not to overtire them. A patient's daily routine should be planned carefully. Activities should be spaced so that there's ample opportunity to participate as well as adequate rest periods in between.

Comfort

A nurse should provide immobile patients with as much comfort as possible. Reposition patients no less than every two hours and use positioning devices such as pillows and wedges to promote proper body alignment and circulation and to reduce issues of skin breakdown.

Non-Pharmacological Comfort Interventions

When the nurse assesses the patient and finds they need something to alleviate a discomfort, they may first think of pharmacological interventions such as an analgesic. The nurse must also consider nonpharmacological interventions to comfort a patient, as these often come with little to none of the commonly experienced drug side effects.

There are many examples of nonpharmacological interventions the nurse may employ before turning to medication. Repositioning a patient who is feeling uncomfortable may be the first step in relieving a cramp or excessive pressure. This may involve getting the patient in or out of bed, sitting in a chair, or ambulating if appropriate. The nurse may also use pillows to prop and position the patient into a more comfortable position in the bed.

A patient may complain of being too hot or too cold. The nurse may look at what the patient is wearing and decide if additional clothing would help or if the removal of clothing items, as appropriate, would assist. Giving the patient their coat, a warm blanket from the floor's blanket warmer, or socks may comfort a cold patient. Many hospitals do not allow fans, as they are an infection control risk, but the nurse may provide other options to the patient who wishes to cool off. If the patient is not on a fluid restriction, ice chips or ice water may be helpful in refreshing them. Removing excessive blankets may cool them off as well.

The nurse can use heat and cold in even more targeted approaches to relieve pain. Application of heat, such as warm washcloths, electric blankets, and warm baths will increase blood flow to the painful area, reduce muscle spasms, slow down peristalsis, relax the smooth muscles, and even decrease stomach acid production.

Cold application, on the other hand, cannot only decrease the spasmodic activities of muscles but also cause vasoconstriction in the areas where it is applied. The application of cold items such as an ice pack, cool washcloth, and ice cubes can decrease inflammation and increase peristalsis. The application of cold items may have a longer-lasting effect than the application of heat in some patients.

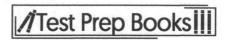

The nurse should not feel uncomfortable offering therapeutic touch where and when appropriate. Most nursing schools train their students in at least the most basic of massage techniques that the nurse may use on clients experiencing muscle tension. Massage should only be applied with the patient's consent and in an appropriate manner. The nurse may use lotion or oil if appropriate to relieve areas of muscle tension. Common areas that become tense include the neck, shoulders, and lower back. By massaging these areas, the nurse may be able to promote healthy blood flow, decrease tension, and maybe even relieve achiness that the client may be experiencing.

Some clients may request alternate therapies for spiritual needs. The nurse may refer the client to the appropriate entity for these interventions. For example, most hospitals offer a clergy that will come to the patient and talk with them. Patients may have spiritual issues they may want to discuss. The clergy and spiritual staff available at the hospital can address those needs, talk with the patient, and pray with them.

The nurse may use certain psychological modalities for relieving a patient's pain or discomfort. Distraction such as music therapy can be helpful in moving the patient's focus off the discomfort, as pain is perceived in the mind and can sometimes be overcome there as well. The nurse may educate the patient about a topic that is troubling them, thus relieving any anxiety they may feel. Simple strategies aimed at relaxation such as controlled, deep breathing may assist a patient in pain. Deep breathing causes the body to take in far more stress-reducing oxygen and release the waste product carbon dioxide, thus making the patient immediately feel better. Breathing techniques are a hallmark of natural childbirth, as the woman focuses on her breathing to work her way through each contraction. Sometimes the simple act of listening to the patient as they voice their concerns may be all it takes to alleviate their apprehension, working through the inner conflict.

There are certain relaxation strategies that may be used on patients when muscle tension is present. These fall mainly into the categories of progressive muscle relaxation, autogenic training, and biofeedback. **Progressive muscle relaxation** techniques will have the patient alternately tighten and then relax different muscle groups. **Autogenic training** involves the patient training their body to respond to verbal commands, often targeted at the breathing rate, blood pressure, heartbeat, and temperature of the body. **Biofeedback** often includes breathing exercises. The goal of all of these relaxation strategies is to promote relaxation and reduce stress.

Whichever nonpharmacological technique the nurse chooses should be selected very carefully, using critical thinking and sound nursing judgment to best serve the patient's need and alleviate their discomfort.

Nutrition and Oral Hydration

A patient admitted to a facility will often have specific nutritional needs, such as a diet modification or restriction. Conditions, such as nausea or vomiting, and equipment, such as nasogastric tubes, can further complicate the goal of maintaining adequate nutrition. The nurse should also be familiar with intravenous (IV) accesses and how to monitor them.

There are several different dietary restrictions that a patient may have depending on their condition. A **cardiac diet**, or **heart-healthy diet**, is for patients with heart conditions. This diet is generally low in sodium, fat, and cholesterol. The nurse will educate the patient about this diet, but it is important for the nurse to ensure the correct meal tray is delivered to the patient. Other dietary restrictions for health reasons include the **renal diet**—for patients with kidney problems or failure—a **diabetic diet**, which focuses on controlling carbohydrate intake, and a **fluid-restricted diet** for patients with heart or kidney failure.

There are cultural and religious considerations to be aware of when it comes to dietary restrictions. Some adherents of the Jewish and Islamic faiths, for example, do not consume pork products. Some Jews also do not consume meat and dairy products in the same meal. Acceptable Jewish meals are referred to as **kosher,** while in the Islamic faith, foods that are acceptable are called **halal.** Some people believe it is wrong to consume any meat and only eat non-animal foods. They are called **vegetarians.** **Vegans** do not consume any animal product of any kind, such as milk or honey.

Some patients may be **lactose intolerant. Lactose** is a sugar found in dairy products that can cause gastrointestinal upset to sensitive individuals. These people may need to abstain from consuming dairy products or take a digestive aid—such as the enzyme lactase—to help them digest the lactose.

There are numerous other dietary restrictions a patient can have for various reasons. The important points for the nurse are to be familiar with the patient's diet order, to ensure the correct tray is delivered, to correct a mistake made by the food service, and to ensure the patient's wishes are respected.

Illness and medications can sometimes bring on side effects of nausea and/or vomiting. The patient experiencing these side effects will likely prefer to abstain from food—called fasting—until the nausea and vomiting subsides. If the nausea and vomiting is short-lived, fasting is not a problem. If the fasting is prolonged, however, the patient will experience nutritional deficits and further complications.

The nurse must always assist the health care team in carefully monitoring all of a patient's **intake and output (I&O)** to ensure adequate nutrition and hydration. Any nausea or vomiting must be recorded, as well as the amount of meals eaten. The intake and output record will be tracked by the health care team and interventions based upon it. There are medications, such as Zofran (ondansetron), that can alleviate nausea and prevent vomiting. In the case of a patient receiving chemotherapy treatments who has constant nausea and trouble eating, there are medicines that can encourage appetite.

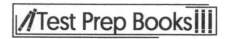

Some patients may have a **nasogastric (NG) tube** placed through the nose, down the esophagus and into the stomach for therapeutic or diagnostic purposes. The nurse ensures patient comfort and monitors the tube for dislodgement or displacement. The tube is usually secured in one nostril of the patient's nose with a strip of tape. Any changes in the tube must be reported to the nurse immediately.

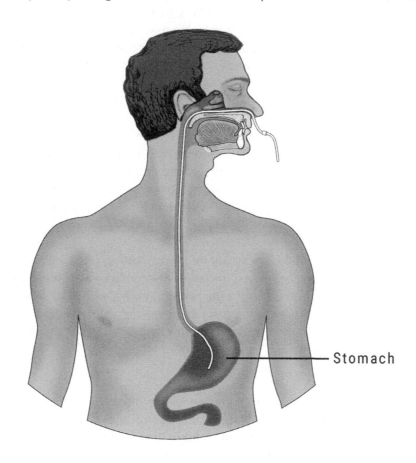

Stomach

The patient who is confused can be even further aggravated by the placement of an NG tube and may need special assistance to prevent disturbing the tube. As a last resort, a method of preserving the tube would be to put physical restraints on the patient, but only if all other options have been exhausted.

Food Nutrients

Carbohydrates

Carbohydrates are **organic** (containing carbon) compounds that are converted into energy for the body. They may be simple, such as refined table sugar, or complex, such as pasta, rice, and fiber.

Fats

Fats are lipid-containing compounds that are necessary for cell wall integrity, energy storage, and protection of all body organs against injury. **Cholesterol** is a body fat that exists in two forms: **low-density lipoprotein (LDL)** and **high-density lipoprotein (HDL)**. LDLs are associated with the formation and progression of **atherosclerosis**, which is a build-up of lipid cells in the vasculature that results in hypertension and cardiovascular disease. Fats are also classified by the configuration of the hydrogen bonds and are classified as **saturated fats**, which are solid at room temperature, or **unsaturated fats**, which are liquid at room temperature. Research indicates that replacing saturated fats with unsaturated fats in the diet facilitates the removal of excess cholesterol from the body. Fats are contained in dairy and animal products, nuts, and vegetable oils. Current recommendations include a consuming a balanced diet that provides unsaturated fats and limited animal fats.

Proteins

Proteins are also organic compounds that contain carbon, hydrogen, and oxygen and form **amino acids**, the building blocks of the protein molecule. There are nine **essential amino acids** that must be consumed because the body cannot synthesize them. A **complete protein** consists of all nine essential amino acids, while an **incomplete protein** is deficient in one or more of the essential amino acids. Proteins are essential for all intracellular processes and as enzymes that facilitate all chemical reactions in the body. Nutritional sources of protein include animal products, dairy products, beans, and tofu.

Minerals/Electrolytes

Mineral/electrolytes are metals and nonmetals, including sodium, potassium, chloride, phosphorous, magnesium, calcium, and sulfur. They are necessary for fluid balance, transmission of nervous impulses, bone maintenance, blood clotting, healthy teeth, and protein synthesis and cardiac-impulse conduction. Minerals and electrolytes are generally consumed in adequate amounts from a balanced diet.

Vitamins

Vitamins are organic compounds that are necessary for blood clotting, immune function, maintenance of teeth, and the action of enzymes. There are two classes of vitamins. **Fat-soluble vitamins**, including A, D, E, and K, can be stored in excess in the body in the event of excessive intake. **Water-soluble vitamins**, including B-complex and C, are not stored in the body and ingested amounts greater than body requirements will be excreted in the urine. Vitamins are present in fruits, vegetables, fish, organ meats, and dairy.

Fiber

Dietary fiber is composed of complex carbohydrates and other plant substances that are not broken down by the digestive enzymes. Fiber can be water soluble or insoluble, and both forms contribute to the normal function of the gastrointestinal system. **Soluble fiber** that is present in oatmeal, blueberries, nuts, and beans facilitates the excretion of cholesterol, controls abrupt increases in blood glucose levels, and contributes to normal bowel function. The **insoluble fiber** that is present in whole grains, the skin and seeds of many fruits, and brown rice improves bowel function and also contributes to a feeling of fullness following food intake, which can lead to modest weight loss.

Water

Making up about 75 percent of the body, water is a vital necessity to human life. Water feeds cells and organs, creates a lubricant around the joints, and regulates body temperature. It is also important to digestion, as water moves food through the intestines.

Dietary Supplements

Dietary supplements contain various nutrients that are intended to compensate for inadequate dietary intake of those elements. These products should be used with care by anyone who also takes prescription medications because adverse interactions between the two are common.

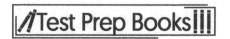

Special Dietary Needs

Weight Control

Weight control requires a balanced diet that is calorie controlled and combined with adequate aerobic exercise. Current research indicates that the consumption of sugar and white flour, rather than dietary fats, is the greatest dietary threat to successful weight management.

Diabetes

Diabetes requires a balanced diet that is carbohydrate controlled. Diabetes may be due to a lack of insulin production by the pancreas or cellular insensitivity to the insulin that is present in the bloodstream. The controlled intake of carbohydrates limits the amount of insulin that is necessary to protect the body against the side effects of chronically elevated blood glucose levels.

Cardiovascular Disease

Cardiovascular disease most often is accompanied by excess fluid volume that is manifested by hypertension and edema. The condition requires a balanced diet that is sodium controlled, with adequate fluid intake.

Hypertension

Hypertension is associated with fluid volume excess, which means that excess dietary sodium and fluid should be avoided.

Cancer

Cancer may affect multiple body systems, which means that the diet should be balanced with additional calories to meet energy needs.

Lactose Sensitivity/Intolerance

Lactose sensitivity/intolerance results from the deficiency of the enzyme **lactase**, which is necessary for the breakdown or digestion of **lactose,** a sugar found in dairy products. This deficiency can result in stomach bloating, nausea, vomiting, and diarrhea following the ingestion of dairy products.

Gluten Free

Gluten-free diets must be free of wheat, barley, and rye in any form. This means that, in addition to bread, all processed foods must be avoided. Gluten intolerance may be a symptom of **celiac disease**, which affects the absorption of food in the small intestine, or an allergic response to wheat gluten; however, it is most commonly due to the lack of a necessary digestive enzyme. Possible manifestations include stomach bloating, diarrhea, fatigue, and weight loss.

Food Allergies

Food allergies can be related to one or several foods for a given patient. The allergic responses can range from mild to life threatening. The diet must be balanced and free of the allergens.

Personal Hygiene

Part of the nurse's regular assessment of the patient includes their level of personal hygiene. This is most important upon their initial admission assessment, as how well they are groomed walking into the facility speaks to how well they take care of themselves on a day-to-day basis at home. The nurse will very quickly be able to make a judgment about how hygienic the patient is when doing the standard head-to-toe assessment.

Components of personal hygiene include evidence of washing themselves, how they care for their feet and nails, how they dress and the cleanliness of their clothes, whether or not they have shaved, if their hair is clean and maintained, and their level of oral hygiene.

Different people uphold themselves, their families, and their households to different standards of cleanliness. Some people are more pristine, while others are slovenlier. There are certain "accepted" standards of cleanliness, but not everyone maintains every single one at all times. The nurse keeps the client's personal hygiene in the context of their physical abilities, state of illness, and cultural context. Some cultures may be used to a lower or higher level of cleanliness, and the nurse keeps this in mind when performing the assessment.

Examples of cultural differences include how often it is acceptable to bathe or shower in a week. Some cultures may stick to a daily routine, while others may think weekly is acceptable. The presence or absence of hair on certain parts of the body on males and females may be different from culture to culture. The tolerance of bodily odor may also vary as to how strong of an odor is present and acceptable. The practice of bathing or showering may be an exclusively private act in some cultures, while in other cultures it is a public, communal activity. The nurse endeavors to understand the cultural context from which their client hails.

Many nurses may dismiss oral hygiene as a low priority compared to their other daily duties with their patients, but in fact, it is a strong indicator of overall health. The oral hygiene practices of the patient should be assessed and observed, and patient education should take place where possible. It is recommended that adults and children brush their teeth twice a day and floss once a day. Mouthwash should be used as needed. All three of these items—toothbrushes, floss, and mouthwash—should be available in the patient admission kits in most facilities. The nurse can go over their use upon patient admission.

Nurses are not allowed to trim fingernails or toenails in most facilities. The main reason for this is patients with **diabetic neuropathy**, a common ailment among diabetics, have little to no feeling in their extremities and are prone to injury. The nurse may assist the patient in keeping their nails clean until such time as they are able to have them trimmed by the appropriate party, whether a licensed podiatrist, the patient, or a trusted family member.

The nurse will assist in other hygienic activities with the patient, depending on their functioning capabilities. Most facilities require one bath per day. This may be an independently taken bath or shower by the patient, an assisted bath, a partial bed bath, or a complete bed bath. The nurse and their assistant will help the patient complete this activity to ensure they remain clean while staying in the facility, as this promotes overall health and wellness.

Perineal care is one item of personal hygiene that the nurse and nursing assistant will ensure is completed regularly. Many patients suffer from bowel and bladder incontinence as well as often having urinary catheters and sometimes rectal tubes for the collection of urine and stool. Maintaining a clean perineal area is vital to preventing infection and preserving skin integrity.

Rest and Sleep

Sleep and rest are essential to optimal health and healing. Patients can have difficulty sleeping. Whenever possible, plan the patient's care routine to correspond with periods when the patient is awake. Care activities should be grouped together when appropriate to avoid disturbing the patient more than necessary. Although patients need adequate rest periods, they should be encouraged to get

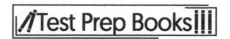

out of bed and participate in activities when they're able, which aids in better rest. For a patient who's unable to leave their bed, encourage them to perform active, range of motion exercises.

Patients in unfamiliar surroundings, or in facilities with constant lighting and noise, can become disoriented to day and night. Provide these patients with as many environmental cues as possible, such as dimming the lights and keeping the noise level low at night, turning the lights on and opening curtains and blinds in the morning, etc. Performing activities of daily living on a set schedule can also help the patient to stay oriented.

Pharmacological and Parenteral Therapies

Adverse Effects/Contraindications/Side Effects/Interactions

Most of the nurse's day-to-day work will involve the administration of pharmacological and parenteral therapies as part of the patient's treatment plan. In general, **pharmacological therapy** has to do with the branch of science in which drugs are created for the use of combatting disease processes. Each of these drugs is administered into the body via pill, patch, or otherwise and has a measurable, desired effect on the body. Parenteral therapies are a specific mode of medication delivery via some other route than the alimentary canal, usually by a needle. This can be intravenous (IV), intrathecal, intraosseous, and subcutaneous, among other routes.

With all medication administration, the nurse must be mindful of the drug's potential adverse effects. As far as pharmacology has come in the past century, no drug has been perfected to the point of not having any potential adverse effect. An **adverse effect** is defined as a negative response to a medication that is not part of the desired effect. The chemical structure of the drug is what usually triggers these adverse effects. Adverse effects are greatly minimized by appropriate dosing for the individual patient.

Some drug side effects are quite obvious. Take, for example, warfarin. Warfarin, or Coumadin, is used to thin out the blood in patients at risk for forming deadly blood clots, such as those with atrial fibrillation. However, if inappropriately dosed and under-monitored, warfarin can cause serious hemorrhaging because of its effect on the body's clotting mechanisms and ability to achieve hemostasis. Patients taking warfarin should be carefully monitored for overdosage and signs of bleeding.

At times, a drug may cause an adverse effect when it is coadministered with some other substance that affects its chemical structure or its ability to be absorbed by the body. Narcotics, for example, should not be taken while drinking alcohol. Alcohol, a depressant, exacerbates the effect of the narcotic, also a depressant, to the point that the patient's drive to breathe and their consciousness may be completely knocked out, causing death.

Another type of adverse effect is an allergic reaction. Depending on the patient's unique immune system's makeup, some drugs may cause the immune system to kick into overdrive, decreasing the desired effect and adding a lot of unwanted effects. Common signs of an allergic reaction include mild reactions such as itching and rash, escalating all the way to a severe reaction such as anaphylactic shock. **Anaphylaxis** involves an inflammation and narrowing of the patient's airway. This makes breathing difficult and presents a life-threatening situation.

The nurse should be aware of common contraindications for a certain drug's use. A **contraindication** is a situation in which it is inappropriate to administer a drug. For example, if a patient is taking a potassium-sparing ACE inhibitor for the management of heart failure, supplementation of potassium should be avoided or only carefully done under the management of the attending physician or nephrologist. This is because the ACE inhibitor causes the body to excrete *less* potassium than it normally does, meaning supplementing potassium puts the patient at risk for hyperkalemia, a life-threatening condition that can cause heart rhythm abnormalities and dysfunction. Another common contraindication to be mindful of is the administration of Coumadin, or warfarin, with another blood thinner such as aspirin. The concurrent usage of these two medications aimed at decreasing the body's own hemostatic response can result in a life-threatening hemorrhage in the patient and should be avoided.

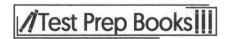

If the nurse ever suspects that the administration of a drug is contraindicated by the usage of another, they should always raise their concern with the ordering physician, the pharmacist on staff, and/or nursing management to confirm. It is a patient safety issue that is worth the extra time to investigate to prevent patient harm.

Adverse effects and contraindications are some of the rarer occurrences in day-to-day pharmacological therapies that the nurse will encounter. More commonly, the nurse will encounter milder, unwanted effects of drug administration called **side effects**. Most drugs have side effects or undesirable effects of administration. For example, a patient put on antibiotics for a respiratory infection may experience gastrointestinal (GI) upset such as stomachache, excessive flatulence, and diarrhea. Antibiotics destroy the native GI tract bacteria as part of their mechanism of action, which is what causes these side effects. Side effects are usually mild enough that the patient can either bear with them until they are finished taking the medication for the original cause, or the doctor may prescribe a counter drug to lessen the side effects of the original drug. As each additional drug carries with it the potential for more side effects, use of more medications should be weighed carefully as to their potential for helping the patient. The clinical judgment of the doctor and nurse and the patient's preference are all considered in these decisions.

Drug interactions are an aspect of pharmacology that the nurse must keep in mind when performing medication administration. A **drug interaction** may occur between many different drugs and substances. These interactions may fall into one of three categories: synergistic, antagonistic, or an interaction in which a whole new action is produced that neither substance could produce on their own.

A **synergistic interaction** is one in which the two concurrently administered substances *enhance* each other's action. Sometimes the prescriber uses the synergistic action of drugs to their advantage when the synergy would be helpful to the patient's condition. In some instances, however, synergy of two drugs is detrimental to the patient. An example of synergistic medications working in the patient's best interest would be the use of multiple antibiotics to treat an infection. Many patients with respiratory infections, such as pneumonia, will be prescribed a combination of different antibiotic therapies for two reasons. One is that the prescriber does not always know the exact causative organism of the infection and wants to wipe it out completely, and two, these combinations of antibiotics have been shown to be more effective than just using one specific antibiotic.

An example of synergistic drugs having an unwanted effect is the combination of multiple blood thinners, such as Coumadin and aspirin, that was mentioned above. In some patients' cases, the combination of the two drugs may be warranted and helpful, while in others it could have a devastating effect on the patient, resulting in a massive bleed.

Antagonistic drug interactions are ones in which the two coadministered substances cancel each other out or greatly decrease each other's potential action. Patients who are taking cholesterol-lowering drugs such as statins, for example, are discouraged from drinking grapefruit juice, as it has an antagonistic action on the statin. The grapefruit essentially absorbs all the statins before the body can, thus canceling out any positive effects they might have had for the patient, rendering them useless.

A nurse who is well versed in pharmacological knowledge, including drug side effects, adverse effects, contraindications, and interactions, will be able to better serve and protect their patients from harm.

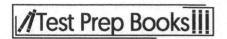

Blood and Blood Products

Blood and blood products are commonly administered during surgery. Depending on the healthcare facility, these products may be administered by the anesthesiologist, circulating nurse, or perfusionist. The administration of blood or blood products is guided by policy set by the healthcare institution. These policies cover everything from blood/blood product order entry to post-transfusion monitoring. It is imperative that the product be checked by two independent personnel, one of whom is the transfusionist. During this independent double-check, the following items are verified: patient name, date of birth, medical record number, patient ABO type, unit ABO type, unit expiration date and time, and presence of consent for blood products.

In the operating room, the most commonly administered blood product is **packed red blood cells (PRBC).** Indications for PRBC transfusion are rapid blood loss, low hemoglobin/hematocrit levels in the presence of coronary artery disease, and hypovolemia due to blood loss. During the preoperative phase, the surgeon may order blood products to be on hold for transfusion. This is common practice for cases where the level of anticipated blood loss is likely to require transfusion, such as open-heart surgery or repair of abdominal aortic aneurysm. The patient may choose to donate his or her own blood several weeks prior to surgery, in order to have his or her own blood available for transfusion, if indicated.

Fresh frozen plasma (FFP), platelets, and **cryoprecipitate** are indicated for coagulation, but work by different mechanisms. FFP, platelets, and/or cryoprecipitate may be on hold for surgery if the patient is on blood thinning agents, such as warfarin. For patients receiving anticoagulation therapy, **prothrombin time/international normalized ratio (PT/INR)** and **partial thromboplastin time (PTT)** are tested to determine need for reversal of the anticoagulation agents. FFP is used for active bleeding to promote coagulation, or to reverse anticoagulation therapy. Liver disease is associated with interruption in blood clotting processes. Patients with known liver disease undergoing major surgery often have FFP on hold in cases intraoperative transfusion of FFP is needed to help control bleeding. Platelets are transfused during surgery if serum lab values reveal thrombocytopenia (low serum platelet levels) and the patient is not showing signs of proper coagulation prior to the end of the procedure. Cryoprecipitate is prepared from plasma and contains fibrinogen and other clotting factors, including von Willebrand and factor VIII. The primary indications for cryoprecipitate transfusion are bleeding and hypofibrinogenemia (low serum fibrinogen level).

In an emergent situation where the patient's ABO is unknown, uncrossmatched, type O negative blood can be obtained from the blood bank. This should only be used when delaying transfusion during crossmatch process is a threat to the patient's life. An instance where uncrossmatched blood may be indicated is an emergency aortic dissection surgery where the patient presents to the emergency department and goes straight to surgery, and the type and crossmatch are not yet completed. The patient could bleed to death before the crossmatch process is completed.

Intraoperative cell salvage is widely used in cases where a high amount of blood loss is anticipated. During intraoperative cell salvage, blood lost into the surgical field is collected via suction into a machine. This machine filters the blood and anticoagulates it by adding **heparin** (an anticoagulation drug) to it. This keeps the blood from clotting prior to transfusion back to the patient's circulatory system. If the amount of blood collected into the chamber is sufficient, and the surgeon determines the need for transfusion, the machine centrifuges and washes the blood. This blood can be transfused back to the patient intravenously. Some patients who would otherwise refuse a blood transfusion (such as a Jehovah's Witness) may consent to intraoperative cell salvage. If intraoperative cell salvage is planned as part of the procedure, it should be discussed with the patient preoperatively.

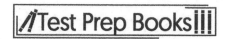

Central Venous Access Devices

One route of pharmacological and parenteral therapy is the use of **central venous access devices**, or **CVADs**. In some patients, access to larger veins to distribute larger amounts and concentrations of medications is necessary. CVADs serve this purpose. A centrally inserted venous catheter or port gives the practitioner access to such vessels as the larger veins of the chest, neck, or groin, if necessary. These central lines can remain in the patient for significantly longer than a peripherally inserted IV access. Central lines avoid the inflammation that occurs because of frequent peripheral IV sticks. Patients with a central line avoid the discomfort of frequent needlesticks when they have a port implanted or a central line placed. Central access is less likely to clot, making them a superior choice in certain patient situations.

CVADs must be carefully monitored for infection. Sterile technique must be observed for dressing changes and at the time of insertion. CVAD infections are costly and difficult to treat, as well as complicating the patient's hospital stay.

Common uses for a central venous catheter include the infusion of multiple rounds of blood products for a trauma patient, withdrawal of blood in a patient requiring frequent blood draws such as a patient in the ICU, and the administration of drugs, including chemotherapy, antibiotics, fluids, and nutritional compounds.

A **peripherally inserted central catheter (PICC) line** is placed in patients requiring frequent and large doses of medications. The PICC line consists of a soft, flexible tube called a **catheter** that is inserted by a specially trained doctor or nurse with the use of an ultrasound machine for guidance. The cephalic, basilic, and brachial veins are some of the more commonly used veins for PICC insertion. The patient will have a chest x-ray performed post insertion to ensure that the PICC line tip is resting in the distal end of the superior vena cava, at the cavoatrial junction.

If the patient with a central venous catheter has intermittent mechanical occlusion that interferes with infusions, they may have what is called **pinch-off syndrome**. This rare occurrence is when the catheter becomes pinched within the body between the first rib and the clavicle, causing the occlusion.

A second type of central venous catheter is an **implanted VAD**. These chambers are implanted into the subcutaneous space of the patient's chest wall. The skin above the device heals, and the port can be accessed easily with a single needlestick. While the chest wall is the most commonly used site, a patient's arm may be used if the chest wall is contraindicated. The catheter, wherever the chamber is located, will terminate in the central vasculature.

Other types of CVADs include nontunneled catheters such as subclavian, jugular, or femoral lines and tunneled catheters such as Hickman's, Broviac's, Groshong's, and small-bore catheters.

With any CVAD, the nurse must always verify placement before using. This is done by verifying a chest x-ray was done post insertion that positively confirmed placement. The nurse may look for the interventional radiology report, operative note, discharge summary, referring MD note, hospital transfer note, or some form of patient-provided documentation before use to verify correct placement and authorization.

Central lines must always be flushed with 10 milliliters of saline before and after the medication is administered to clear the line.

Dosage Calculation

The nurse administering pharmacological or parenteral therapies to the patient will often have the dosages precalculated for them; however, it is vital to have a basic knowledge of how to perform dosage calculations if verification or manual calculations must be done.

The place to start with dosage calculations is a working knowledge of common conversions. The following chart provides a list of conversions for the nurse to know:

- 1 liter is equal to 1000 milliliters.
- 1 gram is equal to 1000 milligrams.
- 1 milligram is equal to 1000 micrograms.
- 1 kilogram is equal to 2.2 pounds.
- 1 teaspoon is equal to 5 milliliters.
- 3 teaspoons is equal to 1 tablespoon.
- 1 kilogram is equal to 1000 grams.
- 30 milliliters is equal to 1 ounce.
- 1 tablespoon is equal to 15 milliliters.

The nurse must also know common abbreviations used in measurements, listed below:

- oz: ounce
- tbsp: tablespoon
- mL: milliliter
- kg: kilogram
- dL: deciliter
- lb: pound
- g: gram
- mg: milligram
- L: liter
- tsp: teaspoon
- mcg: microgram

Commonly encountered units of measurement within nursing include mass, volume, and time. Most hospitals use the metric system. The metric system is an internationally recognized system of measurement that provides one base unit for length, mass, and volume. Length is measured in meters, mass is measured in grams, and volume is measured in liters. Each unit can be expressed as bigger or smaller measurements in increments of 10, 100, and 1000. For example, a kilogram, the prefix "kilo-" meaning "1000," refers to 1000 grams. Other prefixes for the metric system are listed below:

- hecto-: 100
- deca-: 10
- deci-: 0.1
- centi-: 0.01
- milli-: 0.001

Converting smaller metric measurements to larger ones and vice versa requires only moving the decimal point left or right, depending on the difference in tenths, hundredths, or thousandths. For example, if a patient's height is measured as centimeters and the nurse wants to convert it to meters, they simply

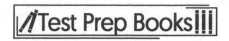

move the decimal point to the left two steps, as a meter is divided into hundredths when it is converted to centimeters. If the patient's measurement is 152 centimeters, the correct conversion to meters would be 1.52 meters.

One of the most frequently used calculations a nurse will need to know is the basic dosage calculation. The nurse will take the desired dose, noted as "D"; divide it by the amount of the drug the nurse has on hand, noted as "H"; multiply this total by the volume in which the drug comes (which could be tablet, capsule, or liquid form), noted as "V"; and they will arrive at the correct dose.

For example, if the nurse has an order to administer 50 milligrams (mg) of Dilantin and has a formulation of 125 mg in 5 mL, how does the nurse set up the equation? The dose, or "D," is 60 mg. The amount on hand, or "H," is 125 mg. The nurse will put D over H, divide 50 by 125, which gives her 0.4 mg. They will then multiply 0.4 times the volume in which the Dilantin is formulated in, which is 5 mL. 0.4 times 5 is 2, so the correct dosage for the patient is 2 mL of Dilantin.

Expected Actions/Outcomes

The nurse will be expected to obtain information about the client's list of prescribed medications, involving the formulary review and consultations with the pharmacist. It is vital that the nurse be able to use critical thinking when expecting certain effects and outcomes of medication administration, including oral, intradermal, subcutaneous, intramuscular, and topical formulations. Over time, the client should be evaluated for their response to their medication regime. This includes a variety of home remedies, their prescription drugs, and any over-the-counter (OTC) drug usage. The response of the client to their medications, whether therapeutic or not, should be evaluated. If adverse reactions or side effects occur, the patient's medications will need to be reevaluated and modified.

Most medical facilities have electronic health record systems that, once the client is registered for the first time, will keep track of their medication record. This will need to be modified with each doctor's visit and hospital stay, of course, but is a helpful tool in recording the client's list of medications.

With all medication administration, the nurse should keep their eye on the expected outcome. Identifying the **expected outcome**, or goal, of the patient's medication regime will assist in keeping the medication list as short and maximally effective as it needs to be. The expected outcome is the overarching goal and principle that will guide the health care team and the patient in their decision-making process.

The nurse should have access to literature that provides information about drugs, including expected outcomes, mode of action in the body, appropriate dosing, contraindications, and adverse effects. A **formulary** is an example of this type of literature that gives an official list of medicines that may be prescribed and any related information on the drug, a helpful tool for nurses. The formulary will give both the generic and the brand name for the drug and is maintained by physicians, nurse practitioners, and pharmacists to ensure it is accurate and up to date. Drugs listed in the formulary have been evaluated for safety and effectiveness by a committee of experts to provide practitioners with those deemed best for patients.

The nurse should use one of the greatest pharmacological references available to them in the health care facility: the pharmacist. Most hospitals have a team of pharmacists on staff whose sole purpose is to oversee the correct dosage, administration, and usage of all the patients' medication needs. Most pharmacists have a doctorate level of education in pharmacy, which the nurse would be wise to make good use of, and often. Pharmacists are often found on the floors, overseeing correct antibiotic and other drug dosages and administration, as well as being stationed in the hospital's pharmacy, which is only a phone call away. If the nurse has a question about a medication's use for a patient, they should not hesitate to contact the pharmacist and consult them and their pharmaceutical knowledge. They are a very helpful and valuable member of the health care team.

The two most common routes of medication administration the nurse will encounter are oral and intravenous. There are, of course, other routes of medication administration that the nurse will need to be knowledgeable and competent in performing. **Intramuscular injections** are the preferred route for vaccinations such as the pneumococcal and influenza vaccines. The deltoid muscle is preferred for most vaccines, but other sites the nurse may use if necessary include the ventrogluteal, dorsogluteal, and vastus lateralis sites.

One important aspect of intramuscular injection is the **Z-track technique**. In this technique, the nurse pulls the skin downward or upward, injects the medication at a 90 degree angle, and then releases the skin. This creates a "zigzag," or Z-shaped, track that prevents the injected fluid from leaking backward into the subcutaneous tissue. Backward leakage of tissue may cause tissue damage, thus the usage of the Z-track technique. The nurse must avoid massaging the site, as this may cause leakage and irritation.

Prescription drugs are those that may only be prescribed by a qualified health care practitioner. They may be obtained with a prescription from the pharmacy, dispensed by a qualified pharmacist. **OTC medications** may be obtained without a prescription, at the discretion of the patient. Home remedies include any sort of tonic or home-prepared solution that the patient makes for themselves at home as a cure for an ailment. These are often made with commonly found household or pantry items. Many home remedies are unproven in their effectiveness but rather anecdotally recommended by a friend or family member, often passed down through the generations. An example of a simple home remedy is lemon juice and honey in hot water as a "cure" for a sore throat. These simple ingredients have medicinal properties that may soothe the sore throat and may be preferred by the patient to an OTC or prescription formulation for sore throats. The nurse should obtain information about any home remedies the patient may be using to get a full picture of their health and wellness habits.

Medication Administration

The nurse observes the six rights of the patient with every medication administration. The patient has the right to 1) the right medication, 2) the right route, 3) the right time frame in which the medication is to be delivered, 4) the right client to whom the medication is to be administered, 5) the right dosage, and 6) the right documentation that the drug has been administered. These rights work to ensure patient safety.

In addition to the rights of the patient, the nurse should ensure that the appropriate physician and pharmacist orders have been given. The nurse should assess the patient for any allergies. This information can be found in the patient's medical record or chart if they have been previously admitted. The allergy information on the patient should include the specific type of reaction they had, whether it was a mild rash or a severe, anaphylactic reaction.

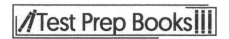

There are several different routes by which a medication can be administered by a nurse, including the following:

Intramuscular

The provider will use an intramuscular injection to ensure rapid absorption of a medication into the bloodstream when the intravenous infusion of the medication is inappropriate or inaccessible. Common sites for intramuscular injection include the deltoid, vastus lateralis, and ventral gluteal muscles.

Z-Tract Injection

When injecting medications capable of causing skin irritation or discoloration in the event of leakage from the injection site, the provider will apply traction to the skin surrounding the injection site with the nondominant hand, insert the needle into the muscle at a 90-degree angle, inject the medication, withdraw the needle, and release the traction on the skin, trapping the injected solution in the muscle.

Subcutaneous Injection

The provider will choose a subcutaneous site to inject medications that will absorb more slowly because of the limited blood supply in the fatty subcutaneous space. Using the nondominant hand, the provider will pinch the skin, insert the needle at a 90-degree angle into the fatty layer just under the skin, inject the medication, and withdraw the needle. It should be noted that for small children and individuals with little subcutaneous fat, a 45-degree angle is recommended to ensure the medication enters the subcutaneous tissue rather than muscle.

Oral/Sublingual/Buccal

The provider understands that the oral, sublingual, and buccal administration routes are appropriate for agents that will be rapidly absorbed into the bloodstream through the mucous membrane of the gastrointestinal tract. In addition, the sublingual and buccal routes are appropriate if the patient is unable to swallow a medication, or when the medication would be poorly absorbed or inactivated in the stomach. The provider is aware that sublingual and buccal medications are provided in tablet, film, and spray forms.

The provider will assist the patient to swallow **oral medications** that will be processed in the stomach or small intestine.

The provider will place **sublingual medications** under the tongue to facilitate rapid absorption of the medication into the bloodstream.

The provider will place **buccal medications** between the cheek and the gum where the medication will be absorbed through the capillary bed.

Topical

Topical medications are applied to the skin, mucous membrane, or body tissue, and may be provided as **transdermal patches**; ointments, lotions, and creams; or powders. The provider will assess the administration site for local reaction, and will rotate the site as appropriate for transdermal patches. In addition, the provider will avoid personal contact with the medications that are commonly absorbed rapidly through the skin.

Inhalation

The provider understands that inhalant drugs are used to deliver the medication directly to the target organ, which results in more rapid and efficient local absorption of the medication, in addition to decreased systemic exposure to the effects of the medication.

The provider will use medication-specific metered dose inhalers, dry powder inhalers, or **nebulizers** to administer inhaled agents that may include antimicrobials and corticosteroids. The licensed provider is also responsible for verifying the patient's understanding of the proper use and administration of these medications.

Instillation (eye-ear-nose)

The provider understands that medications may be **instilled** into the eye, ear, or nose to promote absorption or to treat local irritation of the site.

To instill eye drops, the provider will clear any accumulated secretions, use the nondominant hand to expose the conjunctival sac, instill the prescribed solution into the inner canthus while avoiding any contact with the eye, and use a sterile cotton ball to dry the eyelid.

To instill eye ointment, the provider will clear any accumulated secretions, use the nondominant hand to expose the conjunctival sac, apply the prescribed ointment along the sac from the inner canthus to the outer canthus while avoiding any contact between the eye and the medication container, and use a sterile cotton ball to dry the eyelid.

To instill medications into the ear, the provider will warm the solution to normal body temperature, position the patient with the head turned to the unaffected side, gently pull the ear up and back, instill the medication avoiding contact between the medicine dropper and the ear canal, place a sterile cotton ball loosely in the outer ear and instruct the patient to remain supine for fifteen minutes.

To instill nasal drops, the provider will instruct the patient to gently blow his/her nose, position the patient supine with the head tilted back, and instill the drops while avoiding contact between the inner nares and the medicine dropper.

Intradermal

The provider will use a 1 milliliter tuberculin syringe with a 5/8 inch 25- to 27-gauge needle to inject the prescribed medication into the interior portion of the forearm. The provider must identify the appropriate injection angle for the prescribed treatment; for example, allergy testing requires that the injection is 15-to-20 degrees, while insulin may be injected intradermally at 90 degrees.

Transdermal

The provider understands that **transdermal medications**, which are absorbed through the skin, provide the continuous release of a precise amount of the medication for a specific period of time. When applying a new dose of the medication, the provider will remove remaining residue from the previous dose, verify that the skin is intact and free of irritation, and sign and date the patch. Birth control pills, smoking cessation medications, pain relief agents, and nitroglycerin are some of the medications that are applied transdermally.

Vaginal

The provider understands that vaginal medications, which are available as suppositories, foams, ointments, and sprays, are used to alter the pH of the vagina, treat local infection, and provide comfort.

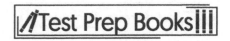

The provider will insert the suppository form into the vaginal vault where it will liquefy as a result of body temperature. The provider will apply the ointment and spray medications according to the manufacturers' directions.

Rectal
Antiemetics, analgesics, and cathartics are commonly available as **suppositories**. The provider will insert the rectal suppository above the internal anal sphincter to prevent displacement.

Injection Site
Site Selection
The provider will select the appropriate injection site with consideration of the age and stature of the patient and the administration requirements of the prescribed medication. The provider is aware that injection sites must be systematically rotated for medications such as insulin that are repeated daily.

Needle Length and Gauge
The provider will select the needle gauge and length that is consistent with the selected injection site and the administration requirements of the prescribed medication.

Medication Packaging
Multidose Vials
The provider will withdraw the calculated amount of medication from the multidose vial using aseptic technique to avoid contamination of the remaining solution.

Ampules
The provider will break the ampule using safety precautions related to glass breakage and withdraw the entire contents into the syringe. The provider will then verify that the syringe contains the calculated volume of medication, replace the needle, and administer the medication according to protocol.

Unit Dose
The provider is aware the patient's medications will most often be provided in single-dose amounts, as opposed to multidose amounts, in order to avoid medication errors.

Prefilled Cartridge-Needle Units
The provider is aware that injectable medications may be provided as prefilled cartridges with attached needles. Depending on the manufacturer, a nondisposable holder will be provided for the cartridge. The provider must verify that the prefilled cartridge contains the calculated dose.

Powder for Reconstitution
The provider will inject the prescribed amount of diluent into the vial, mix the solution, and withdraw the calculated amount of medication.

Six Rights of Medication Administration
The "six rights" must be addressed for every medication dose. The provider will:

- Use two means of identification (ID) to verify the right patient, which can include the patient's verbal report and the agency ID band.

- Verify the prescription and the medication as provided by the pharmacy.

- Compare the route of administration documented in the medication record with the original prescription.

- Verify the time schedule as documented in the medication record.

- Calculate the correct dose and verify the result with another provider as required by agency policy.

- Document the administration of the medication and the patient's response in the medication record according to agency policy.

Parenteral/Intravenous Therapies

Clients requiring intravenous therapies will need to be assessed for the appropriate vein to be used. Selecting the best vein is crucial to ensuring the medication can be delivered safely and effectively. The nurse should always go farthest away from the center of the patient's body first. It may be tempting to go for a thick, juicy vein near the patient's inner elbow first, but using distal veins first is proper procedure. This is because if a vein is blown toward the center of the patient's body, it cannot be used again distally. The only time it is appropriate to use a more proximal vein, such as the antecubital (AC) (located in the fold of the elbow), is in emergent cases. The AC is also a frequent blood draw site for quick draws on stable patients. It is also preferred that the nurse select the patient's nondominant arm. If the patient is left-handed, for example, the right arm is preferred for an IV site.

When selecting an IV site, the nurse should avoid the side of the body where a dialysis catheter is, a side that is paralyzed, and a side where a mastectomy has been performed, if possible.

Education will be needed for the patient who is to receive intermittent parenteral fluid therapy. Fluids are often required for the sake of client hydration and electrolyte needs. An IV is often obtained for this purpose so that it is available when needed.

The patient should be educated about signs of IV infiltration that they will need to report to the nurse. An infiltrated IV is one in which the catheter has dislodged outside of the vein or the vein has blown, and IV fluids and medications are leaking into the interstitial space. Signs of IV infiltration include swelling, coldness, and pain around the IV site. The nurse will not be able to pull back any fluid or blood from the IV catheter as it is dislodged from the correct site of insertion.

Other complications of IV therapy include hematoma around the insertion site; extravasation of a toxic drug into the surrounding tissue; embolus or clot formation; fluid overload in the patient from overadministration; phlebitis, or swelling and inflammation of the vein; and infection around the IV site.

The nurse oversees IV pump function for correct and accurate delivery of IV fluids and medications. IV pumps are prone to breakdown and failure and thus will need close nurse supervision. The nurse monitors the fluid and medication bags above the pump and ensures that the measurements on the machine match up with the actual delivery.

Pharmacological Pain Management

Pain is the most commonly seen symptom in the emergency department, as most emergency situations cases cause patients to have a high level of pain. However, since cases in the emergency department often vary widely in scope and every patient will have a different personal threshold for pain tolerance,

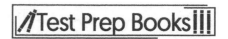

best practices are difficult to develop when it comes to pain management. It is often done on a case by case basis. However, when a patient's pain is not managed in a way that seems appropriate to that individual, it can cause patient and family dissatisfaction in the healthcare organization. As a result, medical staff must try to provide effective and safe pain management options that can make the patient comfortable at the present time, but that also do not cause harm over time. In some cases, like a sprained muscle, ice therapy and time can provide adequate pain management. More serious cases, defined as pain that does not subside after an objectively reasonable period of time for the injury, may require topical, intramuscular, or oral pain medication. These can include stronger doses of common over-the-counter pain medications, or prescription pain medications.

Prescription pain medications, especially opioids and muscle relaxers, are known for causing debilitating addiction, so when prescribing them to a patient, the lowest dose and dosing frequency necessary should be utilized. Additionally, patients should be closely monitored for their reactions to their pain medications. Finally, some individuals who are addicted to prescription pain killers and muscle relaxers may feign injuries in order to receive another prescription. Therefore, all patients' medical histories should be thoroughly evaluated to note their history of pain medication usage. Patients should also be assessed for showing any signs of drug abuse history and withdrawal symptoms (such as damaged teeth, shaking, and agitation).

Procedural sedation allows patients to remain somewhat alert during medical procedures that may be uncomfortable but not unbearably painful, such as resetting bones. Unlike general anesthesia, where patients are completely sedated and do not feel any sensations, procedural sedation allows patients to be somewhat conscious and aware of bodily functions. It can be utilized with or without pain-relieving medications. Practitioner awareness is crucial when administering procedural sedation, especially when pain relief is also utilized. Recently, overuse and improper use of common procedural sedation agents, such as propofol, and common pain relief medications that are often used in conjunction, such as fentanyl, have caused high profile deaths.

Total Parenteral Nutrition (TPN)

Certain patient conditions may warrant the administration of **total parenteral nutrition (TPN)**. **Parenteral**, as mentioned above, entails delivery of medication or nutrition via a route other than the alimentary canal.

TPN is a formulation that provides the patient all their daily caloric and nutritional needs directly into their circulatory system, usually through a CVAD. The CVAD must not be used for any other purpose than the TPN administration, as many interactions between drugs may occur. The tubing of the TPN must be changed every 24 hours with the first bag of formula for the day.

Patients requiring TPN usually have a condition that requires bowel rest, and thus the alternative form of nutrition is required. These conditions include ulcerative colitis, bowel obstruction, congenital GI anomalies, prolonged diarrhea, and short bowel syndrome postoperatively.

TPN is very expensive to prepare, another reason its use should be carefully considered. TPN is known to cause more complications as well as not preserving GI tract function and structure; thus, routine use is not recommended. TPN is a known cause of thrombosis in peripheral veins. Therefore, a CVAD is necessary for its administration.

TPN is composed of water, energy, essential fatty acids, vitamins, and minerals in formulations specific to the patient's needs. **Catabolism**, or the body's ability to break up complex molecules, is factored into TPN preparation.

The preparation of the TPN will vary based on the patient's diagnostic profile. For example, the formulation for a patient with renal failure will have less protein, the formulation for a patient with heart failure will have less fluid, and the formulation for a patient with respiratory failure will have a lipid emulsion that minimizes carbon dioxide production.

At the beginning of a TPN administration, the directions will often include starting it at 50 percent of its prescribed rate to ease the body into getting used to it.

The patient's weight, complete blood count, electrolyte levels, and blood urea nitrogen will be monitored by pharmacists, nutritionists, and other members of the interdisciplinary team responsible for TPN administration. Often the liver will be evaluated for function. Other lab work, including serum albumin, prothrombin time, plasma and urine osmolality, calcium, magnesium, and phosphate, will be monitored for their response to the TPN.

Insulin is often added to the patient's bag based on their blood glucose levels and history of diabetes, as the TPN can cause great fluctuations in glucose levels.

Common complications of TPN administration include glucose abnormalities, hepatic complications, electrolyte imbalances, volume overload, bone demineralization, and gallbladder complications.

Reduction of Risk Potential

Changes/Abnormalities in Vital Signs

One of the most basic nursing skills is obtaining and analyzing **vital signs**. Heart rate, blood pressure, breathing, and temperature are clues that must be interpreted to evaluate a patient's functioning status. Alterations in the vital signs must be carefully monitored to stay on top of the patient's condition and ensure timely and effective interventions take place.

The patient's **heart rate**, measured in beats per minute, tells the nurse a lot about the heart. In an adult, the normal heart rate is 60 to 100 beats per minute.

There are certain points in the body where the pulse can be felt, or **palpated**. Palpable pulse points include the carotid in the neck, the brachial near the elbow, the radial and ulnar on either side of the wrist, the femoral in the groin, the popliteal behind the knee, the posterior tibial behind the ankle, and the dorsalis pedis on top of the foot. The nurse uses these palpable peripheral pulse points to assess and count the heart rate on the patient. The location at which the nurse obtains the pulse is up to their discretion and based on the specific patient's situation. A **radial pulse** is the most commonly used in a stable, uncomplicated patient. A patient who is in critical condition with weakened blood circulation to the periphery of the body may need a femoral or carotid pulse taken, as these are closer to the heart and more detectable in situations of lowered cardiac output. The **brachial pulse** is the one that is measured when blood pressure is taken using an arm cuff.

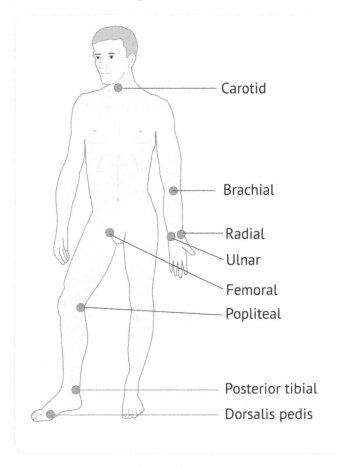

After the location of the pulse is decided and the nurse is palpating with the **two-finger technique**, the nurse will note the quality of the pulse. Qualities of the pulse can be faint, weak, strong, or bounding. The nurse grades the pulse on a scale of +1 to +4, with 1 indicating a faint pulse and 4 indicating a bounding pulse.

A pulse that is greater than 100 is called **tachycardia** and can arise from any number of causes. Exercise can raise the heart rate above 100 but is not considered abnormal or pathological, as it returns to normal at rest. Tachycardia without exercise and accompanied by other symptoms may be suggestive of a disease state at work and should be investigated.

Common causes of tachycardia include anxiety, medication side effects, street drug use, anemia, overactive thyroid, fear, stress, heart attack, or heart failure, among many others.

Bradycardia is the term for a heart rate that is less than 60 beats per minute. In some patients, this may be a normal finding. Patients who are experienced athletes often run bradycardic. This is because they have strengthened their heart through exercise to the point that their heart beats more efficiently with fewer beats, delivering adequate blood supply to the tissues and organs of the body. Bradycardia noted in a patient without a history of bradycardia, accompanied by other troublesome signs such as a decreased level of consciousness and hypotension, should be evaluated for probable causes and treatment.

Bradycardia may be caused by an underactive thyroid, infections of the heart, coronary artery disease, normal aging processes, medications for heart failure and hypertension, and hyperkalemia, to name a few.

The **blood pressure** is a vital sign that indicates how strongly the heart is pushing the blood through the circulatory system. Blood pressure is measured as a systolic number over a diastolic number. The **systolic number** represents the pressure at which the heart chambers are contracted, and the **diastolic number** represents the pressure when the heart chambers are at rest. Blood pressure is measured in millimeters of mercury (mmHg), as that is what the original **sphygmomanometer**, or blood pressure cuffs, used to determine a pressure reading.

In general, normal systolic ranges are between 100 and 120 mmHg, and normal diastolic ranges are between 60 and 80 mmHg. Between 120 and 139 mmHg systolic and 80 and 89 mmHg diastolic is considered **prehypertensive**, and 140 mmHg or greater systolic and 90 mmHg or greater diastolic is considered **hypertensive**.

Blood Pressure Levels	
Normal	systolic: less than 120 mmHg diastolic: less than 80mmHg
At risk (prehypertension)	systolic: 120–139 mmHg diastolic: 80–89 mmHg
High	systolic: 140 mmHg or higher diastolic: 90 mmHg or higher

Like tachycardia and bradycardia, hypertension and hypotension may arise from many different causes. Accompanying symptoms and patient history are key factors to consider when assessing changes in blood pressure.

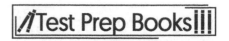

Some patients may run a low blood pressure without any other accompanying symptoms, and that is to be noted as their normal, but no treatment is necessary.

Orthostatic hypotension is a special type of hypotension that occurs when the patient changes position. This occurs most commonly when they change from a seated position to standing. The patient will experience profound dizziness and unsteadiness, which is why orthostatic hypotension may lead to falls, and the patient should be cautioned to change positions slowly. Orthostatic hypotension may be measured by taking the patient's blood pressure first when lying down, then sitting up at the edge of the bed, and then a final reading while they are standing. If they are truly experiencing orthostatic hypotension, their blood pressure readings will trend downward significantly over the course of the three readings. Orthostatic hypotension is often a side effect of medications for hypertension.

A severe form of hypotension is **shock**, in which the body is no longer delivering an adequate supply of blood with its oxygen and nutrients to the vital organs of the body. The patient in shock will need immediate treatment and fluid resuscitation.

Low volume of blood, as occurs with a hemorrhage or a dehydrated state, will lead to low blood pressure. Blood transfusions, fluid resuscitation, and possibly blood pressure-raising medications such as intravenous (IV) dopamine may be necessary to correct hypovolemic hypotension.

A patient's **rate of breathing** should be between 16 and 20 breaths per minute and can be observed and counted simply by looking at the patient's chest for a rise and a fall. **Tachypneic** patients are those who are breathing at a rate greater than 20 breaths per minute. Patients with **bradypnea**, on the other hand, are those who are breathing below 16 breaths per minute.

Apnea is an absence of breathing and may occur during a normal sleep cycle, but prolonged and repeated occurrences of apnea are problematic and may suggest a disease process such as obstructive sleep apnea.

A patient may be tachypneic because of a blood clot, pneumonia or other respiratory infection, anxiety, asthma, chronic obstructive pulmonary disease (COPD), or diabetic ketoacidosis. Patients may be bradypneic because of an overdose of alcohol or narcotics, increased intracranial pressure, obesity, an underactive thyroid, a brain lesion, or many other causes. The nurse will look for accompanying symptoms and read through the patient history to help accurately evaluate the cause of the breathing abnormality.

The body regulates its temperature through a process called **thermoregulation**. The normal body temperature is right around 98.6 degrees Fahrenheit, give or take a degree depending on the patient's own normal.

Hyperthermia is a temperature that is above normal and may indicate an infection-fighting fever or a heat-induced condition such as heat stroke. Excessive sweating, confusion, and decreased level of consciousness may accompany hyperthermia and should be treated by making efforts to get the patient cooled down.

Hypothermia occurs when the body cannot produce enough heat to replace the heat it has lost, such as if a patient is in a harsh, cold environment without adequate warm clothing or a source of heat such as a furnace. Patients who are older, taking certain medications that interfere with the body's ability to regulate its temperature, have spinal cord injuries, are intoxicated with drugs or alcohol, or are very young are particularly susceptible to hypothermia and should take extra caution when exposed to very low temperatures.

Diagnostic Tests

A **diagnostic test** is one in which the result is hoped to assist in making a diagnosis of the patient's condition. The diagnostic test will reveal the patient's strengths and weaknesses and provide the clinician with data about the patient's condition.

There are many different diagnostic tests available for innumerable patient conditions. Different mediums are used to diagnose conditions, including blood work, ultrasound technology, x-rays, procedures that put cameras in the body to visualize internal structures, and more.

A female patient who has discovered a lump in her breasts may be scheduled for a **mammography**. This type of diagnostic procedure is a type of x-ray that visualizes the tissue of the breast. This can help identify lumps that the patient or the practitioner is not able to palpate. The generally agreed-upon guideline for mammography is for it to be performed once every year or two after the age of forty for early breast cancer detection.

Patients with certain heart conditions may have an **echocardiography** performed. An **echo**, as it is commonly referred to, visualizes the structures and chambers of the heart through ultrasonography. An echo technician will use a small probe called a **transducer** to emit sound waves into the chest that create a sonographic image of the heart. Gel is applied to the skin of the chest to allow the transducer to easily glide back and forth as different aspects of the heart are visualized. Clots, holes, and any structural abnormalities will be identified during the echo. The official reading and interpretation of the echo images will be performed by a cardiologist after the tech has taken the images.

The **complete blood count (CBC)** is a type of diagnostic test that requires a small vial of blood to be drawn from the patient. The blood is sent to the lab, and the components of the blood are measured. The CBC measures red blood cells (RBCs), white blood cells (WBCs), hemoglobin, hematocrit, and platelets. This simple test can give the clinician a quick look at the body's oxygen-carrying capacity, immune function, and clotting capability all in one go.

For a patient with symptoms related to the gastrointestinal (GI) tract, the **endoscope** is a handy diagnostic tool to visualize the internal environment of the stomach and intestines. Generally, there are two types of scope: upper endoscopy and lower endoscopy. An **endoscopy** is a procedure in which a flexible tube with a camera, light, irrigation, and instrument ports are inserted for visualization of the GI tract. The patient receiving an upper GI endoscopy will require IV sedation as well as topical anesthetics applied to the throat. Lower endoscopy generally requires anesthesia as well, except for anoscopy and sigmoidoscopy, which do not travel as deeply into the body. Biopsy of tissue may be performed during a scope. As well as diagnosing certain conditions such as colon cancer, peptic ulcers, and other mucosal lesions, the scope may be performed for therapeutic reasons such as removing foreign bodies, hemostasis of bleeding lesions, debulking of tumors, placement of stents, placing a feeding tube, reduction of volvulus, and decompression of a dilated colon. Common hemostatic methods include placing hemoclips, injecting hemostatic drugs, thermal coagulation, variceal banding, and sclerotherapy.

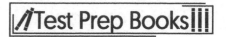

Look at the image of a colonoscopy below:

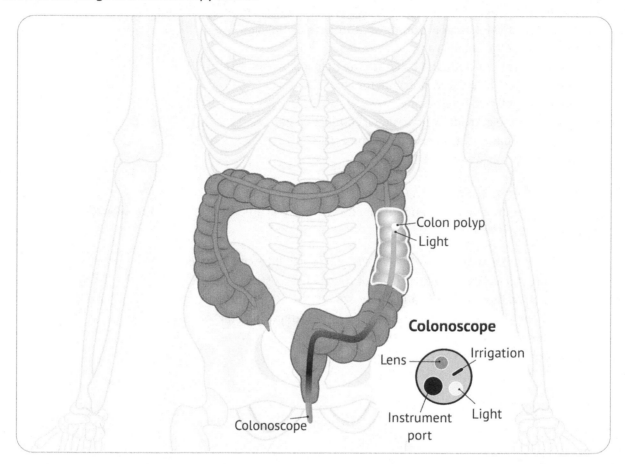

One of the most regularly performed diagnostic tests is the computed tomography scan. It may be referred to as a **CT** or **CAT scan**, but the meanings are all the same: a test in which a region of the body is scanned and images are obtained using radiography. The patient lays on a sliding table that moves them in an out of a circular opening in which the scanner is housed. As the patient moves through the scanner, an x-ray source and x-ray detector spin around the patient in a circular motion, taking images of the inner structures of the patient's body. These images are then sent to a computer, which makes a composite of all the images into 3-D images to be viewed and interpreted by a qualified radiologist. There are variations on how the CT can be taken, including stopping the patient for each scan or slice or keeping the patient in motion for a spiral CT, but the basic concept is the same.

CT scans may be noncontrast or with contrast. With IV or oral contrast, the patient drinks or is injected with a barium-based solution, targeted at whichever body tissues need imaging, and picked up by the x-ray during the scan. Contrast is often contraindicated in patients with renal failure, as their kidneys are unable to metabolize the substance. Contrast CTs are used to visualize tumors and inflammation and assess the vascular system for pulmonary emboli, aneurysms, or aortic dissection, among many other purposes.

Electrocardiography (EGG/ECG)
To perform a standard 12-lead EGG/ECG, the provider will:
- Verify the order and obtain all equipment before approaching the patient.
- Explain the procedure to the patient and assist him/her to a supine position.

- Expose the limbs and the chest, maintaining appropriate draping to preserve patient's privacy.
- Clean the electrode sites with alcohol and remove excess body hair according to agency policy.
- Attach electrodes to appropriate anatomical positions.
- Attach machine cables to the electrodes.
- Enter the patient data and calibrate the machine as necessary.
- Request that the patient does not move or speak.
- Obtain an artifact-free tracing.
- Remove the electrodes and residual conductive gel.
- Return the patient to a position of comfort.
- Submit the tracing for interpretation.

Correct Placement of EKG Leads

The accuracy of the tracing is dependent on correct lead placement; therefore, the provider will position the chest leads as follows:

- V_1 - right sternal border at the level of the fourth intercostal space
- V_2 - left sternal border at the level of fourth intercostal space
- V_3 - centered between V_2 and V_4
- V_4 - the midclavicular line at the level of the fifth intercostal space
- V_5 - horizontal to V_4 at the anterior axillary line
- V_6 - horizontal to V_4 at the midaxillary line

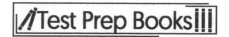

The provider must attach the limb leads to the extremities, not the torso. In addition, the provider must avoid large muscle groups, areas of adipose tissue deposit, and bony prominences when placing the limb leads on the four extremities.

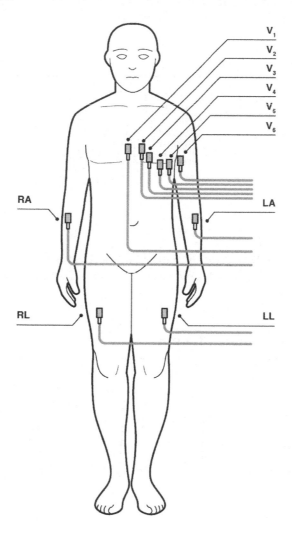

Patient Prep

In order to ensure an accurate tracing, the provider will:

- Explain the procedure to the patient.
- Expose the chest as necessary.
- Clip or shave excess hair as consistent with agency policy.
- Wipe the skin surface with gauze to decrease electrical resistance.
- Remove excess oils with alcohol wipe if necessary.
- Verify that the electrode is intact with sufficient gel.
- Attach the electrodes as appropriate.
- Complete the tracing.

Recognize Artifacts

Artifact is most often the result of patient movement while the tracing is being recorded, and the provider must be able to differentiate between the artifact and lethal arrhythmias. Artifact is most often evidenced by a chaotic wave pattern that interrupts a normal rhythm, as shown in the figure below.

EKG Artifact

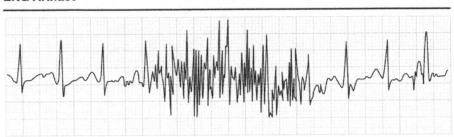

Recognize Rhythms, Arrhythmias

Normal Sinus: The rhythm originates in the sinoatrial (SA) node as indicated by the presence of an upright p wave in lead 2. A p wave precedes every QRS complex, and the rhythm is regular at sixty to one hundred beats per minute.

Normal Sinus Rhythm

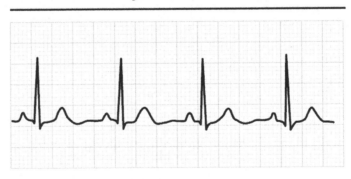

Sinus Tachycardia: The rhythm originates in the SA node as indicated by the presence of an upright p wave in lead 2. A p wave precedes every QRS complex, and the rhythm is regular at a rate greater than one hundred beats per minute.

Sinus Tachycardia

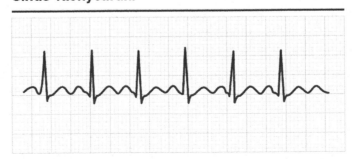

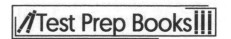

Sinus Bradycardia: The rhythm originates in the SA node as indicated by the presence of an upright p wave in lead 2. A p wave precedes every QRS complex, and the rhythm is regular at less than sixty beats per minute.

Sinus bradycardia

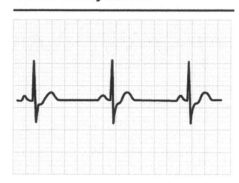

Atrial Fibrillation: The SA node fires chaotically at a rapid rate, while the ventricles contract at a slower but inefficient rate in response to an impulse from an alternative site in the heart. Individual p waves are not visible due to the rapid rate, and the QRS complexes are generally wider than the QRS complexes in the sinus rhythms.

Atrial Fibrillation

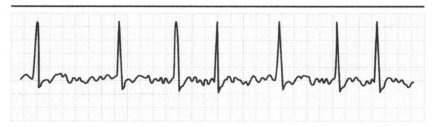

Complete Heart Block: The SA node generates a p wave that is not transmitted to the ventricles. The ventricles respond to an impulse from an alternative site, and the resulting complex has no association with the p wave. This condition requires immediate intervention.

Complete Heart Block

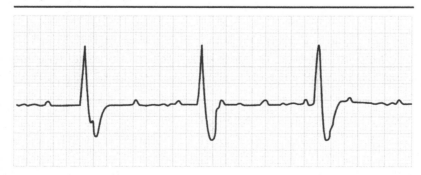

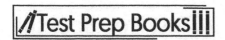

Ventricle Fibrillation: There is only erratic electrical activity resulting in quivering of the heart muscle. Immediate intervention is necessary.

Ventricular Fibrillation

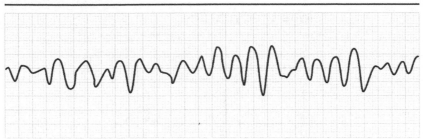

Rhythm Strips

The provider can use a six- to ten-second strip of cardiac activity to identify the heart rate and rhythm. The ECG paper is standardized to measure time from left to right, with each small box equal to four-tenths of a second, which means that each large box is equal to one-fifth of a second and the time elapsed between the black ticks is three seconds. The provider calculates the heart rate by dividing 300 by the number of large squares between two QRS complexes. In the figure below, the heart rate is 300/4 = 75. Alternatively, the provider can identify the heart rate by counting the number of QRS complexes in a ten-second EKG strip and multiplying that result by ten.

The provider will assess the rhythm by comparing the distance between complexes 1 and 2 with the distance between complexes 2 and 3.

Cardiac Rhythm Strip

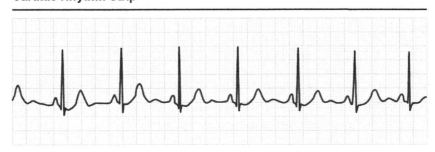

Holter Monitor

The **Holter monitor** is a portable device that is used for monitoring the EKG/ECG. The monitor may be used for routine cardiac monitoring or for diagnosing cardiac conditions that may not be evident on a single EKG/ECG tracing. The provider will attach the leads to the patient's chest, verify the patient's

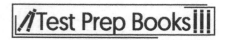

understanding of the process, and provide the patient with a diary with instructions to record all activity and physical symptoms for the duration of the testing period.

Holter monitor with EKG reading

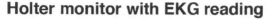

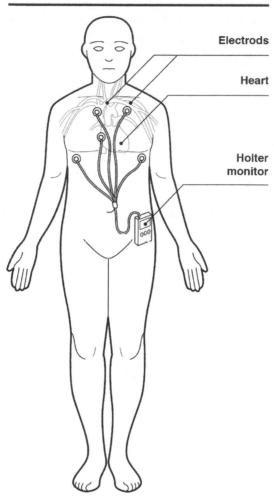

Electrods

Heart

Holter monitor

Cardiac Stress Test

The provider uses the cardiac stress test to identify the patient's cardiac response to the stress of exercise. The cardiac activity is recorded after the patient's heart rate reaches a target rate that is equal to 220 minus the patient's age. There are two forms of the test, which include the treadmill test and the pharmacologic test. Patients who are physically able walk on the treadmill until the target heart rate is achieved. Patients who are unable to tolerate the exercise will receive medications to raise the heart rate to the desired level. The provider will reverse the effects of these medications as soon as the appropriate tracings are obtained.

Vision Test: Color

The most commonly used test for color blindness is the **Ishihara Color Vision Test**, which is a series of circular images that are composed of colored dots. The identification of the numbers embedded in the colored plates is determined by the patient's ability to identify the red/green numbers and background.

There are currently online variations of this test in addition to color testing forms that the provider may use for younger children who are not yet able to identify numbers.

Vision Test: Acuity/Distance

Snellen Chart

The chart contains eleven rows of letters that differ in size from row to row and is viewed from a distance of twenty feet. The resulting numbers, 20/100 for example, indicate that the patient can see objects at a distance of 20 feet that are visible to a person with normal eyesight at a distance of 100 feet.

E Chart

The **E chart** contains nine rows of letters that differ in size from row to row depicting the letter E is alternating positions. The chart is useful for children and others who are not familiar with the English alphabet. The scoring is similar to the Snellen chart.

Jaeger Card

The **Jaeger card** uses six paragraphs in differing font sizes ranging from 14 point to 3 point Times New Roman font to test near vision. The J1 paragraph at 3 point Times New Roman font is considered to equal 20/20 vision per the Snellen chart.

Ocular Pressure

The provider uses a tonometer to touch the surface of the patient's anesthetized cornea in order to record the pressure inside the eye.

Visual Fields

Visual fields are defined as the total horizontal and vertical range of vision when the patient's eye is centrally focused. The provider may use this test to detect "blind spots" or scotomas.

Pure-Tone Audiometry

The patient's pure-tone threshold is identified as the lowest decibel level at which sounds are heard 50 percent of the time.

Speech and Voice Recognition

The **speech-awareness recognition (SAT),** or **speech-detection threshold (SDT)**, is defined as the lowest decibel level at which the patient can acknowledge the stimuli. The test utilizes spondees—two-syllable words that are spoken with equal stress on each syllable—as the stimuli for this test.

The **speech-recognition threshold (SRT),** or less commonly speech-reception threshold, measures the lowest decibel level at which the patient can recognize speech at least 50 percent of the time. This test also may be used to validate pure-tone threshold measurements, to determine the gain setting for a patient's hearing aid, or to provide a basis for suprathreshold word recognition testing.

Suprathreshold word recognition is used to assess the patient's ability to recognize and repeat one-syllable words that are presented at decibel levels that are consistent with social environments. Human-voice recordings are used to present the words, and the patient's responses are scored. The provider may use the results of this test to monitor the progression of a condition such as Meniere's disease, to identify improvement afforded by the use of hearing aids, or to isolate the part of the ear that is responsible for the deficit.

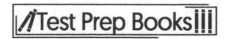

Tympanometry

The provider uses a tonometer to assess the integrity of the **tympanic membrane** (ear drum) and the function of the middle ear by introducing air and noise stimuli into the ear. The provider then assesses the resulting waveform and records the results.

Allergy Test: Scratch Test

The provider applies a small amount of diluted allergen to a small wound created in the patient's skin in order to identify the specific allergens that elicit an allergic response in the patient. The allergist will select up to fifty different allergens for testing, which means that the provider will make fifty small incisions or scratches in the patient's skin arranged in a grid system to facilitate the interpretation and reporting of the test results. The provider will observe the patient closely for a minimum of fifteen minutes following the introduction of the allergen for the signs of an anaphylactic reaction, in addition to signs of a positive reaction. The provider will document all positive results that are evidenced by a reddened raised area that is pruritic.

Allergy Test: Intradermal Skin Testing

The provider may use intradermal injections of the allergen to confirm negative scratch tests, or as the primary method of allergy testing. Using a 26- or 30-gauge needle, the provider will inject the allergen just below the surface of the skin. The provider must closely observe the patient and record results based on the appearance of raised, reddened wheals that are pruritic.

Pulmonary Function Tests

Pulmonary function tests evaluate the two main functions of the pulmonary system: air exchange and oxygen transport. The specific tests measure the volume of the lungs, the amount of air that can be inhaled or exhaled at one time, and the rate at which that volume is exhaled. The tests are used to monitor the progression of chronic pulmonary disorders, including asthma, emphysema, chronic obstructive lung disease, and sarcoidosis.

Spirometry

Spirometry is one of the two methods used to measure pulmonary function. The provider attaches the mouthpiece to the spirometer and instructs the patient to form a tight seal around its edge. The provider will then demonstrate the breathing patterns that are necessary for successful evaluation of each of the pulmonary measurements. The spirometry device calculates each of the values based on the patient's efforts.

Peak Flow Rate

Peak flow rate is defined as the speed at which the patient can exhale. This measure is commonly used to evaluate pulmonary function in patients with asthma.

Tuberculosis Tests/Purified Protein Derivative Skin Tests

Tuberculosis tests/purified protein derivative (PPD) skin tests are screening tests for the presence of Mycobacterium tuberculosis. The provider will use a tuberculin (TB) syringe to inject 0.1 ml of tuberculin purified protein derivative, the TB antigen, into the interior portion of the forearm. The solution forms a small, round elevation or wheal that is visible on the skin surface. The patient must return to the agency for evaluation of the site between forty-eight and seventy-two hours after the injection. The provider will assess the site and document the size of any visible induration or palpable swelling. The provider will not include any reddened areas in that measurement. The provider will refer all results that exceed 5 mm for additional testing and treatment.

Blood Pressure

Technique

To obtain an accurate measurement, the provider will:

- Assist the patient to a seated position.

- Expose the upper arm at the level of the heart.

- Apply the appropriately sized cuff.

- Palpate the antecubital space to identify the strongest pulsation point.

- Position the head of the stethoscope over the pulsation pulse.

- Slowly inflate the cuff to between 30 and 40 mm Hg above the patient's recorded blood pressure (BP). If this information is unavailable, the cuff may be inflated to between 160 and 180 mm Hg.

- Note the point at which the pulse is initially audible, which represents the systolic BP.

- Slowly deflate the cuff and record the point at which the pulse is initially audible as the systolic BP.

- Record the point at which the sounds are no longer audible as the diastolic BP.

Equipment

The **stethoscope** is a Y-shaped, hollow tube with earpieces and a diaphragm that transmits the sound to the earpieces when the provider places the diaphragm against the patient's body.

The **sphygmomanometer** includes the cuff, the mercury-filled gauge, or manometer that records the patient's pressure, and the release valve that regulates the air pressure in the cuff.

Pulse

Technique

To assess the pulse the provider will:

- Expose the intended pulse point.
- Palpate the area for the strongest pulsation.
- Position the middle three fingers of the hand on the point.
- Count the pulse for one full minute.

The provider will identify the pulse points that include the radial artery in the wrist, the brachial artery in the elbow, the carotid artery in the neck, the femoral artery in the groin, the popliteal artery behind the knee, and the dorsalis pedis and the posterior tibialis arteries in the foot.

The provider will assess the pulse rate by counting the number of pulsations per sixty minutes. In addition to the pulse rate, the provider will document the regularity or irregularity and strength of the pulsations.

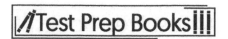

Height/Weight/BMI

Technique

To record an accurate height, the provider must instruct the patient to:

- Remove all footwear.
- Stand straight with the back against the wall.
- Remain still until the height is recorded.

To record an accurate weight, the provider must first zero the scale and then instruct the patient to:

- Remove all heavy objects from the pockets.
- Stand on the scale facing forward.
- Remain still until the weight is recorded.

The **BMI** (body mass index) is equal to:

- Imperial English BMI Formula: $weight\ (lbs) \times 703 \div height\ (in^2)$
- Metric BMI Formula: $weight\ (kg) \div height(m^2)$

For example:

The BMI of a patient who weighs 150 pounds and is 5'6" is equal to:

$$\frac{150 \times 703}{66 \times 66} = \frac{105{,}450}{4{,}356} = 24.2\ or\ 24.0$$

Equipment

Body scales may be mechanical or digital. Some digital scales also provide detailed metabolic information including the BMI in addition to the weight. Other scales can accommodate patients who are confined to bed.

Body Temperature

There are five possible assessment sites for body temperature, including oral, axillary, rectal, tympanic, and temporal. The route will depend on the patient's age and the agency policies. Assessment of oral temperatures requires the provider to verify that the patient has had nothing to eat or drink for five minutes before testing in order to avoid inaccurate readings.

Thermometers may be digital with disposal covers for the probe, wand-like structures that use infrared technology and are moved across the forehead to the temporal area, or handles with disposable cones that measure the tympanic temperature.

Oxygen Saturation/Pulse Oximetry

When every hemoglobin molecule in the circulating blood volume is carrying the maximum number of four oxygen molecules, the **oxygen saturation rate** is 100 percent. The normal oxygen saturation level is 95 percent to 100 percent, and levels below 90 percent must be treated.

The provider measures oxygen saturation noninvasively by the application of a **pulse oximetry device**, which the provider will attach to the patient's finger. The device may be used for continuous or intermittent monitoring of the saturation rate.

The pulse oximeter is a foam-lined clip that attaches to the patient's finger and uses infrared technology to assess the oxygen saturation level, which is expressed as a percentage.

Respiration Rate

The respiratory rate is counted, and the breathing pattern is assessed. The provider should ensure that the patient is unaware that the breathing rate is being counted by leaving the fingers resting on the radial pulse site while the respiratory rate is assessed.

Age-Specific Normal and Abnormal Vital Signs

Age	Temperature Degrees Fahrenheit	Pulse Range	Respiratory Rate Range	Blood Pressure mmHg
Newborns	98.2 axillary	100-160	30-50	75-100/50-70
0 - 5 years	99.9 rectal	80-120	20-30	80-110/50-80
6 - 10 years	98.6 oral	70-100	15-30	85-120/55-80
11 - 14 years	98.6 oral	60-105	12-20	95-140/60-90
15 - 20 years	98.6 oral	60-100	12-30	95-140/60-90
Adults	98.6 oral	50-80	16-20	120/80

Examinations

- **Auscultation** refers to listening to the sounds of body organs or processes, such as blood pressure, using a stethoscope.

- **Palpation** refers to using the hand or fingers to apply pressure to a body site to assess an organ for pain or consistency.

- **Percussion** refers to tapping on a body part to assess for rebound sounds. It may be used to assess the abdomen or the lungs.

- **Mensuration** refers to the measurement of body structures, such as measuring the circumference of the newborn's head.

- **Manipulation** refers to using the hands to correct a defect such as realigning the bones after a fracture.

- **Inspection** refers to the simple observation of the color, contour, or size of a body structure.

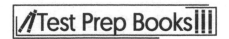

Body Positions/Draping
The provider will use proper draping to maximize the patient's privacy and to facilitate the planned procedures.

Draping Body Position

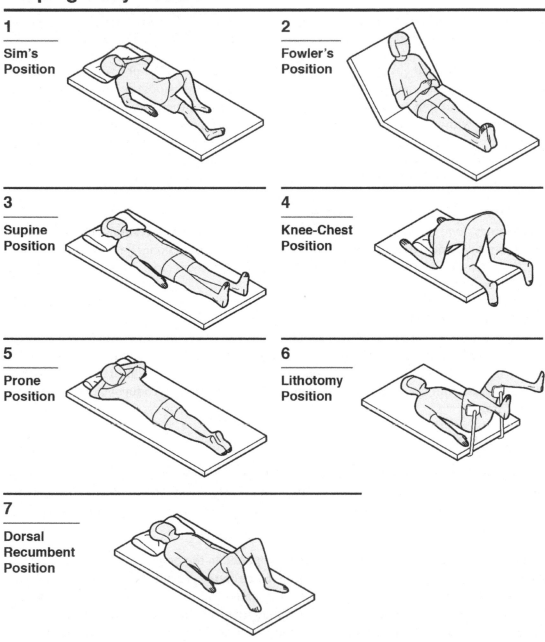

1 Sim's Position

2 Fowler's Position

3 Supine Position

4 Knee-Chest Position

5 Prone Position

6 Lithotomy Position

7 Dorsal Recumbent Position

Pediatric Exam
The purpose of the pediatric exam is to assess the child's growth and development and to provide family counseling regarding behavioral issues, nutrition, and injury protection. In addition, providers screen children for specific conditions at various ages to ensure that appropriate treatment is not delayed. For

instance, newborns are tested for phenylketonuria and hearing loss. Children between three and five years old are tested for alterations in vision, and school-aged children are screened for obesity.

Growth Chart

The **growth chart** is a systematic assessment of a child's growth pattern that can be compared to gender-specific norms.

The head circumference, height, and body weight are measured in children from birth to three years of age. In children older than three, the BMI is measured in addition to height and weight.

The **head circumference** is measured from birth to three years of age. The provider will measure the head circumference by placing a flexible measuring tape around the widest circumference of the child's head, which most commonly is above the eyebrows and the top of the ears. The provider will weigh infants lying down without clothes or diapers, and older children on mechanical or digital scales. To assess an infant's height, the provider will lay the child on a flat surface with the knee straightened and extend the flexible tape from the top of the infant's head to the bottom of the foot. The provider will position older children with their backs to a wall for an accurate measurement of their height.

Pelvic Exam/ Papanicolaou (PAP) Smear

The **pelvic exam** is done to assess the organs of the female reproductive system. The ovaries and the uterus are assessed by palpation, and the cervix is assessed by inspection. The **PAP smear** sample is a screening test for cervical cancer. The sample, obtained from the opening of the cervix, is transferred to glass slides for processing.

Prenatal/Postpartum Exams

The provider performs the prenatal pelvic exam to assess the development of the fetus and the status of the maternal reproductive system. The pelvic exam is done at the first visit, but is not repeated with every visit. In a normal pregnancy, it may not be repeated until the third trimester. The provider performs the postpartum exam to assess the return of the maternal reproductive organs to the nonpregnant state.

Laboratory Values

The nurse will need a savvy knowledge of common lab tests performed, why they are performed, and the normal values that are expected from the tests. These values will indicate if a disease process is at work in a body system. The nurse will need to be able to interpret that abnormality to report it to the ordering physician.

One commonly taken lab test is the **serum electrolyte panel**. In the body, the electrolytes work to maintain healthy cellular functions and metabolism. **Electrolytes** provide the structure in cell walls, generate energy for metabolic activity, transport fluid, cause muscle cell contraction, and even generate electrical impulses in the cardiac cells. Electrolytes that are often measured and assessed in the patient include sodium, potassium, magnesium, phosphorus, chloride, and calcium. The normal values of these electrolytes are listed below:

- Sodium: 135–145 mEq/L
- Potassium: 3.5–5.1 mEq/L
- Magnesium: 1.6–2.6 mg/dL
- Phosphorus: 2.5–4.5 mg/dL

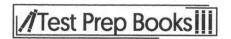

- Chloride: 98–107 mEq/L
- Calcium: 8.5–10.0 mg/L

Values outside of these normal parameters may suggest an electrolyte imbalance. Hyper/hypokalemia, hyper/hyponatremia, hyper/hypomagnesemia, hyper/hypochloremia, hyper/hypocalcemia, and hyper/hypophosphatemia are all conditions that should be immediately reported to the ordering physician if they are newly developed or worsened since the last reading. Signs and symptoms accompanying these electrolyte abnormalities should also be noted and treated as appropriate.

The CBC, as noted earlier in the Diagnostic Tests section, is useful for giving the clinician a picture of the health of the circulatory system. The CBC will show if the patient is anemic, leukemic, or lacking the necessary platelets for clotting and maintaining hemostasis. The following list shows normal, expected values for each component of the CBC:

- Red blood cells: 4–5 million cells/mcL for women, 5–6 million cells/mcL for men
- White blood cells: 4500–10,000 cells/mcL
- Hemoglobin (Hbg): 14–17 gm/dL
- Hematocrit (Hct): 41%–50% for men, 36%–44% for women
- Platelets: 140,000–450,000 cells/mcL
- Mean corpuscular volume (MCV) (the size of red blood cells): 80–95

The **comprehensive metabolic panel (CMP)** is a group of lab values that are often taken together that measure how well the kidneys and liver are functioning and levels of blood sugar, cholesterol, calcium, and protein levels in the body. The electrolytes may be measured using the CMP or as part of a smaller lab test called a **basic metabolic panel (BMP)**. Though it varies based on facility, the CMP generally consists of fourteen separate lab tests, while a BMP may only contain eight separate lab tests. The practitioner will determine which of these tests to perform.

The following are normal levels found on a CMP:

- Blood glucose: 70–110 mg/dL
- Albumin: 3.4–5.4 g/dL
- Alkaline phosphatase: 44–147 IU/L
- Alanine aminotransferase (ALT): 7–40 IU/L
- Aspartate aminotransferase (AST): 10–34 IU/L
- Blood urea nitrogen (BUN): 6–20 mg/dL
- Creatinine: 0.6–1.3 mg/dL
- Total bilirubin: 0.3–1.0 mg/dL
- Total protein: 6.0–8.3 g/dL

The final lab test the nurse will need to be able to interpret is the **arterial blood gas (ABG)** sample. A commonly performed test in patients with respiratory disorders or on mechanical ventilation in the intensive care unit (ICU), this test shows the pH balance, carbon dioxide level, and bicarbonate level in the patient's blood. This test will show how well the patient's respiratory processes are performing. Adjustments to respiratory and other therapies may be made based on it. The arterial sample is usually obtained from the radial, femoral, or brachial arteries. The following are normal ABG ranges:

- Oxygen (O2) saturation (SaO2): 94%–100%
- Arterial blood pH: 7.35–7.45

- Partial pressure of oxygen (PaO2): 75–100 mmHg
- Partial pressure of carbon dioxide (PaCO2): 38–41 mmHg
- Bicarbonate (HCO3): 22–28 mEq/L

Abnormalities in the ABGs could suggest an alkalotic or acidotic state of the patient's blood that will need correction. Reporting abnormal values to the physician and the respiratory therapist will be part of the nurse's expected duties.

Urinalysis

- Physical: The provider will perform a visual assessment of the color and turbidity of the urine sample.

- Chemical: The provider will use the reagent strip to assess the specific gravity, the pH, and the presence and quantity of protein, glucose, ketones hemoglobin and myoglobin, leukocyte esterase, bilirubin, and urobilirubin.

- Microscopic: The provider will separate the urine sediment from the fluid volume to microscopically identify the presence of RBCs, WBCs, epithelial cells, bacteria, yeasts, and parasites.

- Culture: The provider will assess the presence of infectious agents in the urine sample by inoculating the agar plates, incubating sample at body temperature, and observing, and documenting any growth at twenty-four and forty-eight hours after inoculation of the sample.

Hematology Panel

- **Hematocrit (HCT):** The provider will assess the RBC count as defined by the hematocrit by placing the anticoagulated blood sample into the microhematocrit centrifuge and documenting the results.

- **Hemoglobin:** The provider will assess the amount of the hemoglobin protein that is present in the red blood cells by placing the anticoagulated blood sample into the microhematocrit centrifuge and documenting the results.

- **Erythrocyte Sedimentation Rate (ESR):** The provider will assess the ESR, which is a nonspecific indicator of inflammation, by placing the anticoagulated sample in the Westergren tube and recording the height of the settled RBCs after one hour.

- **Automated Cell Counts:** The provider will use the automated device to assess RBC, WBC, and platelet counts by preparing the sample, obtaining, and documenting the results.

- **Coagulation testing/international normalized ratio (INR):** The provider will calculate the INR, which is used to assess blood-clotting levels in patients being treated with Warfarin, according to laboratory protocol after verifying that the sample was not drawn from a heparinized line.

Chemistry/Metabolic Testing

Glucose

The provider will identify the blood glucose sample, which measures the amount glucose in the circulating blood volume, as fasting or nonfasting before processing and documenting the results.

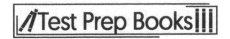

Kidney Function Tests

Kidney function is assessed by measuring the levels of metabolic waste products, **including blood urea nitrogen (BUN)** and creatinine, and by calculating the **glomerular filtration rate (GFR)**, which corresponds with the clearance of waste products from the blood by the kidneys. The provider will process the sample to obtain the BUN and creatinine levels. The provider will then use the creatinine level and the patient's age, body size, and gender to calculate to the GFR according to the agency-approved equation for GFR. There are four equations that may be used to calculate the GFR in adults that include the Modification of Diet in Renal Disease (MDRD), the Study equation (IDMS-traceable version), and the Chronic Kidney Disease Epidemiology Collaboration (CKD-EPI) equation.

Liver Function Tests

Elevated levels of **alanine transaminase (ALT)** and **aspartate aminotransferase (AST),** two liver enzymes, indicate acute/chronic hepatitis, cirrhosis, or liver cancer. Decreased levels of these enzymes may be due to Vitamin B-12 deficiency. Albumin, a protein synthesized by the liver that is necessary for the maintenance of osmotic pressure in the vasculature, is decreased in liver failure due to cirrhosis or cancer. The liver processes bilirubin, a waste product resulting from the normal destruction of old red blood cells, for excretion by the gastrointestinal system; however, elevated levels may be due to liver failure or transfusion reactions. The provider will verify a ten-minute centrifuge time, process the sample, and document results.

Lipid Profile

Excess dietary intact of animal fats can result in elevated total cholesterol **and low-density lipoprotein (LDL)** or "bad cholesterol" levels, while elevated **high-density lipoprotein (HDL)** or "good cholesterol" levels are the result of appropriate nutrition or the effect of cholesterol-lowering medications. Elevated triglycerides levels may result from diabetes, obesity, liver failure, or kidney disease. The provider will verify that the fasting sample was obtained before the administration of **N-Acetylcysteine (NAC)** or Metamizole, if indicated. The provider will then process the sample per protocol within two hours of the venipuncture and document the results.

Hemoglobin A1c

Hemoglobin A1c measures the percentage of the hemoglobin molecules that are coated or glycated with glucose. The **hemoglobin** molecules are located in the red blood cell, which has a lifespan of 110 to 120 days; therefore, the hemoglobin A1c test measures the average blood sugar for a four-month period. The normal A1c level is less than 5.7 percent; levels between 5.7 percent and 6.4 percent indicate prediabetes and levels greater than 6.5 percent indicate diabetes. Elevated HGB A1c levels must be confirmed with additional testing before treatment is initiated. The provider will inform the patient that fasting is not required, process the sample, and document results.

Immunology

Mononucleosis Test

The immune system produces heterophile proteins in response to the presence of the Epstein-Barr virus (EBV), the causative agent of mononucleosis. Specific tests include the analysis of the viral capsid antigen (VCA), the early antigen (EA), or the EBV nuclear antigen (EBNA). The **Monospot test** detects antibodies that are not specific for mononucleosis, leading to false positive and false negative results. In addition, the Monospot test may be insensitive to the heterophile antibodies produced by children with mononucleosis. The provider will freeze the sample if processing is delayed beyond twenty-four hours after preparation.

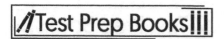

Rapid Group A Streptococcus Test

Identification of the beta-hemolytic bacterium *Streptococcus pyogenes*, the most common cause of acute pharyngitis in adults and children, is obtained by using isothermal nucleic acid amplification technology. The provider will transfer the sample to the testing device adhering to proper wait-times, process the sample, and document the results.

C-Reactive Protein (CRP)

CRP is an indicator of inflammation that is released into the bloodstream in response to tissue injury or the onset of an infection. The provider will verify that all reagents and the serum sample are at room temperature, assess the processed sample for agglutination, and document the results.

HCG Pregnancy Test

Serum levels of **human chorionic gonadotropin** hormone detect the presence of a pregnancy. Elevated levels may indicate a normal pregnancy, either single or multiple, chorionic cancer, or hydatiform mole. The provider will centrifuge the clotted sample for ten minutes at room temperature, and document the results.

H. pylori

There are three testing methods for the *Helicobacter pylori* organism, including histological examination and culture of samples obtained by endoscopic biopsy, the urea breath test (UBT) that measures CO_2 levels on exhalation, and the fecal antigen test that identifies antibodies to the organism. The provider will verify that patient has avoided antibiotics and bismuth preparations for two weeks prior to the testing. The provider will process all samples according to the specific test requirements and document the results.

Influenza

Influenza testing methods include the **Rapid Influenza Diagnostic Test (RIDT)**, and the **Real Time Polymerase Chain Reaction**, and the viral culture, which identify the genetic material of the virus in secretions obtained from a nasal or throat swab. The provider will process all samples according to the specific test requirements and document the results.

Fecal Occult Blood Testing

Occult bleeding is not visibly apparent, which means that detection methods rely on the chemical reaction between the blood and the testing reagents for identification of blood in a sample. For home sample collection with guaiac testing, the provider will instruct the patient to collect three samples on three different days to optimize results. The patient will secure the test card and submit it to the provider for testing. The provider will apply a guaiac solution to the sample to identify a bluish tinge in the test area, which is considered positive for the presence of occult blood.

Potential for Alterations in Body Systems

The nurse will work with patients who are at risk for an alteration in their body systems. The nurse identifies compromising patient situations that have the potential to lead to complications. These complications could include aspiration, skin breakdown, insufficient vascular perfusion, and the devastating problems that may occur when a patient has been sedentary for too long.

There are many conditions that may cause a patient to be at risk for **aspiration**. A patient who has suffered a stroke and has developed **dysphagia**, or difficulty swallowing, is immediately considered at

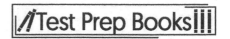

risk for aspiration. This is because the mechanical difficulty they experience when they try to swallow can sometimes lead to leakage of the substance they are trying to swallow into their airway instead of the esophagus. Foreign substances in the airway lead to immediate difficulty breathing and respiratory distress. At this point, aspiration has occurred, and the patient needs emergent intervention to restore proper respiratory faculties.

A client with a feeding tube in place, whether nasogastric (NG) or placed via gastrostomy, is at risk for aspiration. Aspiration is, in fact, one of the most common complications of enteral feedings. The stomach becomes quite full with the feedings, causing gastric contents to reflux, and secretions accumulate in the pharynx where they are then aspirated. The integrity of the upper and lower esophageal sphincters may become compromised over time, contributing to aspiration risk. The patient receiving tube feedings also has the potential to have a weakened swallowing and gag reflex, contributing to aspiration risk. Clients on tube feedings should be carefully monitored for fullness of the stomach and signs of fluid buildup such as wet-sounding coughs and a rattle-like sound when breathing.

Patients who are sedated are at risk for aspiration due to their altered level of consciousness. The head of the bed should remain elevated at least 45 degrees—90 degrees if the patient has recently received an enteral feeding to promote digestion and stomach emptying. Laying the patient flat on their back puts them at risk of aspiration.

All patients who have been immobilized by an illness are at risk for skin breakdown while in bed. The increased pressure on bony prominences that a prolonged period spent in bed creates can easily compromise skin integrity and lead to an ulceration. The nurse works to prevent pressure ulcers by keeping the client on a "turn every two hours" repositioning schedule. Every two hours, the client will be repositioned in bed, from the left side to the right side and then back again. The patient should only be positioned on their back for feedings, as this position can put quite a bit of pressure on the sacrum, an area especially vulnerable to breakdown.

There are many patient situations that may put them at risk for insufficient vascular perfusion. Patients with impaired circulation may be at risk because of hypervolemia, hypovolemia, a low amount of circulating oxygen associated with low hemoglobin counts, low blood pressure, immobilization of a limb, decreased cardiac output as seen in heart failure, and diabetes. After the nurse has identified that the client has a compromise of vascular perfusion, efforts will be made to intervene and restore normal circulation. Early mobility, in which the client is encouraged to get out of bed and get moving as soon as they are able, is vital to maintaining healthy circulation. Compression stockings are commonplace in immobile patients to artificially maintain healthy circulation.

Certain factors put a patient more at risk for developing cancer. A patient who uses tobacco or is exposed to secondhand smoke on a regular basis is at a greater risk for developing cancers of the lung, mouth, esophagus, larynx, and esophagus. Patients with a family history of a certain type of cancer such as breast, colon, ovarian, and uterine are more at risk for developing these types of cancers. The nurse will review and record a client's risk factors for developing cancers when performing the initial admission assessment.

Potential for Complications of Diagnostic Tests/Treatments/Procedures

When a client undergoes a procedure or diagnostic test at the hospital, things do not always go according to plan. The nurse is there to assess the client when they return from their procedure to monitor them for complications. When a complication is noted, the nurse is quick to intervene, alert the attending physician, and take care of the patient to get them stabilized.

One common diagnostic procedure performed regularly at hospitals is the cardiac catheterization. Patients returning from a cardiac catherization are at risk for developing complications such as bleeding and dysrhythmias. Most facilities have protocols and checklists in place postprocedure that the nurse will follow strictly. These checklists include regular vital-sign monitoring, checking the access site for bleeding or hematoma, and cardiac monitoring for dysrhythmias. The client will be made to lay flat for a predetermined amount of time, usually six hours, so that blood flow to the accessed artery is not compromised and the access point can fully heal. Bleeding around the puncture point as well as formation of an aneurysm are other possible complications. Any abnormality will be reported to the cardiologist.

A patient who has a limb with a cast placed will be monitored for compartment syndrome. The nurse pays close attention to the limb, especially the more distal end, to ensure that adequate circulation is maintained and is not cut off by the cast placement. Assessment of pulses, whether radial or ulnar in the upper limbs or dorsalis pedis or posterior tibial in the lower limbs, will be performed to assess that circulation is not compromised.

After any test that involves incision, puncture, or any other access to the client's circulatory system, bleeding and infection are always major risks. Patients with **thrombocytopenia**, or a low platelet count, are at an increased risk for bleeding, as they lack the necessary component for proper hemostasis. Blood pressure monitoring is an excellent way to monitor the patient's hemodynamic status. A lowered blood pressure that is trending downward is an ominous sign that the client may be losing blood internally. Hypotension is the first step toward any sort of shock state and can lead to an interrupted delivery of oxygen to vital organs and tissues. Identifying if the client is bleeding and where the source of the bleed is will require an advanced interventional team such as a rapid-response team, usually headed by an intensivist or ICU doctor.

Along with bleeding, infection is a common complication of invasive diagnostic procedures. The nurse works to prevent infection by performing meticulous handwashing before and after client care, observing infection prevention precautions such as donning gloves and gowns in patients with communicable diseases and disinfecting equipment after use. The disposal of medical supplies in the appropriate receptacle, such as sharps in the sharps container, will assist in the goal of preventing the spread of infections. The nurse takes care to perform certain tasks using an aseptic or sterile technique, such as dressing changes, insertion of urinary catheters, insertion of NG tubes, and obtaining IV accesses.

Potential for Complications from Surgical Procedures and Health Alterations

During the surgical consent process, surgical risks and potential complications are explained to the patient by the surgeon. The risk of complications depends on the type of surgical procedure being performed, as well as the condition and comorbidities of the patient. The perioperative environment predisposes the patient to risk of hypothermia. Per best practice guidelines, the operating room temperature should be kept between sixty-eight and seventy-three degrees Fahrenheit. Depending on the procedure, the patient may be partially clothed or fully naked. If the procedure is one hour or greater in duration, thermoregulation measures should be taken to prevent hypothermia. These measures can include warming blankets and warm intravenous fluid administration. Methods for monitoring patient temperature in the perioperative environment include temporal, esophageal,

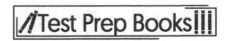

bladder, rectal, and via thermodilution catheter, which is inserted into the pulmonary artery. Hypothermia places the patient at greater risk for developing surgical site infection (SSI). Although the signs of SSI may not be apparent for several weeks postoperatively, steps in preventing SSI are implemented in the preoperative period. The **Joint Commission's Surgical Care Improvement Project (SCIP)** outlines standards around preoperative antibiotic prophylaxis and other measures to decrease risk of SSI. Major surgical procedures involving the vascular system, such as abdominal aortic aneurysm repair and open-heart surgical procedures, present the risk for high amounts of blood loss. Hemodynamic changes often occur as a result of blood loss. Hemodynamic changes during the surgical procedure can include hypotension, hypertension, cardiac arrhythmias, and decreased oxygen saturation. Changes in hemodynamic stability can create the need for blood transfusion. Blood loss can lead to cardiac complications, especially in those with coronary artery disease. Patients with cardiac disease are at risk for **myocardial infarction (MI)** due to the surgical process. In vascular procedures, the clamping of vessels can release calcified areas or plaque into circulation, which can cause an MI or a stroke. **Venous thromboembolism (VTE)** is another potential complication from surgery. VTE prophylaxis measures are implemented preoperatively to reduce this risk. Depending on the patient, these measures can include application of **sequential compression devices (SCDs)** to bilateral lower extremities. SCDs work by creating mild, intermittent compression to the extremities to prevent pooling of blood while the patient is not ambulatory. The physician may choose to order a medical VTE prophylaxis protocol. For example, the patient may receive enoxaparin (Lovenox), a blood thinner, for a set number of doses postoperatively.

A rare yet life-threatening complication of surgery is **malignant hyperthermia (MH).** MH is a genetic disorder that presents after exposure to anesthetic gases and/or paralytic drugs. Since MH is a genetic disorder, the preoperative interview should include questions that assess family history of MH and complications of anesthesia. If the patient indicates a history of MH or a family history of difficulty with anesthesia, the perioperative team should be prepared for MH crisis and discuss this risk with the entire perioperative team. Symptoms of MH crisis include muscle rigidity, tachycardia, rising body temperature, and rising levels of **end-tidal carbon dioxide (ETCO2).**

Finally, death is a potential complication of the surgery process. Risk of surgical death is related to the type of surgery and patient comorbidities. Adverse perioperative events such as dissecting a major blood vessel can also lead to death. Emergency procedures generally carry a higher risk of death than routine procedures.

System Specific Assessments

The nurse will need to be skilled in doing body system–specific assessments on clients who have undergone a diagnostic procedure or a treatment. The nurse needs to be able to use sound nursing judgment and critical thinking to hone in on the system they need to examine based on the client's condition.

Knowledge of peripheral pulse assessment is necessary to evaluate the patient's circulatory status. Strong pulses at a normal rhythm are good; faint pulses that are either too fast or too slow are worrisome and need further evaluation. Pulses are graded on a scale of 0 to 4, 0 being absent, 1 being weak, 2 being normal, 3 being increased volume, and 4 being a bounding pulse. The pulse is assessed and documented with further action being taken if necessary.

Another way to evaluate the health of the circulatory system is to assess for and grade edema. **Edema**, a fluid accumulation in the peripheral tissues of the body, can get to a point where, when pushed down upon with a finger, the impression stays in the skin. These impressions can be graded by their depth, ranging from +1 to +4 as shown in the diagram below.

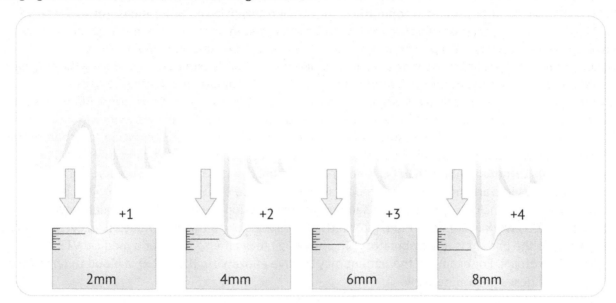

The neurological system may need specific evaluation requiring the nurse's keen assessment skills. The nurse will start by evaluating the client's level of consciousness, which is measured by interviewing the client and their knowledge of who they are, where they are, and the time. A client oriented to all three of these components is said to be **oriented times three**, while a client who only knows their name, for example, is only **oriented times one**. Commonly, this is noted in the nurse's notes as "**A&OX3**" or something similar. The "A" stands for "alert," as opposed to obtunded, drowsy, sleepy, difficult to arouse, and other altered levels of consciousness.

Other components of the neurological assessment include assessment of the cranial nerves, usually used on stroke assessments, motor and sensory function, pupillary response, reflexes, cerebellar function, and vital signs.

The following are the **"Five P's" of Neurovascular Assessment:**

- Pain
- Pulse
- Pallor
- Paresthesia
- Paralysis

The nurse can assess the client's musculoskeletal system by testing for bilateral strength and equality of movement. Muscular strength can be graded on a 0 to 5 scale. A patient with no visible muscle contraction is graded as a 0, a patient who has visible contraction but still no movement is graded as a 1, a patient that is contracting and trying to move but cannot overcome gravity is graded as a 2, the same without the ability to push against resistance is a 3, the same with only a limited effect of resistance on their effort is a 4, and finally, a full contraction with movement that can overcome elevated levels of resistance is a 5.

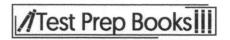

Diabetic patients have a constant battle maintaining a healthy level of blood sugar. The nurse taking care of a diabetic patient keeps a close eye on not only the patient's blood sugar but also their diabetic medications, the fluids they are receiving, and their mealtime habits. The classic symptoms of hyperglycemia are **polydipsia** and **polyuria**, where the patient drinks copious amounts of fluid and produces massive amounts of urine. Hypoglycemia symptoms reflect the interruption of blood glucose to the brain, resulting in neurological symptoms such as confusion, lowered level of consciousness, slurred speech, lightheadedness, and dizziness.

Therapeutic Procedures

The nurse will need to be able to assess a client who has recently undergone a therapeutic procedure, apply their knowledge regarding the procedure, educate the client about aftercare, and monitor the patient postprocedure, observing the proper precautions.

Many therapeutic procedures will use anesthesia, whether local, regional, or general. **Local anesthesia** includes topical and injected anesthetics such as lidocaine and benzocaine and are common in minimally invasive procedures such as external biopsies, removals of skin lesions and moles, and dental surgeries. A **regional anesthetic** only provides analgesia to a certain part of the body and includes epidural, spinal, or paravertebral nerve blocks. **General anesthesia** renders the patient completely unconscious using medical gas or IV transfusion.

There are four stages of anesthesia: induction, excitement, surgical anesthesia, and emergence. The anesthetist carefully monitors the patient as they travel throughout these stages, maintaining them in the appropriate state of consciousness while the procedure occurs. During these stages, the client is closely monitored using pulse oximetry, blood pressure readings, measurement of heart rate and rhythm, and body temperature. The patient airway will be monitored, especially if under general anesthesia and an artificial airway is being used such as an endotracheal tube.

All three levels of anesthesia come with their own potential complications. With local anesthetics, the patient may get too high off of a dose, or the anesthetic may be administered too rapidly. Potential complications of a local anesthetic include excitability, seizure activity, depression of the central nervous system, and respiratory and cardiac distress. Regional anesthetics can cause headache, soreness at the injection site, infection, bleeding, bruising, and low blood pressure. General sedation complications range from mild to severe, including sore throat, fatigue, and dizziness, all the way to malignant hyperthermia, respiratory arrest, cardiac arrest, and cerebrovascular accident or stroke.

Before and after the procedure, the nurse will assess the client's knowledge of the therapeutic intervention being performed, answer questions within their scope of practice, refer to the performing physician where appropriate, and educate the patient regarding the procedure. Each facility will have client education literature that can be accessed and printed out for the client and nurse's use. Informed consent will need to be obtained for most serious interventions, so this information will be useful to have on hand to answer the client's questions.

The nurse will ensure that the patient's preoperative orders are followed, such as the observance of NPO (nothing by mouth), in which the patient is not to eat or drink anything preprocedure. Any medications that are required before the procedure will be administered and documented in a timely manner. Many procedures have a pre- and postprocedure checklist that the nurse will ensure gets filled out.

The nurse will need to identify the client before and after the procedure following the two-identifier technique. Usually this involves having the client state their name and date of birth, along with a scanning of their identification band for additional identification.

The client who is to go home following a procedure will need home care instructions, such as taking care of an incision site. The nurse will educate the patient about their posthospital care. Usually, if an incision is present, there will be specific instructions as to how to keep the site clean, when the client can shower and bathe again, and how to do dressing changes. Follow-up appointments will be made to ensure the client's progress and healing.

Methods of Collection
Blood
For a venipuncture process, the provider will:

- Identify the patient, review the order, and label the collection tubes.
- Assess the nondominant hand to identify a vein that is straight and palpable.
- Wash hands and apply PPE.
- Clean the selected site with an alcohol swab per agency policy.
- Inspect the test-specific vacuum tubes and needles to verify that:
  - The tube is securely sealed and vacuum has been maintained.
  - Appropriate additives such anticoagulants or other fixatives that may be required to maintain the sample are present in the tube.
  - The chosen needle size is appropriate to the selected vein.
- Complete the venipuncture per agency policy.
- Apply pressure and a sterile dressing to the venipuncture site.
- Submit the sample for processing per agency policy.

The provider will use a capillary/dermal puncture to obtain blood from small children or when only a small volume of blood is necessary as in finger-stick puncture for blood glucose analysis.

Urine
The provider can collect a random urinalysis any time the patient voids.

To obtain a midstream/clean catch urine sample, the provider will instruct the patient to first clean the urinary meatus with the appropriate antiseptic solution, void without collecting the initial volume, and then deposit the remaining output into the container.

Before beginning the collection of a timed twenty-four-hour collection, the provider must obtain a storage container containing any necessary preservative from the laboratory, and confirm the accommodations for refrigeration of the sample if required. The first time the patient voids, the provider will discard the specimen and record the time. All urine collected in the following twenty-four-hour period will be collected by the provider and stored in the prepared container at the prescribed temperature.

Catheterization may be used to obtain a sterile specimen. The provider will pass the sterile catheter into the bladder to drain the urine into a sterile container, which must then be labeled and transported to the lab according to agency policy.

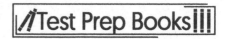

The pediatric urine collector is a plastic pouch attached to a foam adhesive backed base. The provider will verify that the skin around the urinary meatus is clean, dry, and free of powder or lotions. The provider will adhere the adhesive section of the collection device over the urinary meatus and replace the patient's diaper.

Fecal Specimen
The provider will place the fecal specimen in a clean, leak-proof, properly labeled container, and promptly transport the sample to the laboratory for processing.

Sputum Specimen
The sputum specimen must contain sputum, not saliva, and it is best obtained early in the morning.

Throat Swab
After assisting the patient to a seated position in a chair or bed, the provider will use sterile swabs to remove the sample from the back of the throat while avoiding contact with the uvula and tongue. The provider will then break the tips of the swabs and secure them in the labeled collection sleeve, transport the sample to the lab according to agency policy, and document the sample collection time and site.

Genital
The provider will position the patient according to the site being sampled. The provider will use sterile swabs to sample the top of the vaginal vault for a vaginal swab, the center of the cervical os for a cervical swab, or the urinary meatus for a urethral swab. The provider will then break the tips of the swabs and secure them in the labeled collection sleeve, transport the sample to the lab according to agency policy, and document the sample collection time and site.

Wound
The provider will position the patient according to the site being sampled. The provider will remove and discard the existing dressing, use sterile swabs to obtain the sample from the center of the wound, then break the tips of the swabs and secure them in the labeled collection sleeve. Once the swabs are secured, the provider will dress the wound, ensure that the sample is delivered to the laboratory, and document the wound assessment and the sample collection time and site.

Nasopharyngeal
The provider will position the patient in a seated position with the head tilted back. After verifying the patency of the nares, the provider will insert the sterile swab 3 to 4 inches into the nasopharynx, rotate the swaps to obtain the sample, remove the swabs, break the tips of the swabs to secure them in the labeled collection sleeve, transport the specimen to the laboratory, and document the collection site and time.

Physiological Adaptation

Alterations in Body Systems

Nurses must have the ability to assess a client for alterations in their body systems. This is an inevitable occurrence, as a body system alteration is precisely the reason the client is at the hospital in the first place. The nurse will identify the body system alteration and draw up a plan of care based on their findings.

Intake and output are items that are closely monitored by the nurse to discover if an alteration in a body system has occurred. There are several types of drainage a client may experience that fall into the category of input and output. The nurse measures the drainage where appropriate and notes its appearance. Color, quantity, consistency, and any other notable characteristics are observed and documented. Types of drainage the nurse may encounter in client care include feeding tube drainage, respiratory secretions, drainage from a chest tube, rectal tube output, and urinary catheter output.

Clients with cancer may be put on radiation therapy to target and destroy cancerous tumors. This client may develop alterations in certain body systems as a result. The client is likely to become quite fatigued, as their energy is sapped by the intensity of the therapy. Weakness often accompanies fatigue. They may experience skin reactions such as a rash. The skin may become red, looking like a sunburn. The skin above the targeted location for radiation absorbs a bit of the radiation, which is why the reaction occurs. Other radiation therapy side effects may be specific to the area in which the therapy is targeted. If therapy occurs near the stomach or abdomen, for example, stomachache, nausea, vomiting, and diarrhea may occur.

If the nurse is caring for a woman who is pregnant, they will be mindful of certain body alterations associated with the prenatal period. One such complication is high blood pressure during pregnancy, called *preeclampsia*. The woman's blood pressure is carefully monitored during the prenatal period to watch for the development of this condition, which could lead to complications for both the mother and the baby. Gestational diabetes is another prenatal complication of which the nurse is mindful. Somewhere between twenty-four and twenty-eight weeks, pregnant women are screened for gestational diabetes by performing the oral glucose tolerance test (OGTT). This glucose screening will identify if the woman is at risk, and treatment will follow if necessary.

Patients who are developing an infection will often have some telltale symptoms that the nurse will be watchful for. The classic signs of a localized infection on the outer surface of the body will be redness, inflammation, heat, and swelling. If the infection is systemic, within the body, the patient may have a fever, increased WBC count (or decreased if the infection has been prolonged), prodromal malaise, fatigue, chills, elevated heart rate, and even altered level of consciousness and orientation. Some infections will have specific symptoms related to the organ or tissue of the body affected. For example, a urinary tract infection (UTI) will cause the patient to have pain or burning while urinating, called *dysuria,* possibly blood in the urine, and frequent urges to void. A respiratory infection, on the other hand, will have respiratory-specific symptoms such as cough, difficulty breathing, and adventitious breath sounds on lung auscultation.

Having a basic knowledge of how an infection works, from start to finish, is advantageous to the nurse when trying to understand what is going on within the client's body. The causative organism must enter the body through some entryway: respiratory tract, break in the skin, urinary tract, IV access, GI tract,

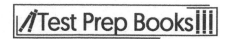

and so on. The organism then goes through what is called the "incubation period," which refers to the time that elapses between the organism entering the body and when symptoms actually begin occurring. During the incubation period, the organism is usually multiplying until it starts to have a noticeable effect on the body. Some pathogens will have a longer incubation time, while others will have shorter. Depending on the pathogen, there may be some communicability of the disease involved, in which the disease can be spread from one person to another. Therefore, observing universal precautions is vital to prevent the spread of disease. Meticulous handwashing by the nurse and all members of the health-care team, as well as patients and family, is vital.

A full-blown infection occurs when the body's natural defenses cannot overcome the organism effectively and symptoms occur, compromising overall body function. The patient may have an elevated WBC count on the CBC, indicating the body is bolstering its immune defenses to try and overcome the infection. The final stage of the infection is when the body's immune system plus the help of medication and therapeutic interventions destroy the organism, restoring the body to natural, normal functioning ability.

Patient education is an important aspect of care that the nurse diligently performs when body system alterations occur. Helping the patient understand what is going on in their body and answering their questions is an excellent way to reduce anxiety and promote calm and understanding. Anxiety, the nurse knows, only causes additional stress in the body, which will not be conducive to healing.

When educating the patient, the nurse will talk about the body system alteration they are experiencing, using their knowledge of pathophysiology, anatomy, and physiology as well as incorporating lessons about the pharmacological interventions being used on the patient. Discussion of risk factors related to the body alterations and side effects of medication is important to include. The nurse will discuss factors that will promote healing, such as the patient getting adequate rest and early mobility. The nurse will encourage the patient to call on the health-care team whenever a need arises, whether the need is for the nurse's aide, the nurse, or the physician. The patient should be encouraged to ask their questions and raise their concerns, as they are an important member of the health-care team. The nurse will include information about helpful resources that the client may access such as community groups for the client's specific condition or illness, social services, and community meal or ride programs.

The following detail the basics of the body systems and their normal functions:

Integumentary

The skin or **integumentary** body system is the largest organ of the body in surface area and weight. It is composed of three layers, which include the outermost layer or epidermis, the dermis, and the hypodermis. The thickness of the epidermis varies according to the specific body area. For example, the skin is thicker on the palms and the soles of the feet than on the eyelids. The dermis contains the hair follicles, sebaceous glands and sweat glands. **Melanin** is the pigment that is responsible for skin color.

The main function of the skin is the protection of the body from the outside environment. The skin regulates body temperature, using the insulation provided by body fat and the secretion of **sweat**, which acts as a coolant for the body. **Sebum** lubricates and protects the hair and the skin, and melanin absorbs harmful ultraviolet radiation. Special cells that lie on the surface of the skin also provide a barrier to bacterial infection. Nerves in the skin are responsible for sensations of pain, pressure, and temperature. In addition, the synthesis of Vitamin D, which is essential for the absorption of calcium from ingested food, begins in the skin.

Vernix caseosa is a thick, protein-based substance that protects the skin of the fetus against infection and irritation from the amniotic fluid from the third trimester until it dissipates after birth. Several childhood illnesses, such as measles and chicken pox, are associated with specific skin alterations. Acne related to hormonal changes is common in adolescents, and the effects of sunburn are observed across the life span. In the elderly, some of the protections provided by the skin become less effective; decreases in body fat and altered sweat production affect cold tolerance, loss of collagen support results in wrinkling of the skin, and decreased sebum secretions lead to changes in hair growth and skin moisture content.

Musculoskeletal

The **musculoskeletal system** consists of the bones, muscles, tendons, ligaments, and connective tissues that function together, providing support and motion of the body. The layers of bone include the hard exterior compact bone, the spongy bone that contains nerves and blood vessels, and the central bone marrow. The outer compact layer is covered by the strong **periosteum membrane**, which provides additional strength and protection for the bone. **Skeletal muscles** are voluntary muscles that are capable of contracting in response to nervous stimulation. Muscles are connected to bones by **tendons**, which are composed of tough connective tissue. Additional connective tissues called **ligaments** connect one bone to another at various joints.

In addition to providing support and protection, the bones are important for calcium storage and the production of blood cells. Skeletal muscles allow movement by pulling on the bones, while **joints** make different body movements possible.

The two most significant periods of bone growth are during fetal life and at puberty. However, until old age, bone is continually being remodeled. Specialized cells called osteoclasts break down the old bone, and osteoblasts generate new bone. In the elderly, bone remodeling is less effective, resulting in the loss of bone mass, and the incidence of osteoporosis increases. These changes can result in bone fractures, often from falling, that do not heal effectively. Muscle development follows a similar pattern with a progressive increase in muscle mass from infancy to adulthood, as well as a decline in muscle mass and physical strength in the elderly.

Nervous

The two parts of the nervous system are the **central nervous system**, which contains the brain and spinal cord, and the **peripheral nervous system**, which includes the ganglia and nerves. The cerebrospinal fluid and the bones of the cranium and the spine protect the brain and spinal cord. The nerves transmit impulses from one another to accomplish voluntary and involuntary processes. The nerves are surrounded by a specialized **myelin sheath** that insulates the nerves and facilitates the transmission of impulses.

The nervous system receives information from the body, interprets that information, and directs all motor activity for the body. This means the nervous system coordinates all the activities of the body.

The fetal brain and spinal cord are clearly visible within six weeks after conception. After the child is born, the nervous system continues to mature as the child gains motor control and learns about the environment. In the well-elderly, brain function remains stable until the age of eighty, when the processing of information and short-term memory may slow.

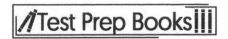

Cardiovascular, Hematopoietic, and Lymphatic

The **cardiovascular system** includes the heart, the blood vessels, and the blood. The heart is a muscle that has four "**chambers**," or sections. The three types of blood vessels are: the **arteries**, which have a smooth muscle layer and are controlled by the nervous system; the **veins**, which are thinner than arteries and have valves to facilitate the return of the blood to the heart; and the **capillaries**, which are often only one-cell thick. Blood is red in color because the red blood cells (RBCs) that carry oxygen contain hemoglobin, which is a red pigment.

The deoxygenated blood from the body enters the heart and is transported to the lungs to allow the exchange of waste products for oxygen. The oxygenated blood then returns to the heart, which pumps the blood to the rest of body. The arteries carry oxygenated blood from the heart to the body; the veins return the deoxygenated blood to the heart, while the actual exchange of oxygen and waste products takes place in the capillaries.

The fetal cardiac system must undergo dramatic changes at birth as the infant's lungs function for the first time. Cardiovascular function remains stable until middle age, when genetic influences and lifestyle choices may affect the cardiovascular system. Most elderly people have at least some indication of decreasing efficiency of the system.

The **hematopoietic system**, a division of the **lymphatic system**, is responsible for blood-cell production. The cells are produced in the bone marrow, which is soft connective tissue in the center of large bones that have a rich blood supply. The two types of bone marrow are red bone marrow and yellow bone marrow.

The **red bone marrow** contains the stem cells, which can transform into specific blood cells as needed by the body. The **yellow bone marrow** is less active and is composed of fat cells; however, if needed, the yellow marrow can function as the red marrow to produce the blood cells.

The red bone marrow predominates from birth until adolescence. From that point on, the amount of red marrow decreases, and the amount of yellow marrow increases. This means that the elderly are at risk for conditions related to decreased blood-cell replenishment.

The **lymphatic system** includes the spleen, thymus, tonsils, lymph nodes, lymphatic vessels, and the lymph. The **spleen** is located below the diaphragm and to the rear of the stomach. The **thymus** consists of specialized lymphatic tissue and lies in the mediastinum behind the sternum. The **tonsils** are globules of lymphoid tissue located in the oropharynx. The **lymphatic vessels** are very small and contain valves to prevent backflow in the system vessels. The vessels that lie in close proximity to the capillaries circulate the lymph. **Lymph** is composed of infectious substances and cellular waste products in addition to hormones and oxygen.

The main function of the lymphatic system is protection against infection. The system also conserves body fluids and proteins and absorbs vitamins from the digestive system.

The spleen filters the blood in order to remove toxic agents and is also a reservoir for blood that can be released into systemic circulation as needed. The thymus is the site of the development and regulation of white blood cells (WBCs). The **tonsils** trap and destroy infectious agents as they enter the body through the mouth. The lymphatic vessels circulate the lymph, and the lymph carries toxins and cellular waste products from the cell to the heart for filtration.

There is rapid growth of the thymus gland from birth to ten years. The action of the entire system declines from adulthood to old age, which means that the elderly are less able to respond to infection.

Respiratory

The **respiratory system** consists of the airway, lungs, and respiratory muscles. The airway is composed of the pharynx, larynx, trachea, bronchi, and bronchioles. The lungs contain air-filled sacs called **alveoli**, and they are covered by a visceral layer of double-layered pleural membrane. The **intercostal muscles** are located between the ribs, and the **diaphragm**—the largest muscle of the body—separates the thoracic cavity from the abdominal cavity.

On **inspiration**, the airway transports the outside air to the lungs, while the **expired air** carries the carbon dioxide that is removed by the lungs. The alveoli are the site of the exchange of carbon dioxide from the systemic circulation with the oxygen contained in the inspired air. The muscles help the thoracic cavity to expand and contract to allow for air exchange.

The respiratory rate in the infant gradually decreases from a normal of thirty to forty breaths per minute, until adolescence when it equals the normal adult rate of twelve to twenty breaths per minute. Pulmonary function declines after the age of sixty because the alveoli become larger and less efficient, and the respiratory muscles weaken.

Digestive

The **digestive system** includes the mouth, pharynx, esophagus, stomach, small intestine, large intestine, and sigmoid colon. The entire system forms a twenty-four-foot tube through which ingested food passes. Digestion begins in the mouth, where digestive enzymes are secreted in response to food intake. Food then passes through the **esophagus** to the **stomach**, which is a pouch-shaped organ that collects and holds food for a period of time. The **small intestine** begins at the distal end of the stomach. The lining of the small intestine contains many **villi,** which are small, hair-like projections that increase the absorption of nutrients from the ingested food. The **large intestine** originates at the distal end of the small intestine and terminates in the rectum. The large intestine is four feet long and has three segments, including the **ascending colon** along the right side, the **transverse colon** from right to left across the body, and the **descending colon** down the left side of the body, where the sigmoid colon begins.

The enzymes of the mouth, stomach, and the proximal end of the small intestine break down the ingested food into nutrients that can be absorbed and used by the body. The nutrients are absorbed by the small intestine. The large intestine removes the water from the waste products, which forms the stool. The muscle layer of the large intestine is responsible for **peristalsis**, which is the force that moves the waste products through the intestine.

The function of the digestive system declines more slowly than other body systems, and the changes that most often occur are the result of lifestyle issues or medication use.

Urinary

The **urinary system** includes the kidneys, ureters, bladder, and urethra. The **kidneys** are a pair of bean-shaped organs that lie just below and posterior to the liver in the peritoneal cavity. The **nephron** is the functional unit of the kidney, and there are about 1 million nephrons in each of the two kidneys. The **ureters** are hollow tubes that allow the urine formed in the kidneys to pass into the bladder. The urinary **bladder** is a hollow mucous lined pouch with the **ureters** entering the upper portion, and the **urethra**

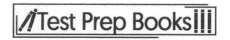

exiting from the bottom portion. The urethra is a tubular structure lined with mucous membrane that connects the bladder with the outside of the body.

In addition to the formation and excretion of the waste product urine, the nephron of the kidney also regulates fluid and electrolyte balance and contributes to the control of blood pressure. The ureters allow the urine to pass from the kidneys to the bladder. The bladder stores the urine and regulates the process of urination. The urethra delivers the urine from the bladder to the outside of the body.

The lifespan changes in the urinary system are more often the result of the effects of chronic disease on the system, rather than normal decline.

Reproductive

The major organs of the female reproductive organs include the uterus, cervix, vagina, ovaries, and fallopian tubes.

The **uterus** is a hollow, pear-shaped organ with a muscular layer that is positioned between the bladder and the rectum. The uterus terminates at the **cervix**, which opens into the **vagina**, which is open to the outside of the body. The **ovaries**, supported by several ligaments, are oval organs 1- to 2-inches long that are positioned on either side of the uterus in the pelvic cavity. The **fallopian tubes**, which are 4 inches long and .5 inches in diameter, connect the uterus with the ovaries.

The male reproductive organs include the penis, scrotum, testicles, vas deferens, seminal vesicles, and the prostate gland. In addition to the urethra, the **penis** contains three sections of erectile tissue. The **scrotum** is a fibromuscular pouch that contains the testes, the spermatic cord, and the epididymis. The pair of **testes** is suspended in the scrotum and each one is approximately 2 inches by 1 inch long. The **vas deferens** is a tubular pathway between the testes and the penis, and the **seminal vesicles** are small organs located between the bladder and the bowel. The **prostate gland** surrounds the proximal end of the urethra within the pelvic cavity.

The main function of the male reproductive system is the production of sperm. Unlike the female, beginning at puberty, several million immature sperm are produced every day in the testes. The sperm are transported through the vas deferens to the penis, and the prostate gland and seminal vesicles contribute fluids that support the activity of the sperm after ejaculation.

At puberty, egg maturation, menses, and sperm production begin, and the secondary sex characteristics appear. Female fertility declines at thirty years of age, and the maturation of eggs in the ovaries ceases at **menopause**, which occurs at fifty years of age. Sperm production continues from puberty until death; however, after sixty years of age the ability of the sperm to travel to the fallopian tube to fertilize an egg is decreased.

Endocrine

The glands of the **endocrine system** include the pituitary, thyroid, parathyroid, adrenal, and reproductive glands, as well as the hypothalamus, the pancreas, and the pineal body. The function of the system is to synthesize and secrete hormones that control body growth, sexual function, and metabolism, which is the production and use of energy by the body. The **thyroid** gland, located on either side of the trachea, regulates energy production, or the rate at which the body uses ingested food to support body functions. The **parathyroid,** located on the upper margin of the thyroid gland, regulates calcium levels by the activation of Vitamin D, which increases intestinal absorption of calcium, and by regulating the amount of calcium that is stored in the bones or excreted by the kidneys. The **adrenal** glands, located on the upper margin of the kidneys, consist of the adrenal cortex and the adrenal medulla. The hormones secreted by the adrenal cortex are necessary for life and include: **cortisol,** or **hydrocortisone**, which regulates the breakdown of proteins, carbohydrates, and fats for energy production and the body's response to stress; **corticosterone**, which works with cortisol to regulate the immune system; and **aldosterone**, which contributes to blood-pressure control. The **adrenal medulla** secretions, including **adrenaline**, regulate the body's reaction to stress known as the **fight-or-flight response**. The ovaries secrete **estrogen** and the testes secrete **testosterone**, which regulate sexual maturation and function. The **pancreas**, located in the right upper quadrant of the abdomen, secretes the **insulin** that regulates blood sugar, in addition to other hormones that regulate water absorption and secretion in the intestines. The **pineal gland**, located in the center of the brain, secretes melatonin, which regulates the circadian rhythm or sleep cycle.

The nervous system connects each of these glands to the hypothalamus and the pituitary gland. The **hypothalamus** senses alterations in hormone secretions in all of these organs and conveys those messages to the **pituitary gland**, which then stimulates each specific organ to either increase or decrease secretion of the relevant hormone. This feedback system is necessary for **homeostasis**.

Sensory

The **sensory organs** include the eyes, ears, nose, tongue, and skin, and they contain special receptor cells that transmit information to the nervous system. The eyes receive and process light energy. The ears process sound waves and also contribute to the maintenance of equilibrium. The nose senses odors and the tongue senses taste. The skin responds to tactile stimulation, including pain, hot, cold, and touch. Internal organs also sense pain and pressure. The brain is responsible for processing all of these sensations.

The senses of touch and smell are active in the fetus and continue to mature after birth. Touch is especially important for infants. The elderly experience a decline in the acuity of all of the senses; however, eyesight and hearing are most commonly affected due to the effects of chronic diseases such as hypertension and diabetes.

Respiratory Problems

Some patients experiencing respiratory issues may receive supplemental oxygen. Oxygen can be administered in several different ways. The most common and minimal administration technique is via nasal cannula. The oxygen will flow through the nasal cannula into the patient's nose, and the tubing will be connected into either a mobile oxygen tank or an oxygen supply on the wall of the patient's room. Depending on the facility, there will often be a respiratory therapy team in charge of caring for patients' respiratory issues.

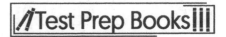

The picture demonstrates oxygen being administered via **nasal cannula**. The two prongs are placed into the nostrils of the patient.

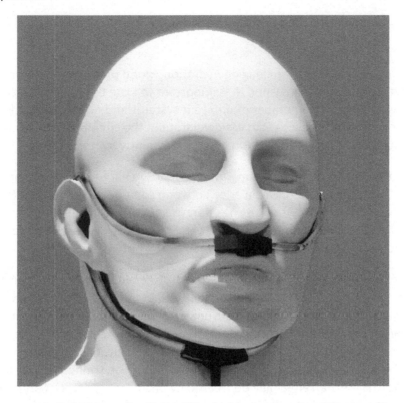

Part of the nurse's normal vital signs collection will include oxygen saturation readings. This is especially important in patients receiving supplemental oxygen and/or with identified respiratory issues. Normal values are generally considered to be 93 to 100 percent, but some patients with COPD may have a baseline saturation in the high 80s.

It is important that the aide understand the flow rate of supplemental oxygen that the patient is receiving. A typical rate is 2 to 4 liters per minute (LPM). The nurse should look for signs of **hypoxia**—a lack of oxygen in the body. These include decreased level of consciousness, shortness of breath, bluish lips or blueness of the extremities/nail beds (**cyanosis**), or unresponsiveness. Any change in respiratory status or suspected issues with oxygen administration should be reported to the nurse or respiratory therapist immediately.

Finally, the nurse must be familiar with IV (intravenous) accesses. IVs are used to administer medicine and fluids. Signs that an IV access is compromised are redness around the site, patient discomfort, bruising, and leakage. Any changes in IV access, IV pump alarms, and patient complaints should be reported to the nurse immediately.

Fluid and Electrolyte Imbalances

Electrolytes are minerals that, when dissolved, break down into ions. They can be acids, bases, or salts. In the body, different electrolytes are responsible for specific cellular functions. These functions make up larger, critical system-wide processes, such as hydration, homeostasis, pH balance, and muscle contraction. Electrolytes typically enter the body through food and drink consumption, but in severe cases of imbalance, they may be medically-administered. They are found in the fluids of the body, such as blood.

Key electrolytes found in the body include the following:

Sodium and Chloride

Sodium (Na+) is mainly responsible for managing hydration, blood pressure, and blood volume in the body. It is found in blood, plasma, and lymph. It is important to note that sodium is primarily found outside of cells and is accessed by a number of different systems and organs to tightly regulate water and blood levels. For example, in cases of severe dehydration, the circulatory and endocrine systems will transmit signals to the kidneys to retain sodium and, consequently, water.

Sodium also affects muscle and nerve function. It is a positively-charged ion and contributes to **membrane potential**—an electrochemical balance between sodium and potassium (another electrolyte) that is responsible for up to 40 percent of resting energy expenditure in a healthy adult. This balance strongly influences the functioning of nerve impulses and the ability of muscles to contract. Healthy heart functioning and contraction is dependent on membrane potential.

Sodium is available in large quantities in the standard diets of developed countries, especially in processed foods, as it is found in table salt. Consequently, sodium deficiencies (**hyponatremia**) are possible, but rare, in the average person. Hyponatremia can result in endocrine or nervous system disorders where sodium regulation is affected. It can also result in excessive sweating, vomiting, or diarrhea, such as in endurance sporting events, improper use of diuretics, or gastrointestinal illness. Hyponatremia may be treated with an IV sodium solution. Too much sodium (**hypernatremia**) is usually a result of dehydration. Hypernatremia may be treated by introducing water quantities appropriate for suspending the sodium level that is tested in the patient's blood and urine.

Chloride (Cl-) is a negatively-charged ion found outside of the cells that works closely with sodium. It shares many of the same physiologic responsibilities as sodium. Any imbalances (hypochloremia and hyperchloremia) are rare but may affect overall pH levels of the body. Chloride imbalances usually occur in response to an imbalance in other electrolytes, so treating a chloride imbalance directly is uncommon.

Potassium

Potassium (K+) is mainly responsible for regulating muscular function and is especially important in cardiac and digestive functions. In women, it is believed to promote bone density. It works in tandem with sodium to create membrane potential. Potassium is a positively-charged ion and is usually found inside cells. It plays a role in maintaining homeostasis between the intracellular and extracellular environments.

Potassium is found in all animal protein and animal dairy products and in most fruits and vegetables. Low potassium levels (hypokalemia) may be caused by dehydration due to excessive vomiting, urination, or diarrhea. In severe or acute cases, hypokalemia may be a result of renal dysfunction and may cause lethargy, muscle cramps, or heart dysrhythmia. It may be treated by stopping the cause of potassium loss (e.g., diuretics), followed by oral or IV potassium replenishment.

High potassium levels (hyperkalemia) can quickly become fatal. Hyperkalemia is often the result of a serious condition, such as sudden kidney or adrenal failure, and may cause nausea, vomiting, chest pain, and muscle dysfunction. It is treated based on its severity, with treatment options ranging from diuretic

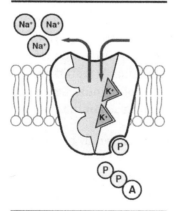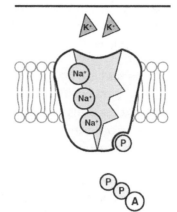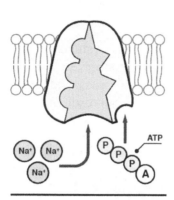

use to IV insulin or glucose. IV calcium may be administered if potentially dangerous heart arrhythmias are present.

1.

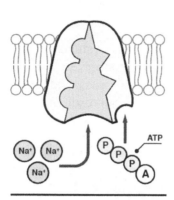

The sodium-potassium pump binds three sodium ions and a molecule of ATP.

2.

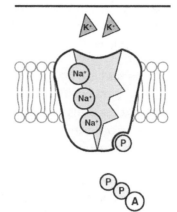

The splitting of ATP provides energy to change the shape of the channel. The sodium ions are driven through the channel.

3.

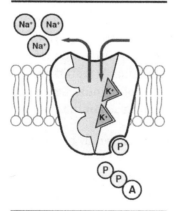

The sodium ions are released to the outside of the membrane, and the new shape of the channel allows two potassium ions to bind

4.

Release of the phosphate allows the channel to revert to its original form, releasing the potassium ions on the inside of the membrane

Calcium and Phosphorus

Calcium (Ca++) is plentiful in the body, with most calcium stored throughout the skeletal system. However, if there is not enough calcium in the blood (usually available through proper diet), the body will take calcium from the bones. This can become detrimental over time. If enough calcium becomes present in the blood, the body will return extra calcium stores to the bones. Besides contributing to the skeletal structure, this electrolyte is important in nerve signaling, muscle function, and blood coagulation. It is found in dairy products, leafy greens, and fatty fishes. Many other consumables, such as fruit juices and cereals, are often fortified with calcium.

Low calcium levels (**hypocalcemia**) can be caused by poor diet, thyroid or kidney disorders, and some medications. Symptoms can include lethargy, poor memory, inability to concentrate, muscle cramps, and general stiffness and achiness in the body. Supplementation can rapidly restore blood calcium levels. In cases where symptoms are present, IV calcium administration in conjunction with an oral or IV vitamin D supplement may be utilized.

High calcium levels (**hypercalcemia**) is usually caused by thyroid dysfunction but can also be the result of diet, limited mobility (such as in paralyzed individuals), some cancers, or the use of some diuretics. Symptoms can include thirst, excess urination, gastrointestinal issues, and unexplained pain in the abdominal area or bones. Severe or untreated hypercalcemia can result in kidney stones, kidney failure, confusion, depression, lethargy, irregular heartbeat, or bone problems.

There is an intricate balance between calcium levels and the levels of phosphorus, another electrolyte. Phosphorus, like calcium, is stored in the bones and found in many of the same foods as calcium. These electrolytes work together to maintain bone integrity. When too much calcium exists in the blood, the bones release more phosphorus to balance the two levels. When there is too much phosphorus in the blood, the bones release calcium. Therefore, the presence or absence of one directly impacts the presence or absence of the other. Indicators of hypocalcemia and hypercalcemia usually also indicate low levels of phosphorus (**hypophosphatemia**) and high levels of phosphorus (**hyperphosphatemia**), respectively.

Magnesium

Magnesium (Mg^{++}) is another electrolyte that is usually plentiful in the body. It is responsible for an array of life-sustaining functions, including hundreds of biochemical reactions such as oxidative phosphorylation and glycolysis. It is also an important factor in DNA and RNA synthesis, bone development, nerve signaling, and muscle function. Magnesium is stored inside cells or within the structure of the bones. It can be consumed through leafy greens, nuts, seeds, beans, unrefined grains, and most foods that contain fiber. Some water sources may also contain high levels of magnesium.

Low levels of magnesium (**hypomagnesemia**) are primarily caused by chronic alcohol or drug abuse and some prescription medications and can also occur in patients with gastrointestinal diseases (such as celiac or Crohn's). Symptoms of hypomagnesemia include nausea, vomiting, depression, personality and mood disorders, and muscle dysfunction. Chronically depleted patients may have an increased risk of cardiovascular and metabolic disorders.

High levels of magnesium (**hypermagnesemia**) are rare and usually result in conjunction with kidney disorders when medications are used improperly. Symptoms include low blood pressure that may result in heart failure. Hypermagnesemia is usually treated by removing any magnesium sources (such as salts or laxatives) and may also require the IV administration of calcium gluconate.

Magnesium imbalance can lead to calcium or potassium imbalance over time, as these electrolytes work together to achieve homeostasis in the body.

Hydration is critical to fluid presence in the body, as water is a critical component of blood, plasma, and lymph. When fluid levels are too high or too low, electrolytes cannot move freely or carry out their intended functions. Therefore, treating an electrolyte imbalance almost always involves managing a

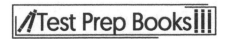

fluid imbalance as well. Typically, as fluid levels rise, electrolyte levels decrease. As fluid levels decrease, electrolyte levels rise. Common tests to determine electrolyte fluid imbalances include basic and comprehensive metabolic panels, which test levels of sodium, potassium, chloride, and any other electrolyte in question.

Hemodynamics

A crucial part of patient assessment and monitoring is their hemodynamic profile. **Hemodynamics** are the forces that cause blood to circulate throughout the body, originating in the heart, branching out to the vital organs and tissues, and then recirculating back to the heart and lungs for reoxygenation and pumping. There are at least three different aspects of hemodynamics that can be focused on: the measurement of pressure, flow, and oxygenation of the blood in the cardiovascular system; the use of invasive technological tools to measure and quantitate pressures, volumes, and capacity of the vascular system; and the monitoring of hemodynamics that involves measuring and interpreting the biological systems that are affected by it.

Hemodynamics can be assessed using noninvasive or invasive measures. Noninvasive measures would include the nurse's assessment of the patient's overall presentation, heart rate, and blood pressure. Invasive measurements would include inserting an arterial blood pressure monitor directly into an artery or the insertion of a Swan-Ganz catheter. The **Swan-Ganz catheter**, also known as **a pulmonary artery catheter (PAC)** or **right-heart catheter**, is threaded into the patient's subclavian vein, down the superior vena cava, right up to the PA. This type of catheter is used quite commonly in ICU patients. PACs give information about the patient's cardiac output and preload. **Preload** is obtained by estimating the **pulmonary artery occlusion pressure (PAOP)**. Another way to assess preload is determining the **right ventricular end-diastolic volume (RVEDV)**, measured by fast-response thermistors reading the heart rate. There is some question as to whether the use of PACs helps patients or not. Some studies suggest that the use of PACs does not reduce morbidity or mortality but rather increases these occurrences. Their use, therefore, should be weighed carefully according to the physician's discretion.

There are many different parameters to consider when assessing a patient's hemodynamics. Blood pressure is the measurement of the systolic pressure over the diastolic pressure, or the pressure in the vasculature when the heart contracts over the pressure when the heart is at rest.

Mean arterial pressure (MAP) shows the relationship between the amount of blood pumped out of the heart and the resistance the vascular system puts up against it. A low MAP suggests that blood flow has decreased to the organs, while a high MAP may indicate that the workload for the heart is increased.

Cardiac index reflects the quantity of blood pumped by the heart per minute and per meter squared of the patient's body surface area.

Cardiac output measures how much blood the heart pumps out per beat and is measured in liters.

Central venous pressure (CVP) is an estimate of the RVEDP, thus assessing RV function as well as the patient's general hydration status. A low CVP may mean the patient is dehydrated or has a decreased amount of venous return. A high CVP may indicate fluid overload or right-sided heart failure.

Pulmonary artery pressure measures the pressure in the PA. An increase in this pressure may mean the patient has developed a left-to-right cardiac shunt, they have hypertension of the PA, they may have worsening complications of COPD, a clot has traveled to the lungs (pulmonary embolus), the lungs are filling with fluid (pulmonary edema), or the left ventricle is failing.

The **pulmonary capillary wedge pressure (PCWP)** approximates the **left ventricular end-diastolic pressure (LVEDP).** This number, when increased, may be a result of LV failure, a pathology of the mitral valve, cardiac sufficiency, or compression of the heart after a hemorrhage, such as cardiac tamponade.

The resistance that the pulmonary capillary bed in the lungs puts up against blood flow is measured via pulmonary vascular resistance (PVR). When there is disease in the lungs, a pulmonary embolism, hypoxia, or pulmonary vasculitis, this number may increase. Calcium channel blockers and certain other medications may cause the PVR to be lowered because of their mechanism of action.

A **hemodynamic measurement** used to assess RV function and the patient's fluid status is the RV pressure. When this number is elevated, the patient may have pulmonary hypertension, failure of the right ventricle, or worsening congestive heart failure.

The **stroke index** measures how much blood the heart is pumping in a cardiac cycle in relation to the patient's body surface area.

Stroke volume (SV) measures how much blood the heart pumps in milliliters per beat.

The **systemic vascular resistance parameter** reflects how much pressure the vasculature peripheral to the heart puts up to blood flow from the heart. Vasoconstrictors, low blood volume, and septic shock can cause this number to rise, while vasodilators, high blood levels of carbon dioxide (hypercarbia), nitrates, and morphine may cause this number to fall.

The following is a list of commonly measured hemodynamic parameters and their normal values:

- Blood pressure: 90–140 mmHg systolic over 60–90 mmHg diastolic
- Mean arterial pressure (MAP): 70–100 mmHg
- Cardiac index (CI): 2.5–4.0 L/min/m^2
- Cardiac output (CO): 4–8 L/min
- Central venous pressure (CVP) or right arterial pressure (RA): 2–6 mmHg
- Pulmonary artery pressure (PA): systolic 20–30 mmHg (PAS), diastolic 8–12 mmHg (PAD), mean 25 mmHg (PAM)
- Pulmonary capillary wedge pressure (PCWP): 4–12 mmHg
- Pulmonary vascular resistance (PVR): 37–250 dynes/sec/cm^5
- Right ventricular pressure (RV): systolic 20–30 mmHg over diastolic 0–5 mmHg
- Stroke index (SI): 25–45 mL/m^2
- Stroke volume (SV): 50–100 mL/beat
- Systemic vascular resistance (SVR): 800–1200 dynes/sec/cm^5

Illness Management

There are certain client situations that indicate a worsening of their illness. The nurse needs to be prepared to identify this worsening and report it immediately to the attending practitioner. A solid knowledge of disease processes must be applied when managing patients' illnesses. The nurse must also be able to educate the patient regarding their condition and the management thereof. Certain interventional skills such as gastric lavage may be required for management of the patient's illness.

Any patient condition that involves a sudden compromise of airway, breathing, or circulation must be reported immediately. Swift intervention is needed to prevent long-term damage or fatality. Airway,

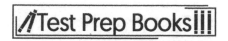

breathing, and circulation are referred to as the patient's **"ABCs"** for short, and their management is at the top of the nurse's assessment checklist.

In addition to addressing the patient's ABCs, the nurse will also prioritize their care based off Maslow's hierarchy of needs. The nurse will recall that, according to this hierarchy, the patient must have physiological needs, such as hunger and thirst, met before higher priorities such as safety, esteem, and self-actualization may be met.

Determining the type of illness is key to creating a strategy to manage it. The client may suffer from chronic diseases such as heart failure, COPD, or diabetes. They may be engaged in a battle with mental illnesses such as anxiety, depression, and bipolar disorder. Depending on the client's unique profile, the nurse will identify their needs and determine a care plan that will assist them in managing their illness effectively.

A change in the client's baseline functioning status is any symptom, blood test, or behavior that trends significantly different from their normal. Some clients have abnormalities as their normal, such as a low blood pressure, low pulse oxygenation, heart dysrhythmia such as prolonged QT segment, or a "normal" level of confusion in dementia patients. The nurse goes off their initial assessments of the patient as well as the patient's medical record and family reports to determine if a notable change is taking place and needs reporting.

The nurse closely monitors the patient's response to interventions that are intended to be therapeutic. The patient may have an unexpected and unwanted response to medications and other therapies. Side effects, adverse reactions, and allergic responses all fall into this category of unwanted response to a pharmacological therapy. A patient receiving mechanical ventilation via an endotracheal tube may become agitated and aggressive, as this type of therapy can be highly irritating. The nurse sees this unwanted response and uses tools such as sedation, within the ordered parameters, to soothe the patient and return them to the therapeutic response.

Using their knowledge of pathophysiology, the nurse works to effectively manage the client's care and prevent complications. Using the example of the patient with diabetes, the nurse knows that tight management of blood glucose is a high priority. The nurse knows that these patients, depending on the cause of their diabetes, have a tough time using the body's insulin to regulate glucose in the bloodstream. The nurse monitors the client's intake at mealtimes, measures blood glucose regularly, administers diabetic medications in a timely manner so they will have maximal effectiveness, and keeps a close eye on the patient when they must be NPO or off the floor for procedures, as these are prime occasions for the patient to have a hypoglycemic event.

The nurse must manage not only one client's illness but often is working to manage an entire caseload of clients all at the same time, depending on what type of unit they are working in. Caseloads of patients require exceptional time management and organizational skills from the nurse. The nurse must be able to prioritize client needs effectively to meet them in a timely manner.

Client education performed by the nurse is a way the nurse may enable the patient to become independent in their own illness management. The patient can then feel more comfortable making informed decisions and speaking up about their care. The nurse answers the client's questions, addresses their concerns, and informs them about therapies and medications. Part of this patient education is assessing what specific education the patient needs. Some clients are very much informed about their condition and treatment modalities, while others may be health-care illiterate, meaning they do not know very much about their condition or their options in managing it. Based on the nurse's assessment of the client's educational needs, the nurse will formulate their educational plan.

There are certain cases of client illness in which the nurse will need to perform gastric lavage. *Lavage* means a cleaning or rinsing out, while *gastric* refers to the stomach. The patient will be placed in high Fowler's position while an NG tube is inserted. This tube is carefully measured from the nose of the client to their earlobe and then to the tip of the xiphoid process. This point is then marked on a piece of tape. Water-soluble gel is applied to the tip of the tube before insertion for lubrication. The client will be instructed to look upward to create a hyperextension of the neck. The tube is advanced into the nares until resistance is met at the nasopharynx. The nurse expects that the client's gag reflex will kick in as well as watering of the eyes. The client will take small sips of water to open the epiglottis at which point the nurse will then be able to advance the tube all the way down to the stomach. Placement is assessed via pH test of aspirated gastric contents from the tube and/or obtainment of chest x-ray. The nurse will secure the NG tube using tape to the client's nose and a safety pin to the client's gown. After correct placement is confirmed, the nurse may use the tube to lavage the client's stomach. This will be done according to the ordering gastroenterologist's preferred method but usually includes the instilment of a solution, clamping of the tube for a determined amount of time, and then removal of the fluid later.

Medical Emergencies

In the event of a medical emergency, there are specific steps to take depending on the situation. There will be written policies for these types of emergencies in the workplace that are used for patients, staff, and/or visitors.

Below are some examples of medical emergencies:

- Choking
- Unresponsive or unconscious person or patient
- Excessive bleeding
- Head injury
- Broken bones
- Severe burns
- Seizures
- Chest pain
- Difficulty breathing
- Allergic reactions that cause swelling and/or breathing difficulties
- Inhalation or swallowing of a toxic substance
- Accidental poisoning

Choking

If someone is choking, the victim will most likely grab at their throat, or they may have a cough that eventually stops, indicating blockage of the airway. If the airway is blocked, they will need the Heimlich maneuver to be performed immediately. Oftentimes people cough and may leave the room to get a drink or to avoid disrupting others. It is best to follow that person to ensure they are not choking.

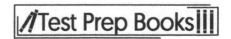

When someone is choking and conscious, the responder, or person at the scene who witnesses and intervenes, should:

- Ask the victim if they are choking and tell them help is here.
- Assist the victim to a standing position.
- Stand behind the victim and wrap the arms around the victim's waist.
- With the hands just above the victim's belly button, place the hand in a fist with the thumb against the victim's stomach.
- Place the other hand on top of the fisted hand.
- Thrust quick, hard, and upward on the victim's stomach.
- Continue this until the food or object comes out of the victim's mouth.
- Do *not* swipe the victim's mouth with one finger, as this could push the blockage further down the airway.

If the victim is still choking and goes unconscious:

- Lower the victim to the floor, shout for help, and have someone call 911.
- Begin cardiopulmonary resuscitation (CPR) by following the basic life support steps until emergency medical services (EMS) arrives.

Unconsciousness or Unresponsiveness

First, try to arouse the person by shaking or tapping them. If they are indeed unresponsive, call for help, have someone call 911, and proceed to:

- Make sure the patient is lying flat and place a backboard under them for CPR.
- Follow basic life support (BLS) protocol.
- Look and listen for breathing (chest rise).
- Check for a pulse in radial artery (wrist).
- If patient is breathing, stay with them until EMS arrives. If there is a pulse but no breathing, begin rescue breaths. Give one breath every five or six seconds. Check pulse every two minutes.
- If no pulse, begin CPR and continue until EMS arrives.
- Direct someone else to get the **automated external defibrillator (AED)** as CPR is continued.
- CPR: Thirty chest compressions then two breaths, repeat for two-minute cycles.
- Chest compressions should be firm and deep, to the rhythm of the disco song "Stayin' Alive," about one hundred beats per minute. This ensures adequate perfusion of organs with blood since the heart is not pumping on its own.
- When the AED arrives, turn it on and follow the prompts for use.

If the patient recovers, turn them onto their left side and continue to monitor them until EMS arrive. Healthcare workers will be trained and certified on BLS, CPR, and AED use.

Excessive Bleeding

Call for help and call 911. Then:

- Have the patient sit down or lie down.
- Use a towel or shirt to hold continuous pressure on the bleeding area.

- Elevate the area above their heart. For example, if the leg is bleeding, have the patient lie down and put their leg on a chair.
- Talk to the patient and monitor their responsiveness. Stay with them until EMS arrives.

Head Injury

Concussions, contusions, and skull fractures are all common types of traumatic brain injuries. **Concussions** occur when the brain is jarred against the skull, usually during sports, hard contact with another person, or hitting the head on the ground. Concussions can cause mental confusion and lead to disruptions in normal brain functioning. The effects of a concussion can show up immediately, or they may not show up for hours or days. Normally, concussions do not cause a loss of consciousness, so it is important to pay attention to other possible symptoms. Another type of traumatic brain injury is a contusion, which is a bruise on the brain. This bruise can swell in the brain and cause a hematoma, or bleeding in the brain. The following list includes symptoms of traumatic brain injuries:

- Confusion
- Depression
- Dizziness or balance problems
- Foggy feeling
- Double vision or changes in vision
- Tiredness
- Headache
- Memory loss
- Nausea
- Sensitivity to light
- Trouble remembering and concentrating

If a patient has a known head injury, or they stated that they hit their head, stay with the patient and call for a supervisor. Monitor the patient for mild symptoms from the list above. If the symptoms are not serious, the patient may require a visit from the physician. If the patient is elderly or has other serious health issues, hospitalization may be required to rule out more serious consequences from the head

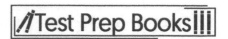

injury. The pie chart below depicts the leading causes of traumatic brain injury, with falls being the largest percentage.

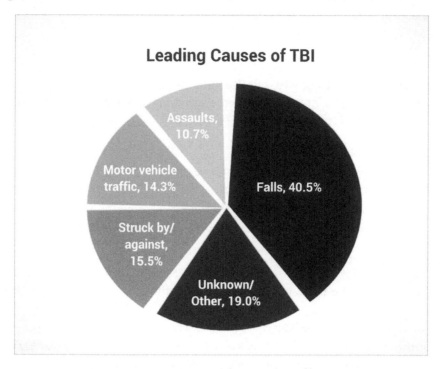

Symptoms of a head injury that are more serious and require immediate emergency treatment include:

- Unequal pupils
- Convulsions
- Fracture of the skull or face
- Inability to move legs or arms
- Clear or bloody fluid coming from the ears, nose, or mouth
- Loss of consciousness
- Persistent vomiting
- Severe headache
- Slurred speech and distorted vision
- Restlessness and irritability

If any of the above symptoms appear after a head injury, call for help and call 911.

Broken Bones (Compound Fractures)

A **compound fracture** is a fracture in which the bone is protruding through the skin. Other symptoms include pain, swelling, deformity in the fractured area, and bruising. This is the most serious type of fracture and requires immediate attention. The following comprises first aid for fractures:

- Call for help and call 911, especially if a fracture in the head, back or neck is suspected.
- Don't move the patient unless they are in danger of further injury.
- Keep the injured area still and stay with the patient.
- Treat any bleeding by holding pressure with a towel or gauze.

- Look for signs of shock in the patient (shallow, fast breathing, or feeling faint) and lay them down with their feet elevated.
- Wrap ice packs in a towel and ice the injured area.
- Wait for EMS to arrive.

Burns

Burn injuries can range from mild to severe, but the initial treatment for all burns is the same. **First-degree burns** affect the top layer of the skin, **second-degree burns** affect two layers, and **third-degree burns** affect all three layers. Call for an emergency response if:

- The burn is through all the skin layers.
- The person is a baby or elderly and the burn is severe.
- The hands, feet, face, or genitals are burned.
- The burn is larger than two inches or is oozing.
- The burn is charred and leathery, or has white, brown, or black patches.

Initial treatment for all burns includes:

- Remove the source of the burn, put out the fire, smother the burning area, or have the person stop, drop, and roll.
- Remove any hot or burned clothing.
- Remove clothing that is tight and remove jewelry (burns can swell very quickly).
- Hold the burned area under cool, running water for twenty minutes.
- Use two cold cloths if running water is not available. Alternate holding them on the area every two minutes.
- Do not put ice on the burn.
- Keep the patient warm by covering the rest of the body.
- Wrap or cover the burn loosely with gauze, or a use a sheet for large areas.
- If EMS has been called, stay with the patient and keep them warm until help arrives.

Seizures

Seizures have many symptoms depending on the type of seizure. Some symptoms include jerking motions, shaking, unconsciousness, stiffness, and blank staring. If someone is having a violent seizure, the steps to follow include:

- Protect the victim's head by moving hard objects out of the way and placing a blanket under their head.
- Loosen clothing around their neck.
- Do not try to hold them down and do not try to put something in their mouth.
- Get help to control bystanders so that the victim has some space.
- When the seizure is over, have the victim lie on their side and make sure their airway is open.
- Call 911 if the seizure lasts more than five minutes, if the victim has other medical conditions, or if the person has never had a seizure before.
- People with known epilepsy may have seizures that are short and frequent, so calling 911 may not be necessary.

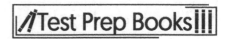

Chest Pain

Chest pain can be a symptom of a heart attack or other serious heart or lung condition. Prompt attention is necessary so that the person can be treated before serious heart damage or death occurs. Chest pain can also be a result of a lung infection, excessive coughing, broken ribs from an injury, anxiety, indigestion, or muscular injury. If the patient has not fallen or does not have any outward physical signs of injury to the chest area, assume that the chest pain is cardiac related. When someone complains of chest pain, do the following:

- Have the person sit down and ask where the pain is located.
- Call for the supervisor immediately.
- Assess if they have any injuries on or near their chest.
- Call 911 (if not in a medical facility) if the pain lasts more than a few minutes, or they have the following symptoms:
- Pain in the arms, shoulders, back and chest
- Difficulty breathing
- Fatigue
- Nausea
- Sweating
- Dizziness
- If there is oxygen available, a respiratory therapist or nurse will place a nasal cannula in their nose and give between two and four liters of oxygen.
- If available and the person is not allergic or taking any blood-thinner medication, the nurse will have the person chew a regular-strength aspirin. Aspirin helps the blood flow to the heart.
- Stay with the person until EMS arrives.
- If the person becomes unconscious, follow BLS guidelines and initiate CPR.

Difficulty Breathing

Breathing difficulties or shortness of breath can be caused by many factors, such as asthma, bronchitis, pneumonia, heart conditions, pulmonary embolism, anxiety, or exercise. People may occasionally have shortness of breath because of an underlying condition that is being monitored by a physician. They may take medication for this symptom and be able to continue to live relatively normal lives. However, if a person has sudden difficulty catching their breath, and it is not relieved with rest, change of position, or their inhaler medication, immediate attention is required. Do the following if a person begins to struggle with breathing:

- Call for help and have the person sit up in their chair or in their bed.

- Instruct the person to try to take slow breaths, inhaling though their nose and exhaling out of their mouth.

- Continue to talk to them reassuringly and soothingly. Anxiety can actually make breathing even more difficult.

- If their breathing becomes easier and they seem to calm down, have a physician see them as soon as possible, especially if this is something new for this person.

- If breathing continues to be difficult, call 911 (if not in medical facility).

- Place oxygen on the patient with a mask or nasal cannula, if available.

- Stay with the patient until help arrives and monitor their level of consciousness and breathing rate.

Allergic Reactions

Allergies can cause many symptoms from mild to severe. Some examples of mild symptoms might include itching, redness on the skin, hives, sneezing, runny nose, and itchy eyes. Wheezing may occur and may be treated with a prescribed inhaler. Life-threatening allergic reactions include swelling of the tongue or throat, difficulty breathing, and **anaphylaxis**, which is a systemic reaction. Anaphylaxis is rare but can lead to death if it is not recognized and treated quickly. Allergies to foods, medications, latex, and insect bites can cause anaphylaxis. Normally a person who has serious allergic reactions will have an **epinephrine pen**, or "epi-pen," with them at all times, to be administered in case of a reaction. If the following symptoms associated with anaphylaxis are observed outside of a medical facility, call 911. Otherwise, report any of the following symptoms to the nurse:

- Difficulty breathing
- Swollen tongue or throat tightness
- Wheezing
- Nausea and vomiting
- Fainting or dizziness
- Low blood pressure
- Rapid heart beat
- Feeling strange or sense of impending doom
- Chest pain

Call 911 even if an epi-pen has been administered for the allergic reaction. Reaction symptoms can continue to occur or can reoccur later.

Poisoning

Poison can be something eaten, inhaled, or absorbed in excess, or exposure to toxic substances. This type of emergency can happen to patients and employees. If there is an accidental poisoning and the person is awake and alert, call the poison-control hotline at 1-800-222-1222. Stay on the phone with poison control and stay with the victim. Try to have the following information available for the responders:

- Weight and age of the victim
- The label or bottle of the substance taken
- The time of exposure to the substance (how long it has been)
- The address of where the victim is located

If the person goes unconscious or is not breathing, call 911.

Many chemical labels, such as cleaning supplies, have warning labels and instructions for dealing with toxic exposure. The eyes may need to be flushed with water, for example. Read labels but also call for help. In healthcare facilities, protocols for chemical spills or exposure exist so that clean up and injury can be dealt with quickly. Always follow the policy provided by the facility or workplace.

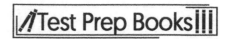

Pathophysiology

Pathophysiology refers to changes in the body due to a disease process. The patient's history of chronic and acute disease is discovered during the preoperative patient interview and chart review. Understanding the pathophysiology of the patient's disease process (or processes) empowers the nurse to know if assessment findings are congruent with the disease process or if findings are indicative of something else. For example, if a patient has 2+ pitting edema with a history of CHF, the nurse may suspect the edema is secondary to a CHF exacerbation and investigate further by auscultating lung sounds and consulting with a cardiologist. It is also important for the nurse to consider the pathophysiological processes associated with the patient's scheduled procedure. The nurse should note that although the scheduled procedure may be minor, the patient's diagnosis may be quite serious. If the patient is having a PowerPort insertion, the surgery process is minor. However, the patient may have a diagnosis of stage IV lung cancer, and this is quite serious. Understanding this, the nurse may allow more time for the patient to verbalize feelings and provide emotional support for the patient.

Unexpected Response to Therapies

There are a vast multitude of unexpected responses that may occur during a patient's therapy. With every desired effect, there are many undesired effects that may develop. The nurse works with the health-care team to prevent, watch for, and treat unexpected patient responses right away.

One of the most dangerous complications for a woman who has just given birth is a **postpartum hemorrhage**. This occurs when the uterus continues to bleed excessively, losing more than 500 mL after the baby has been delivered. An accompanying signal of postpartum hemorrhage is a drop in the hematocrit by more than ten percentage points. A postpartum hemorrhage may be primary, occurring shortly after childbirth, or secondary, occurring within twelve weeks' postpartum. Postpartum hemorrhage arises from many different causes, including abnormal uterine contractility, placental complications, injury due to caesarean section or uterine rupture, or congenital coagulation disorders.

The nurse assesses the mother for potential postpartum hemorrhage by taking vital signs, massaging the uterine fundus, and preventing bladder distention by encouraging the mother to empty her bladder regularly. Heart rate and blood pressure readings will let the nurse know whether the mother is hemodynamically stable or not. Massage of the uterine fundus encourages continued uterine contractions and prevents bleeding associated with a boggy fundus. *Boggy* means that the uterus is soft, not firm as when palpating a contracted muscle. Bladder distention can cause a displacement of the woman's uterus, which can interfere with proper contractions.

A patient receiving total parenteral nutrition (TPN) is at risk for the unexpected development of a **pneumothorax**. When the physician is inserting the catheter that will deliver the TPN, there is a potential for the catheter to enter the pleural space, causing air, fluids, or blood to leak into the pleural cavity. The potential development of pneumothorax, hemothorax, and hydrothorax is one of many reasons why checking the placement of lines in patients is a crucial first step to take before using them.

Observing a sterile technique when placing central lines, dialysis catheters, and other invasive devices into patients is critical. The nurse, as part of the health-care team, works to ensure that a proper sterile technique is observed each time a sterile procedure is to occur. This helps to prevent infections from happening in patients during the placement of such lines. The nurse also supervises the process of disposing sharps such as needles into the proper sharps receptacle, placed in each patient's room in most facilities. Needlesticks from contaminated syringes can spread blood-borne infections such as HIV/AIDS, hepatitis B, and hepatitis C.

NCLEX Practice Test #1

1. A nurse is interviewing with their hospital's case management team to become a case manager. Which of the following role descriptions does NOT fit that of a case manager?
    a. Mediator between patient and other health care providers
    b. Referring patient to community resources
    c. Liaison to insurance companies to ensure coverage and cost-effective care
    d. Administering the patient's daily medications

2. A nursing student is interested in becoming a case manager. Which of the following will be required to attain this nursing role?
    a. Additional case management training, certification, and clinical hours
    b. Passing the NCLEX licensure exam
    c. Graduating with an associate's or baccalaureate degree in nursing
    d. Obtaining the required clinical hours before graduating with a nursing degree

3. A case manager is handling the case of a patient who has only a high school degree level of education and does not know much about medical terminology. Which of the following case manager roles is most important in this situation?
    a. Advocate
    b. Translator
    c. Mediator
    d. Manager

4. There is an interruption in the patient's care when their case is shifted from one health care environment to another in a way that causes ambiguity over who is responsible for care. What is this called?
    a. Continuity of care
    b. Fluidity of care
    c. Fragmentation of care
    d. Division of care

5. Which model of care seeks to promote continuity of patient care across their health journey, ensuring proper case coordination, proactivity, and patient-centeredness?
    a. Community health model
    b. Public health model
    c. Patient-managed care
    d. Patient-centered medical home

6. The nurse gets a report on their caseload of patients for the day and feels overwhelmed by how sick the patients are, knowing they will keep them very busy today. Which aspect of patient assignment is illustrated in this situation?
    a. Patient demographic
    b. Patient acuity
    c. Staffing issues
    d. Scope of practice

7. A nurse manager is assigning teams of patients to the night staff. Which of the following is a nurse-sensitive indicator of nursing performance?

    a. Meal tray delivery

    b. Vital sign accuracy

    c. Relaying of patient messages

    d. Pressure ulcer management

8. A nurse is delegating a task to a certified nursing assistant (CNA). Which of the following factors must the nurse consider?

    a. The school the CNA received their training from

    b. Other team members the CNA associates with

    c. Strengths and weaknesses of that CNA

    d. What time the CNA gets off work

9. When delegating a task to a CNA, the nurse uses which of the following tools to make their decision?

    a. Standardized checklist

    b. Personality test

    c. Drug test

    d. Solicited opinions about the staff member

10. Which key factor of supervision entails investigating whether a task was done and how well it was done?

    a. Professional behavior

    b. Delegation

    c. Follow-up

    d. Exit interview

11. What part of supervision involves the nurse giving the staff member tips for a better performance, using utmost respect and professionalism?

    a. Delegation

    b. Follow-up

    c. Documentation

    d. Coaching

12. When assessing a patient and establishing priorities of care using the M-A-A-U-A-R acronym, the nurse knows that healthcare problems such as safety, skin integrity, infection, and other medical conditions go with which letter of the acronym?

    a. R

    b. M

    c. U

    d. A

13. When establishing priorities for the patient, the nurse considers Maslow's hierarchy of needs. Which level must be attained first before moving higher on the pyramid?

    a. Esteem

    b. Physiological

    c. Love

    d. Safety

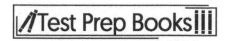

14. The nurse is obtaining the patient's height and weight and the patient willingly steps on the scale without much prompting. Which type of consent was given?
    a. Verbal
    b. Written
    c. Implied
    d. Assumed

15. Which type of law deals with misdemeanors and felonies?
    a. Criminal law
    b. Constitutional law
    c. Common law
    d. Stationary law

16. A state board of nursing has a set amount of continuing education requirements that the nurse must fulfill each year to maintain their license. Which type of law is this?
    a. Statutory law
    b. Administrative law
    c. Constitutional law
    d. Common law

17. A nurse is charged with negligence. Which type of offense is negligence?
    a. Intentional tort
    b. Libel
    c. Slander
    d. Unintentional tort

18. Which of the following is a nurse legally mandated to report?
    a. Marital status
    b. Gunshot wounds
    c. Religious beliefs
    d. Urinary tract infections

19. Which of the following items rules a person out for being an organ donor?
    a. Elderly
    b. Overweight
    c. Substance abuse
    d. Resolved case of depression

20. The school nurse notices that a kindergartener seems to have trouble making certain letter sounds when they talk. Which type of referral would be appropriate in this circumstance?
    a. Dietician
    b. Social services
    c. Physical therapist
    d. Speech therapist

21. Which of the following is the best way to prevent the spread of infection?
    a. Keeping the mouth covered when coughing or sneezing
    b. Disinfecting shared patient equipment
    c. Practicing proper hand hygiene
    d. Avoiding contact with infectious patients

22. What are the correct steps to follow when using a fire extinguisher?
    a. Pull the pin, Squeeze the handle, Aim the nozzle, Swirl around the fire
    b. Pull the pin, Aim at the base of the fire, Squeeze the handle, Sweep from side to side
    c. Squeeze the handle, Aim at the base of the fire, Pull the pin, Sweep from side to side
    d. Stand back, Pull the pin, Squeeze the handle, Sweep from side to side

23. When preparing to transfer a patient from their bed to a wheelchair, what is the first step to take?
    a. Ensure that the bed is locked.
    b. Inform the patient about what is going to happen.
    c. Get another staff member to help.
    d. Have the patient sit up in bed.

24. When attempting to lift something heavy, which of the following should not be done?
    a. Keep the legs straight and bend over to use back muscles.
    b. Spread legs apart and bend at the knees.
    c. Stand close to the object.
    d. Use only feet and legs to turn.

25. An aide is caring for a patient in their home. Which of the following items should the aide recognize as a fire hazard?
    a. Multiple electrical cords plugged into a power strip
    b. A pack of matches on a coffee table
    c. A potholder lying on the stove
    d. A toaster left out on the counter

26. Of the following patients, which one has the highest risk for skin injury?
    a. An elderly woman in an assisted-living facility who ambulates with a cane
    b. An eighty-year-old man in the hospital recovering from hip surgery
    c. A seventy-year-old man hospitalized for pneumonia
    d. An elderly woman who is incontinent of stool, and who is showing signs of confusion

27. Which of the following is not a preventative measure for pressure-ulcer formation?
    a. Padding bony areas on the body
    b. Repositioning the patient at least every two hours
    c. Keeping the patient in a sitting position while in their bed
    d. Changing soiled linens and clothing promptly

28. An aide is caring for a patient with a known respiratory infection. The patient is on droplet precautions. What is the minimum PPE required when caring for this patient?
    a. Gloves, gown, N-95 respirator
    b. Gown, eyewear, gloves, and a disposable mask
    c. Gloves and a disposable mask
    d. Disposable mask, sterile gloves, and eyewear

29. During lunchtime in the dining area, an aide notices a patient grabbing their throat. What should the aide's first action be?
    a. To call for help
    b. Have the patient stand up
    c. Ask the patient if they are choking
    d. To try to open the patient's mouth

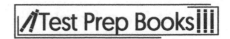

30. Of the following tasks, which one is not considered "dirty"?
    a. Changing a diaper
    b. Assisting with oral care
    c. Changing a wound dressing
    d. Helping a patient get dressed

31. An aide enters a patient's room in response to the call light and sees a fire behind the television. What is the aide's first action?
    a. Activate the fire alarm.
    b. Use the nearest fire extinguisher.
    c. Move the patient to a safer location away from the room.
    d. Smother the fire with a blanket.

32. Which of the following is not a risk factor for falls in the elderly?
    a. Using a cane to walk
    b. Inadequate lighting in a room
    c. Muscle weakness
    d. Slower reflexes

33. When performing HS oral care for a patient with dentures, which action should the nurse take?
    a. Remove the patient's dentures, clean them with cool or tepid water, place them in a denture cup with cool or tepid water or denture cleaning solution, and leave the cup on the bedside table within the patient's reach.
    b. Remove the patient's dentures, clean them with hot water, place them in an empty denture cup, and leave the cup on the bedside table within the patient's reach.
    c. Remove the patient's dentures, wrap them in a paper towel, and place them on the bedside table within the patient's reach.
    d. Remove the patient's dentures, clean them with cool or tepid water, wrap them in a washcloth, and leave them by the sink until the patient is ready for AM care.

34. A nurse is providing AM care to a patient who has suffered a stroke and has right-sided weakness. When dressing the patient, which action should the nurse take?
    a. Before dressing the patient in the new clothing, the nurse should remove all of the patient's old clothing to prevent cross contamination.
    b. The nurse should first undress and redress the patient's upper body, then undress and redress the patient's lower body.
    c. When removing the patient's pants, the nurse should remove the pants from the left leg first and then the right leg.
    d. When redressing the patient in clean pants, the nurse should place the left leg in the pants first and then the right leg.

35. A nurse is assisting a diabetic patient with breakfast. The patient is scheduled for heart surgery in the afternoon. Which breakfast tray is appropriate for this patient?
    a. Coffee, apple juice, lime gelatin, and clear broth
    b. Coffee with sugar substitute, oatmeal, scrambled eggs, and bacon
    c. Coffee with sugar, grits, egg white omelet, and a cup of fresh fruit
    d. This patient should not receive a breakfast tray.

36. A patient is experiencing diarrhea and complaining of lightheadedness when standing. The patient is normally able to ambulate to the bathroom without assistance. What's the first action a nurse should take?

    a. Encourage the patient to drink lots of fluids to prevent dehydration.
    b. This is normal, and the nurse should do nothing.
    c. Provide the patient with additional washcloths, soap, and towels for perineal care.
    d. Place the call bell within reach and instruct the patient to call for assistance before getting out of bed.

37. A nurse is providing AM care to a comatose patient. The patient has been immobile for several weeks and is at risk for muscle atrophy and contractures. What action should the nurse take in caring for the patient?

    a. Passive range of motion exercises should be done with the patient.
    b. Perineal care should be provided, but a full bed bath should be avoided due to the patient's risk for pressure sores.
    c. Before providing oral care, the head of the patient's bed should be flat, and the patient's head should be turned to the side to prevent aspiration.
    d. The patient should be encouraged to do active range of motion exercises while lying in bed.

38. Studies have shown that which of the following practices has the most positive impact on patients?

    a. Personalized comfort measures in their post-operation room, such as a favorite snack or book
    b. Internet and television access during their clinical stay
    c. An attentive communication style between their nurses and physicians
    d. Visible operation and safety checklists that staff members regularly check and notate

39. Which of the following are vulnerable populations at high risk of being abuse and neglect victims?

    a. Men, women, and children
    b. Immigrants, women, and minority races
    c. Children, women, and the elderly
    d. Children, pets, and immigrants

40. A nurse is planning the daily care schedule for an older patient with limited mobility. The patient has physical therapy at 10:00 am and occupational therapy at 2:00 pm. Which schedule is most appropriate?

    a. The nurse will provide AM care at 8:00 am and afternoon care at 3:00 pm.
    b. The nurse will provide AM care at 8:00 am and afternoon care at 4:00 pm.
    c. The nurse will provide AM care at 9:00 am and afternoon care at 4:00 pm.
    d. The nurse will provide AM care at 9:00 am and afternoon care at 3:00 pm.

41. A nurse is caring for a patient who doesn't have pressure sores but is at risk for them due to immobility. How often should the patient be repositioned?

    a. Because the patient doesn't have pressure sores, it's not necessary to reposition them.
    b. The patient only needs to be repositioned when they express discomfort.
    c. The patient should be repositioned at least once every two hours.
    d. The patient should be repositioned each time perineal care is provided.

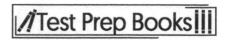

42. Maya eats a nutrient-rich, balanced diet and exercises vigorously for 30 minutes each day. However, she has gained almost 25 pounds over the course of four months. She has also started growing facial hair and has noticed purple stretch marks on her abdomen and breasts. She visits her primary care provider seeking insight as to what is causing these issues. Maya's blood pressure is 135/90 at the appointment. Maya's physician refers her to an endocrinologist, believing she is showing signs of which of the following?

    a. Hypertension

    b. Gestational diabetes

    c. Chronic kidney disease

    d. Cushing's syndrome

43. Mary is a seven-year-old in second grade. She has been absent from school nine days in one month. When Mary's teacher asks her why she has been absent or contacts her parents to ask about the absences, they all simply say she was sick and don't provide any additional information. Mary looks extremely frightened when asked about her absences. She regularly comes to school in large, baggy clothing that smells unpleasantly, and her hair always looks dirty. She falls asleep often in class, and one day her teacher saw her crying as she prepared to leave for home. Mary's teacher is probably concerned that Mary is dealing with which of the following issues?

    a. She is suffering from a hormonal imbalance or disorder

    b. She is too emotional

    c. She is having a mental breakdown

    d. She is being abused or neglected by a caregiver

44. Which of the following options correctly names the type of common medication used to treat anxiety and depression?

    a. Antipsychotics

    b. Selective serotonin reuptake inhibitors (SSRIs)

    c. Dopamine reuptake inhibitors

    d. Homeopathic options

45. Psychosis is a common side effect of which of the following?

    I. Schizophrenia

    II. Methamphetamine, cocaine, or LSD use

    III. Bipolar Disorder

    IV. HIV antiviral medications

    a. II ad IV only

    b. I and II only

    c. I, II, and III

    d. All of the above

46. Jack and Jill are two nursing students who are on rotation in their county's emergency department. One afternoon, a woman comes into the waiting area and collapses on the floor. She says she cannot breathe and rambles about feeling blindsided. She begins thrashing on the floor and starts to sob. Upon reviewing her intake forms, Jack and Jill notice that the woman's health insurance shows she is employed, and she has not had any notable medical or mental health issues. However, she keeps mentioning that her partner has left her. Jack says, "I think she must have an undiagnosed anxiety disorder; we should look into medication options." Jill disagrees with him, saying that this seems more like which of the following?
    a. A situational crisis
    b. A case of cocaine abuse
    c. A case of intimate partner violence
    d. A nonemergency situation that they should send to the scheduling department

47. Which of the following statements is correct?
    a. Self-destruction ideation is characterized by thoughts of harming oneself, while global destruction ideation is characterized by thoughts of harming others.
    b. Suicidal ideation is characterized by thoughts of harming oneself, while homicidal ideation is characterized by thoughts of harming others.
    c. Internal ideation is characterized by thoughts of harming oneself, while external ideation is characterized by thoughts of harming others.
    d. Intrinsic ideation is characterized by thoughts of harming oneself, while extrinsic ideation is characterized by thoughts of harming others.

48. Middle school student Johnny stores an epinephrine injection pen in his locker, lunch bag, and pencil case. Johnny likely suffers from which of the following?
    a. Homicidal ideation
    b. Narcolepsy
    c. Depression
    d. A severe allergy

49. Which of the following is a commonly used anticoagulant that works by blocking the body's ability to adhere platelets together?
    a. Paxil
    b. Coumadin
    c. Heparin
    d. Aspirin

50. Which of the following is a commonly used anticoagulant that works by preventing the activation of thrombin?
    a. Paxil
    b. Warfarin
    c. Heparin
    d. Aspirin

51. What are the blood vessels called that carry blood back to the heart from the rest of the body?
    a. Capillaries
    b. Arteries
    c. Ventricles
    d. Veins

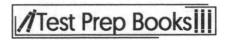

52. The nurse is taking a manual blood pressure reading from a patient who is seated in an armchair. Which of the following body positions should the nurse ask the patient to change in order to get the most accurate reading?
   a. Crossed legs
   b. Holding remote with hand not getting blood pressure reading
   c. Resting head on head rest
   d. Slouching

53. The nurse heard the doctor telling the patient how he needed to change his diet and get more exercise to better manage his diabetes. The nurse knows that the patient did not want to hear this and that the patient has been vocal in the past about not needing to change anything about his lifestyle. The nurse senses that the patient feels angry and frustrated by his conversation with the doctor. The patient is very agitated when the nurse comes to collect vital signs and tells her that he thinks she is lazy. Which defense mechanism is the patient displaying?
   a. Intellectualization
   b. Undoing
   c. Reaction formation
   d. Displacement

54. The nurse walks into the room where the patient is clutching his chest, sweating, and appears short of breath. The patient reports he is experiencing chest pain that is crushing and severe, with some pain in his left arm as well. The nurse knows that this type of chest pain is most likely associated with which following medical condition?
   a. Myocardial infarction
   b. Gastroesophageal reflux
   c. Pneumonia
   d. Pleuritis

55. The action created by a drug is known as what?
   a. Pharmacology
   b. Side effect
   c. Adverse reaction
   d. Intended effect

56. Which assessment technique would the nurse employ to obtain subjective data?
   a. Auscultation
   b. Palpation
   c. Percussion
   d. Patient interview

57. Which statement best describes the evaluation phase of the nursing process?
   a. Subjective, objective, and psychosocial data are gathered in this phase.
   b. Nursing diagnoses are formulated during the evaluation phase.
   c. Evaluation happens across the continuum of the nursing process.
   d. This phase often begins with educating the patient on expected outcomes.

58. A patient is admitted with prolonged vomiting, greater than three days. The nurse knows this patient will need what type of therapy to counteract a dangerous result of prolonged vomiting?
    a. Intravenous (IV) fluids
    b. Antibacterial medications
    c. Anti-nausea medications
    d. Physical therapy

59. The nurse walks into a patient's room and witnesses the patient violently convulsing with rigid muscles. The patient is completely unconscious. The nurse immediately recognizes this is what type of seizure?
    a. Myoclonic
    b. Absence
    c. Grand Mal
    d. Tonic

60. The nurse looks for which of the following signs that the patient is having an allergic reaction after administering a drug?
    a. Aching and stiffness
    b. Coughing and fever
    c. Fever and chills
    d. Itching and rash

61. The nurse knows that which type of the following electrolyte supplements is contraindicated if the patient is on an ACE inhibitor such as lisinopril?
    a. Magnesium
    b. Calcium
    c. Potassium
    d. Sodium

62. When administering a blood-thinning drug such as warfarin, the nurse will be mindful of which type of synergistic drug that could put the patient at risk for excessive bleeding?
    a. Aspirin
    b. Lasix
    c. Lisinopril
    d. Protonix

63. When preparing a patient for the insertion of a central venous access device (CVAD), the nurse explains that the benefits of a CVAD include all except which of the following?
    a. Easier-to-obtain frequent blood draws
    b. Administration of large amounts of medications and fluids
    c. Decreased peripheral sticks and peripheral inflammation
    d. Decreased risk of infection

64. Before using a patient's newly placed PICC line, the nurse knows which test must be performed?
    a. CT scan
    b. Chest x-ray
    c. MRI
    d. Ultrasound

65. Which of the following CVADs is an example of a nontunneled catheter?
    a. Groshong's
    b. Subclavian
    c. Small-bore
    d. Hickman's

66. The nurse has a patient who reports that he is 155 pounds. The nurse needs to record the patient's weight in kilograms. Knowing that 1 kilogram is equal to 2.2 pounds, the nurse then calculates the patient's weight to be what in kilograms?
    a. 60 kg
    b. 70 kg
    c. 341 kg
    d. 300 kg

67. The patient has an order for 240 mg of Tylenol for her pediatric patient. Tylenol comes in 160 mg per 5 mL. How many milliliters does the nurse administer to the patient?
    a. 7.5 mL
    b. 5 mL
    c. 12.5 mL
    d. 10 mL

68. Which of the following will provide the nurse with lists of medications, generic and brand names, and expected outcomes and is maintained by an expert panel of medical practitioners?
    a. Patient medication list from home
    b. Facility procedure manual
    c. Formulary
    d. Electronic health record

69. When giving an intramuscular injection of the pneumococcal vaccine, the nurse selects the deltoid muscle as the site of injection. What technique can the nurse use to avoid leakage of the injected fluid into the subcutaneous tissue?
    a. Aspiration
    b. Injection at a 45 degree angle
    c. Z-track
    d. Massaging the site

70. When administering a medication, the nurse observes all except which of the following rights?
    a. Right medication
    b. Right medical facility
    c. Right time frame
    d. Right person

71. Which term refers to a route of medication administration other than through the gastrointestinal tract?
    a. Parenteral
    b. Enteral
    c. Motor
    d. Buccal

72. The nurse is having her annual tuberculosis exam, or Mantoux test, performed. This test, which entails the injection of TB proteins or antigens, involves which route of administration?
    a. Subcutaneous
    b. Intrathecal
    c. Intradermal
    d. Sublingual

73. The nurse is assessing a patient's IV access site and finds it to be cool and swollen. The IV pump is beeping, and fluid appears to be leaking around the site. The nurse suspects which of the following IV therapy complications?
    a. Clot formation
    b. Fluid overload
    c. Infection
    d. Infiltration

74. The nurse is administering total parenteral nutrition (TPN) to the patient for the first time. He knows that he should administer the medication at which of the following rates?
    a. Slowly, at 50 percent of the prescribed dosage
    b. Quickly, at double the prescribed dosage
    c. Quickly, at three times the prescribed dosage
    d. Slowly, at 25 percent of the prescribed dosage

75. The nurse needs to assess a normal, uncomplicated patient in the doctor's office for a yearly physical. Which is the best spot to assess for this patient's pulse?
    a. Radial
    b. Femoral
    c. Popliteal
    d. Carotid

76. The patient reports that he feels dizzy and lightheaded when he stands up after sitting for a long time. What would be the appropriate intervention performed by the nurse to assess the cause of these symptoms?
    a. Taking the patient's temperature
    b. Observing the patient's rate of breathing and effort of breathing
    c. Assessing bilateral radial pulses and comparing strength
    d. Lying/sitting/standing blood pressure readings

77. The nurse is educating a female client who is to undergo a mammography. Which of the following statements would not be appropriate regarding mammography education?
    a. "This test allows the practitioner to visualize small lumps that they may not have been able to palpate."

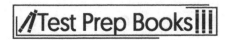

b. "It is recommended that you get a mammography once every year after the age of forty for early detection of breast cancer."

c. "The mammography is a type of computed tomography used to visualize the breast tissue."

d. "This test takes x-ray images of the breast tissue, identifying any masses that may be cancerous."

78. A patient is admitted to the hospital from the emergency department with stomach pain and blood emesis. The nurse knows that which of the following tests is likely to be performed on the patient based on their symptoms?

a. Sigmoidoscopy

b. Upper endoscopy

c. Anoscopy

d. Colonoscopy

79. Which of the following lab values suggests the client is experiencing hypokalemia?

a. 3.2 mEq/L

b. 3.5 mEq/L

c. 5.0 mEq/L

d. 5.5 mEq/L

80. Which of the following terms refers to a state in which the client has a lower than normal count of platelet cells?

a. Neutropenia

b. Anemia

c. Thrombocytopenia

d. Leukopenia

81. The nurse in the ICU takes over for a patient who has been experiencing a respiratory acidosis. The nurse checks the daily labs and finds which of the following values that suggests the patient is still acidotic?

a. 7.38 pH

b. 7.25 pH

c. 7.42 pH

d. 7.48 pH

82. The nurse knows that all except which of the following factors put a patient at risk for aspiration?

a. Difficulty swallowing and weakened gag reflex

b. Liver failure

c. Weakened upper and lower esophageal sphincter reflexes

d. Enteral feedings

83. The nurse is assessing a patient for possible risk factors for developing cancer. The patient reports a longtime smoking habit that she has struggled to kick. The nurse knows that this risk factor puts the patient most at risk for developing all except which of the following cancers?

a. Larynx

b. Esophagus

c. Lung

d. Breast

84. The nurse caring for a patient postcardiac catheterization will perform which specific intervention to monitor for the development of life-threatening dysrhythmias?
    a. Keep the patient flat on their back for at least six hours postprocedure.
    b. Take regular vital signs, especially heart rate and blood pressure.
    c. Regularly observe the patient's ECG via cardiac monitoring, according to facility protocol.
    d. Regularly observe the incision site, looking for bruising, swelling, and redness.

85. A patient reports to the nurse that he is feeling anxious and dizzy, and his heart is racing. Which system-specific assessment will the nurse perform to investigate these symptoms?
    a. Assess the circulatory system by grading the patient's pitting edema.
    b. Obtain and compare bilateral peripheral pulses.
    c. Assess the patient's level of consciousness and motor and sensory function.
    d. Compare the patient's muscular strength bilaterally by having him push against resistance.

86. A patient is in the outpatient clinic for a same-day mole removal. The nurse knows which type of anesthetic is most appropriate for this type of procedure?
    a. Nerve block
    b. Local
    c. Regional
    d. General

87. The nurse assesses drainage from a client's chest tube for all except which of the following?
    a. Consistency
    b. Quantity
    c. Heart rate
    d. Color

88. The nurse is caring for a client who recently underwent radiation therapy to his abdomen. Based on the location of the radiation, the nurse expects which of the following side effects?
    a. Diarrhea
    b. Fatigue
    c. Trembling
    d. Muscle aches

89. A woman who has entered her twenty-fourth week of pregnancy is preparing to take the oral glucose tolerance test, which will screen for which condition of pregnancy?
    a. Hyperemesis gravidarum
    b. Preeclampsia
    c. Iron-deficiency anemia
    d. Gestational diabetes

90. The nurse has a client who has recently undergone abdominal surgery with a large incision site. The nurse knows that which of the following is *not* a sign that the wound has become infected?
    a. Redness
    b. Coolness
    c. Heat
    d. Swelling

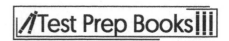

91. When reviewing their knowledge of the stages of infections, the nurse knows that which period precedes the first symptoms of the infection?
    a. Prodromal period
    b. Colonization of organism
    c. Incubation period
    d. Convalescent period

92. The nurse is looking over the patient's lab values for the day. He notices that one lab parameter has gone up significantly, signaling a possible infectious process at work. Which lab parameter is he likely drawing this conclusion from?
    a. Blood urea nitrogen
    b. Hematocrit
    c. Neutrophils
    d. Sodium level

93. A patient needs invasive hemodynamic monitoring as they are being admitted to the ICU for hemorrhagic shock. The nurse will expect an order for which type of line to be inserted?
    a. PICC line
    b. Port-a-cath
    c. Dialysis catheter
    d. Right-heart catheter

94. Which of the following hemodynamic parameters is measured in beats per minute per meter squared of the patient's body surface area?
    a. Cardiac index
    b. Cardiac output
    c. Mean arterial pressure
    d. Stroke volume

95. The nurse notices a patient's medication list contains a drug that is likely to lower her pulmonary vascular resistance. Which type of medicine is the nurse likely looking at to draw this conclusion?
    a. Diuretic
    b. Morphine
    c. Nitrate
    d. Calcium channel blocker

96. A patient with a Swan-Ganz catheter in the ICU is being assessed by the nurse for the first time during the shift. The nurse notices which number on the hemodynamic profile is abnormal and needs further investigating?
    a. Mean arterial pressure: 75 mmHg
    b. Cardiac output: 2L/min
    c. Central venous pressure: 5 mmHg
    d. Pulmonary capillary wedge pressure: 6 mmHg

97. As the nurse is receiving reports on her patients for the day, she knows that which patient will take top priority in being assessed and treated?
    a. 33-year-old female who is nauseous and needs an antiemetic administered
    b. 49-year-old female who is scheduled for a cardiac catheterization and needs to sign the informed consent
    c. 55-year-old male who is being discharged later today and has a question about his care at home
    d. 78-year-old male who is complaining of shortness of breath

98. The doctor has ordered a nasogastric (NG) tube to be placed by the nurse for gastric lavage. After placing the NG, the nurse expects which of the following tests to be performed to confirm the placement of the tube?
    a. Aspiration of laryngeal secretions for pH testing
    b. Chest radiograph
    c. Abdominal ultrasound
    d. Manual palpation of the gastric body for the catheter tip

99. A client has just had a catheter placed in their chest for the purpose of total parenteral nutrition (TPN) administration. The chest x-ray shows that the catheter has slipped and caused a leakage of air into the pleural space. What is this condition called?
    a. Pneumothorax
    b. Hemothorax
    c. Hydrothorax
    d. Pneumonia

100. The nurse is caring for a woman who is three hours postpartum. The nurse takes all except which of the following actions to prevent and monitor for postpartum hemorrhage?
    a. Massage the uterine fundus.
    b. Obtain regular vital signs, including heart rate and blood pressure.
    c. Ensure that the woman avoids bladder distention.
    d. Encourage the woman to perform her Kegel exercises.

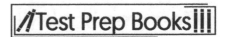

NCLEX Answer Explanations #1

1. D: The case manager no longer performs the role of the floor nurse who administers daily medications. As a case manager, the nurse is a mediator between the patient and other health care providers and a liaison to insurance companies to ensure affordable and cost-effective care. The case manager also connects the patient to community resources through referrals.

2. A: To become a case manager, the nurse needs to fulfill requirements beyond their initial nursing degree. These requirements include case management–specific training, clinical hours following the case management team, and passing a case management certification exam. The initial passing of the NCLEX, clinical hours required for the nursing degree, and the nursing degree itself are all required before beginning case management training.

3. B: The case manager must act as a translator for the patient, translating complicated medical jargon, legal speak, and insurance terminology into a language the patient can easily understand. This translator role goes back to the case manager's overarching role as communicator. The patient must understand what is going on in their plan of care to be an active and successful participant in the care team. Choice *D*, the managerial role of the case manager, has to do with the paperwork side of the patient's case. Choice *A*, the advocate role, occurs when the case manager is communicating with other members of the health care team besides the patient. Choice *C*, mediating, happens between the case manager and the other teams involved.

4. C: Fragmentation of care occurs when the patient's case is shifted from one health care environment to another, in such a way that ambiguity over who is responsible for the patient's overall case results. This leads to errors and prolonged inaction as well as patient frustration. Continuity of care is the opposite of fragmentation of care and is the ideal. Continuity of care means the plan of care stays consistent across many different health care environments that the patient may find themselves in. Choices *B* and *D*, fluidity and division, are not terms used for these concepts.

5. D: The patient-centered medical home (PCMH) is a model of care that promotes wellness for the patient through proactivity, care coordination, and patient-centered planning. PCMH is a model that seeks to combat fragmentation of care and the problems that come with it. The other three terms are not applicable to the description, though community and public health organizations do play a role in promoting community wellness.

6. B: The nurse is noticing how sick the patients are, which refers to acuity. High-acuity patients, or patients who are very sick, present a heavy workload for a nurse's day. The charge nurse who makes the patient assignments takes into account the acuity of the patients they assign to team nurses. Charge nurses try to give out balanced, equitable workloads to nurses to prevent overload and burn-out. Patient demographics, staffing needs, and scope of practice are not the aspects of patient assignment being looked at here.

7. D: One nursing-sensitive indicator of nurse performance is the prevention and management of hospital-acquired pressure ulcers (especially in non-ambulatory patients). When nursing floors are understaffed, or patients are high acuity and burdensome to the nurse, patient care may suffer, providing less time and attention to patients' needs. Meal trays are often delivered by the food management team, vital signs are often obtained by CNAs, and the relaying of messages is handled by the floor secretary. These three items are not nurse-sensitive indicators in most healthcare settings. In other words, nurses' performance is not directly measured by these tasks.

8. C: The nurse must consider the strengths and weaknesses of a particular CNA before delegating a task to them. This will best assist the nurse in making a sound decision. The school that the CNA received their training from, the other staff members they associate with, and what time they get off work are irrelevant to their performance as a CNA. The nurse must be aware of and careful of their own personal bias and prejudice when deciding to whom to delegate tasks. Each person must be judged fairly based on their merit, attitude, and performance.

9. A: When deciding on whether to delegate a task to a CNA or not, the nurse may use a standardized checklist as a tool that will assist them in making this decision. The checklist may include items such as whether the CNA has been properly trained and certified for the specific task. A drug test and personality test are not appropriate for a simple task delegation. Basing one's judgment of the CNA on what other people say about them is not valid or appropriate. The nurse must stay objective and fair when deciding about delegating a task.

10. C: The key task in supervision is the follow-up, where the nurse investigates whether the task was done, whether it was done in a timely manner, and whether it was done correctly. Without follow-up, a type of evaluation, the process is incomplete. Professional behavior is always required of a nurse, regardless of the situation. Delegation has already been performed and is the reason why the supervision is required in the first place. An exit interview is performed when an employee leaves a company and is not part of the supervision of a delegated task.

11. D: Sometimes the supervising nurse must coach the staff member to whom they have delegated a task to ensure a better performance the next time. The nurse should use the utmost professionalism and respect during these encounters, ensuring the staff member is receptive and the criticism is constructive. Follow-up is investigating that the task was done. Delegation is handing out a task to an appropriate staff member. Documentation needs to occur following each task that is performed, and the delegating nurse needs to ensure this is performed for all care activity.

12. A: The letter "R" in the acronym M-A-A-U-A-R stands for the *risks* of healthcare problems such as compromised skin integrity, infection, and other medical conditions. M is for mental status changes and alterations. U is for unaddressed and untreated problems requiring immediate attention. A is for acute pain, acute urinary elimination concerns, and abnormal laboratory and diagnostic data.

13. B: The patient's physiological needs must be met first and foremost, before any other level of the hierarchy can be addressed. Maslow's description of the physiological needs include hunger, thirst, breathing, sleep, and homeostasis. Safety is the next level; it addresses morality, family, and security of the body. Love comes next in Maslow's hierarchy, involving relationships with family and friends. Esteem is one level higher than love, involving self-esteem, confidence, achievement, and respect of others.

14. C: The patient has given implied consent. There is neither verbal nor written confirmation of consent; rather, both parties silently agree without a formal conversation about the topic. Assumed is not a term used for consent, though both parties are assuming that consent is given. Written consent involves a signed legal document by the patient and usually follows a conversation about the plan of care or procedure with the physician performing it. Verbal consent is given by the patient, affirming verbally their consent to the procedure to be done.

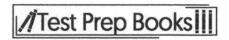

15. A: Criminal law has to do with the arrest, prosecution, and incarceration of those who commit misdemeanors and felonies. Constitutional law has to do with the laws set forth by the Constitution of the United States of America. Common law is based on legal precedents. Stationary is not a term used to describe laws. Stationary sounds similar to "statutory," which has to do with laws passed down by legislative bodies such as a state's legislature. There are statutes criminalizing certain acts, such as assault.

16. B: Administrative law is the type of law given by administrative bodies such as a state's nursing board. Constitutional law is specific to the United States Constitution and does not rule on nursing administrative issues. Common law is based on legal precedents. Statutory law involves legislative bodies such as a state's legislature.

17. D: Negligence, along with malpractice, is a type of unintentional tort. Intentional torts include false imprisonment, batter, and assault. Libel and slander, in which false statements are made as a form of defamation, both fall under the category of intentional tort.

18. B: Nurses are legally mandated to report gunshot wounds, dog bites, communicable disease, neglect, and abuse. Marital status, religious beliefs, and urinary tract infections are not legally mandated items for the nurse to report.

19. C: Substance abuse, as well as chronic disease, alcohol abuse, and communicable diseases potentially rule out a person from being an organ donor. A strict list of criteria must be met for organ donation to occur. These criteria ensure the health and viability of the organs and tissues to be donated. Age, weight, and previous psychiatric illness do not necessarily rule a person out for organ donation.

20. D: The nurse could appropriately make a speech therapy referral in this child's case, connecting the child and the child's family to needed services. The other three options of a dietician, physical therapist, and social services are not appropriate for this specific scenario.

21. C: All of the answer choices are types of standard precautions, but research has shown that proper hand hygiene using soap and water or alcohol-based hand rub (if appropriate) is the best way to prevent the spread of germs.

22. B: Use the acronym PASS to answer this question. The pin should always be pulled first. Choices *A*, *C*, and *D* are not listed in the correct order or with the correct wording. The correct directions and order are: Pull the pin, Aim at the base of the fire, Squeeze the handle, and Sweep from side to side.

23. B: Anytime a task or procedure is about to occur, the patient should be informed first. All of the other options are part of the procedure, but the first step is to explain the task to the patient. Another staff person may not be needed, the patient may not be able to sit up in bed on their own, or they may wonder why they are being asked to sit up.

24. A: When lifting a heavy object, the lower back should not be strained; therefore, bending over and using the back muscles should be avoided. Choices *B*, *C*, and *D* should be done when lifting. Stand close to the object, bend at the knees with legs apart, and use feet and legs to turn if needed.

25. C: Anything flammable that is on top of a stove should be moved off of the stove surface to avoid a fire if the burners are turned on. Keep in mind that this patient is in their own home. All of the other choices are acceptable and pose no immediate fire hazard. Multiple cords should be plugged into a power strip, and a toaster left on the counter is not a hazard. The pack of matches on the table could be a hazard, but the patient is still living independently and may still be capable of using matches correctly. If there are no children in the home, the matches are not of immediate concern.

26. D: An elderly woman who is incontinent with stool will need frequent linen changes and cleansing of her bottom. The constant moisture has a very high potential for causing skin breakdown. In addition to her bottom, she is showing signs of confusion, which means she may become agitated and unaware of her surroundings, leading to potential bruises or tears on her extremities from the bed. The other patient scenarios described are also at risk for skin injury. However, with the information given, *D* is the patient with the highest risk.

27. C: Keeping a patient in a sitting position in their bed puts extra pressure on their coccyx and bottom due to gravity; therefore, this option is not a preventative measure for pressure-ulcer formation. Choices *A*, *B*, and *D* are interventions that should be done to help prevent pressure ulcers.

28. C: Gloves and a disposable mask are all that are required for droplet precaution; however, additional PPE may be used if desiring extra protection. The key word in this question is *minimum*. Choice *A* is not correct because an N-95 mask is not required. Choice *D* is not correct because sterile gloves are not needed and eyewear is optional. Choice *B* would give the most coverage for protection but it is not the minimum PPE required.

29. C: The first thing to do is to check to see if the patient is choking. They may nod their head if they are asked about choking, and they will not be able to talk. If the person is choking, help them stand up so that the Heimlich maneuver can be started. Choice *A*, calling for help, would not be necessary unless the person becomes unconscious or if help is needed with the Heimlich. Choice *D* is incorrect because it is not appropriate to look in the person's mouth for a lodged piece of food, as the nurse could make the obstruction worse, as well as waste precious time.

30. D: Helping a patient get dressed is not considered a dirty task unless the clothing is soiled with any bodily fluid. *A*, *B*, and *C* are all tasks that involve bodily fluids and are considered dirty. Clean tasks should be performed first, followed by dirty tasks.

31. C: Use the acronym RACE to answer this question. The information given in the question leads to the fact that the patient is in the room, and that there is probably an electrical fire. The first action should be to rescue the patient by removing them from the room. Next, activate the fire alarm and then contain the fire by closing the door to the room. Extinguish the fire with the appropriate extinguisher if available. Choice *D*, smothering the fire, is not appropriate for an electrical fire.

32. A: Use of a cane is not a risk factor for falls in the elderly. A cane would actually benefit a person by giving them extra stability when walking. Poor lighting is a risk factor because it could cause someone to stumble over items on the floor or cause an imbalance by bumping into unseen furniture. Muscle weakness and slower reflexes are also risk factors for falls in the elderly.

33. A: The patient's dentures should be removed, cleaned with cool or tepid water, and then stored in a denture cup with cool or tepid water (or denture cleaning solution) within the patient's reach. For Choice *B*, dentures should never be cleaned with or stored in hot water since hot water can damage them. In Choice *C*, a patient's dentures should never be stored in a paper towel because they could accidentally be thrown away. Dentures should always be stored in a denture cup. In Choice *D*, if a patient is unable to put their own dentures in their mouth, or the patient doesn't wish to keep them within reach, storing them by the sink is acceptable. However, they should never be stored in a

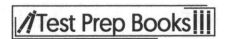

washcloth. A washcloth can be used to handle dentures while cleaning them to prevent accidental damage, but dentures should always be stored in a denture cup.

34. C: When dressing a patient with a weakness or paralysis on one side, the weak side should always be undressed last and redressed first. In Choice *A*, unless the patient has soiled his clothes, it's unnecessary to remove all of their clothes prior to redressing them. The patient should be covered up as much as possible to avoid discomfort and/or overexposure. For Choice *B*, the order of the upper- and lower-body dressing is unimportant as it relates to the patient's right-sided weakness. There might be a valid reason to start with the upper body, but it isn't related to the right-sided weakness. In Choice *D*, this is the opposite order. The nurse should place the right leg (the weak side) into the pants first.

35. D: A patient scheduled for surgery in the afternoon would be NPO (nothing by mouth) status, so they would not be allowed to have any food or beverage. Choice *A* is an example of a clear liquid diet, which would not be appropriate for a patient with an upcoming surgery. This diet is more appropriate for a patient post-surgery, before progressing to a regular diet. Choice *B* is an appropriate diet for a diabetic patient, but this patient is scheduled for surgery in the afternoon and should be NPO. Finally, Choice *C* is an example of a heart-healthy diet, which may be appropriate for the patient after being cleared to eat solid foods post-surgery.

36. D: The *first* action the nurse should take is to give the call bell to the patient and instruct them to call for assistance. If a patient is experiencing lightheadedness, they're at risk for a fall. Patient safety is the number one priority. In Choice *A*, if not contraindicated, the patient should be encouraged to drink lots of fluids, but this is not the first action the nurse should take. In Choice *B*, the findings should be reported to the nurse; however, the nurse should not leave the room before placing the call bell within reach of the patient and instructing them to call for assistance before getting out of bed. In Choice *C*, the patient might require additional supplies for perineal care, but this isn't the first action the nurse should take.

37. A: "Muscle atrophy" is the weakening of a muscle, and a "contracture" is the shortening of a muscle. Both conditions are due to immobility. Therefore, passive range of motion exercises (unless contraindicated) should be done with the patient. In Choice *B*, patients at risk for pressure sores can have full bed baths, but the nurse must thoroughly dry the patient's skin to prevent breakdown. For Choice *C*, the nurse would be expected to provide oral care to the patient, and the patient's head should be turned to the side (if possible) to prevent aspiration. However, unless contraindicated, the head of the patient's bed should be elevated for oral care. For Choice *D*, active range of motion exercises are those performed by the patient independently. A comatose patient is unable to perform active range of motion exercises, so passive range of motion exercises must be performed by the nurse.

38. C: Patients respond favorably to positive intrapersonal communication between their attending nurses and physicians. The other options may be nice for patients, but studies indicate that nurse and physician relationships have the most impact on a patient's overall experience.

39. C: Children, women, and the elderly are vulnerable populations due to tendencies to be physically weaker than their attackers, possibly disabled, unable to communicate, or dependent in some other way.

40. B: Older patients need time to rest between activities, so adequate rest intervals should be allotted when planning a patient's schedule. Providing AM care at 8:00 am would give the patient time to rest before going to physical therapy and providing afternoon care at 4:00 pm would give the patient time to rest after returning from occupational therapy. In Choice *A*, providing afternoon care at 3:00 pm doesn't give the patient an adequate rest period after occupational therapy. For Choice *C*, providing AM care at 9:00 am doesn't give the patient time to rest before physical therapy. In Choice *D*, providing afternoon care at 3:00 pm again doesn't give the patient an adequate rest period after occupational therapy.

41. C: Even if no pressure sores are present, all immobile patients should be repositioned at least once every two hours. For Choice *A*, the patient should be repositioned at least once every two hours to prevent pressure sores from developing. Again in Choice *B*, an immobile patient should be repositioned at least once every two hours. However, if the patient expresses discomfort, the nurse can reposition the patient even if they were repositioned less than two hours ago. For Choice *D*, while it might be appropriate to coordinate care in this manner, again the patient should be repositioned at least once every two hours whether or not any other care is being provided.

42. D: Cushing's syndrome is characterized by weight gain, purple stretch marks (striae), facial hair growth in women, and high blood pressure. Cushing's syndrome is also associated with the classic signs of a "moon face" or "buffalo hump", which are caused by fat deposits on the face, neck, and upper back. Caused by excessive cortisol in the body which can be the result of overproduction within the body or by long term use of corticosteroids.

43. D: All the signs that Mary is showing, such as poor hygiene, absenteeism, withdrawn behaviors, and crying before going home are red flags for abuse and neglect.

44. B: Selective serotonin reuptake inhibitors (SSRIs) are a class of drugs that can treat both anxiety and depression symptoms. Therefore, brand names of this drug, such as Prozac®, Zoloft®, and Lexapro®, may be prescribed to individuals who are suffering from anxiety, depression, or a combination of both.

45. C: Schizophrenia and bipolar disorder are mental disorders in which hallucinations and delusion (key components of psychosis) are common. These characteristics can also result from mind-altering drugs, specifically methamphetamines, cocaine, and LSD. Antiviral medications used to treat HIV do not normally cause psychosis.

46. A: The patient is having many symptoms of panic, such as struggling to breathe, having difficulty controlling her emotions, and acting agitated. However, she mentions that her partner just left, and there are no other indicators of previous physical or mental health problems in her history. This is a good clue that the patient's partner's leaving is a very stressful event for her and a situational crisis that is likely causing these acute, short-term behaviors. Jack and Jill can help this patient by providing comfort, support, and counseling to help her reach a place where they can calmly discuss treatment options needed, if any.

47. B: Suicidal ideation is characterized by recurrent thoughts of suicide, ranging from passive ideation to active ideation. Homicidal ideation is characterized by thoughts or plans to kill another person or a group of people.

48. D: Severe allergies can be life-threatening and lead to anaphylaxis. An epinephrine injection pen is the first line of defense if a person comes into contact with an allergen to which he or she has a serious or life-threatening reaction.

49. D: Aspirin works by inhibiting platelet aggregation to prevent clot formation. Paxil® is used to treat anxiety and depression. Coumadin® (warfarin) works by blocking Vitamin K dependent clotting factors. Heparin enhances the effect of antithrombin III to inhibit thrombin activation.

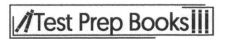

50. C: Heparin works by enhancing the effect of antithrombin III which prevents the activation of thrombin and thus prevents fibrinogen from being converted to fibrin. It is important to note that heparin does not get rid of pre-existing clots, it helps prevent clot expansion and formation of new clots. Paxil® is used to treat anxiety and depression. Coumadin® (warfarin) works by blocking Vitamin K dependent clotting factors. Aspirin works on platelet aggregation.

51. D: The blood vessels that carry blood back to the heart are called veins. Capillaries are where arteries and veins meet to exchange oxygen and carbon dioxide at the tissue level. Arteries carry blood away from the heart to the tissues of the body. Ventricles are a type of blood pumping chamber in the heart, although there are also ventricles in the brain that serve a different purpose.

52. A: The nurse should politely ask the patient to uncross her legs to get the most accurate blood pressure reading. Crossed legs can affect the blood pressure reading, since blood vessels can be compressed. Holding a remote, slouching, and resting the head will not compress any major arteries or veins, thus will not affect the blood pressure reading, so there is no need for the nurse to correct these positions.

53. D: The patient is displaying displacement, in which he is taking his negative feelings toward the doctor and expressing them toward the nurse, unreasonably. Reaction formation is when a person feels negatively but reacts positively. Intellectualization is when a person focuses on minute details of the situation rather than coping with the negative emotions associated with it. Undoing is when a person has done something wrong and acts excessively in the opposite way to redeem themselves of prior wrongdoing.

54. A: The chest pain described is most likely cardiac in origin, so the patient could be experiencing a myocardial infarction, or heart attack. Chest pain associated with gastroesophageal reflux is more often described as a burning sensation, without the other symptoms described. Pneumonia and pleuritis may both cause the patient to have a different type of chest pain, in which a sharp, stabbing sensation is felt upon breathing.

55. A: The nurse should review the pharmacology, or the action created by a drug, of the patient's current medications. Knowing the pharmacological effects of these medications and those of the scheduled preoperative medications can help keep the patient safe. Side effects and adverse reactions are included in the pharmacology. The intended effect does not include possible side effects or adverse reactions.

56. D: The patient interview adds subjective assessment data to the nurse's findings. Auscultation, palpation, and percussion yield objective assessment data.

57. C: The final phase of the nursing process is evaluation; however, evaluation happens across the continuum of the nursing process, not just at the end. The nurse frequently evaluates the effectiveness of care plans, adjusts as necessary, and reevaluates. Data is collected during the assessment phase. Nursing diagnoses are formulated in the diagnosis phase. The implementation phase often begins with educating the patient on expected outcomes.

58. A: One of the most serious side effects of prolonged vomiting is dehydration, thus the patient needs fluids to restore him back to a more normal, hydrated status. Antibiotics may be used in a case of severe bacterial infection, but not likely in this case. Anti-nausea medication will likely be used to stop the vomiting but will do nothing to fix the resulting dehydration. Physical therapy is not typically necessary for such a case unless the patient was bedridden for a long time, which does not seem to be the case here.

59. C: This type of seizure with muscle rigidity, convulsions, and unconsciousness is called a grand mal seizure. An absence seizure involves a brief loss of consciousness where the patient may stare into space. A myoclonic seizure involves the body making jerking movements. A tonic seizure is characterized by rigidity and stiffness of the muscles.

60. D: Itching and the development of a rash are signs that the patient is having an allergic reaction to a medication. These two symptoms are signs that the body's inflammatory response has been kicked into overdrive because of a drug allergy. The other symptoms listed are not commonly associated with an allergic reaction.

61. C: Patients on lisinopril are at risk for hyperkalemia; thus, the supplementation of potassium is to be done under careful clinical supervision or not at all. Lisinopril causes the body to hold on to more potassium than usual, and in renal-compromised patients, the risk for hyperkalemia is ever present. The other three electrolytes mentioned can cause toxic states in the body in low and high concentrations but not as life threatening as the cardiac disturbances a hyperkalemic state can bring about.

62. A: The platelet-aggregation inhibitor, aspirin, has the potential to work synergistically with warfarin in a way that would increase the patient's risk for bleeding. Synergistic drugs work together in ways that enhance each one's individual effectiveness, sometimes for the patient's good but sometimes to the patient's detriment. Lasix, lisinopril, and Protonix are other frequently used drugs that would not work synergistically with warfarin in any significant hemostatic way.

63. D: Though there are many benefits to the CVAD, it still poses a risk for infection to the patient, even more so than a peripheral device, as it is more centric to the patient's circulatory system and vital organs. The CVAD has many benefits, including being able to provide easy access for blood draws; the capacity to deliver large amounts of blood, drugs, and fluids to the patient; and decreasing peripheral sticks and the inflammation that goes along with those. The use of the CVAD must be carefully decided, weighing the pros against the cons.

64. B: The patient must have a chest x-ray to confirm correct placement of the PICC line. Correct placement will show that the PICC line tip is resting in the distal end of the superior vena cava, right at the cavoatrial junction. The other three imaging studies are not routinely ordered to confirm PICC line placement.

65. B: A subclavian catheter is an example of a nontunneled central venous access device. Jugular and femoral lines are other examples of nontunneled catheters. Examples of tunneled catheters include Groshong's, small-bore, Hickman's, and Broviac's.

66. B: The correct conversion of the patient's weight is 70 kilograms. This answer is found by dividing the weight in pounds, 155, by the number of kilograms that are found in a pound, 2.2, which gives the nurse the correct answer. The other three answers are incorrect.

67. A: The correct answer is 7.5 mL. The answer is obtained by using the desired dose divided by the amount on hand multiplied by the volume, or the D/H x V formula. By taking the desired dose (240 mg), dividing it by the amount on hand (160mg), and multiplying it by the volume the drug is formulated in (5 mL), the nurse will then arrive at the correct dose of 7.5 mL.

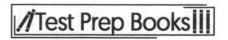

68. C: The formulary is an excellent tool the nurse can access that will give them up-to-date information about drugs, their safety and effectiveness, and their generic and brand names and is maintained and updated by a team of experts. The patient medication list is a separate document and is not used for broad medication reference. The facility procedure manual will give the nurse information about how to respond to a fire and other such facility information but not information in reference to medications. The electronic health record is a document used specifically in reference to the patient but not for general informational purposes.

69. C: The Z-track technique is used to avoid medication leakage into the subcutaneous tissue. The nurse pulls the skin downward or upward, injects the medication at a 90 degree angle, and then releases the skin to create the zigzag track. Aspiration is a technique that may be used to ensure the nurse has not accidentally accessed a vein or artery when injecting but is not necessary for routine injections into the deltoid where there are no large vessels. Massaging the injection site may cause leakage and irritation.

70. B: Right medical facility is not part of the six patient medication administration rights. The six rights are the following: right medication, right route, right time frame, right patient, right dosage, and right documentation.

71. A: *Parenteral* is the term that refers to any route outside of the gastrointestinal tract, also referred to as the *alimentary canal*. *Motor* is not a viable answer choice. *Enteral* also refers to the GI tract or intestines. *Buccal* refers to the cheeks, or inner oral cavity.

72. C: The Mantoux test, or annual tuberculosis test most nurses must undergo as part of facility policy, involves an intradermal injection of the TB proteins or antigens. The dermal layer of the skin is accessed, as opposed to a subcutaneous injection, which goes deeper into the skin. An intrathecal injection goes into the spinal canal. *Sublingual* refers to a route of administration of a drug that will go under the tongue.

73. D: The IV appears to have become dislodged, causing an infiltration of the surrounding tissues. This is marked by coolness and swelling of the site. The leaking of the fluid also suggests an infiltration of the IV site. A clot in the line would cause an obstruction to IV fluids and medications but not swelling of the surrounding tissue. Fluid overload would present systemic symptoms in the patient rather than localized swelling and coolness. An infected site would be warm rather than cool.

74. A: The TPN should be administered slowly, at 50 percent of the prescribed dosage, when beginning therapy. TPN comes with many possible complications as the body adjusts to this different source of nutrition, so starting slowly is recommended. The other three answers are incorrect.

75. A: The nurse assessing a stable, uncomplicated patient will most likely go for the radial pulse. The femoral pulse, found in the groin, would be an invasion of the patient's privacy and not appropriate for this type of routine checkup. The popliteal pulse, found behind the knee, would be an unusual and hard-to-reach spot for a routine pulse assessment. The carotid pulse is reserved for emergency situations such as cardiac arrest to assess for pulselessness before starting cardiopulmonary resuscitation (CPR).

76. D: The nurse should assess for orthostatic hypotension by performing lying/sitting/standing (LSS) blood pressure readings. If the readings trend downward significantly, up to twenty points in mmHg on the systolic side, the patient probably has orthostatic hypotension. Assessing for the patient's temperature and rate of breathing and comparing bilateral radial pulses can all be performed for the sake of having additional data but do not follow the symptoms this specific patient reported.

77. C: The mammography test is a type of x-ray, not computed tomography. While CT scans may be performed, x-rays are the gold standard for early detection of breast cancer. The patient is recommended to get the test once every year after the age of forty for early breast cancer detection. The test can pick up masses that may not be manually palpable to the patient or the practitioner.

78. B: Based on the symptoms of stomach pain and bloody emesis that the patient reported, they will likely be scheduled for an upper endoscopy. An upper endoscopy, also called an esophagogastroduodenoscopy (EGD), visualizes the internal mucosa of the upper gastrointestinal (GI) tract. A sigmoidoscopy visualizes the sigmoid portion of the colon. An anoscopy is performed to visualize the area just inside the anus. A colonoscopy is performed to assess and intervene within the entire colon, usually used for early detection of colon cancer.

79. A: A normal range for serum potassium is between 3.5 and 5.1 mEq/L; thus, 3.2 is the correct answer. 3.5 and 5.0 mEq/L suggest a normal serum potassium. A level of 5.5 mEq/L suggests a hyperkalemic state. The nurse should report hypokalemia and will prepare to administer potassium supplementation if ordered by the physician.

80. C: Thrombocytopenia means that there are a lower than normal number of platelets in the blood. The term comes from the root word "thrombocyte." The prefix "thrombo-" means clot, and the suffix "-cyte" means cell. These cells are responsible for the body's ability to stop bleeding by forming a clot. Neutropenia and leukopenia are used interchangeably referring to a lowered white blood cell count. *Neutrophils,* the root work for *neutropenia,* are the largest portion of the white blood cells. If the neutrophils are significantly lowered, then leukopenia results, thus the interchangeability of the words. Anemia refers to a lower than normal count of red blood cells and reduces the body's ability to carry and deliver oxygen.

81. B: The patient with a pH value of 7.25 is still very much acidotic and needs further therapy to return them to normal. The other values listed fall in the normal range of 7.35 to 7.45 or in the alkalotic range, which is greater than 7.45.

82. B: Liver failure is not a direct correlation with a patient's risk for aspirating. A weakened gag or swallow reflex, weakened upper and lower esophageal sphincters, and enteral feedings are all risk factors for aspiration. Patients with these risk factors should be monitored carefully during feeding times and have the head of their bed kept elevated to between 45 and 90 degrees while receiving feedings.

83. D: Breast cancer is not usually highly correlated to smoking cigarettes, although there is some evidence that smoking does not help a person's risk of avoiding breast cancer. Cancers of the mouth, throat, esophagus, and lungs are all closely correlated with a smoking habit due to their contact with the toxic inhaled smoke. The nurse notes the patient's risk factor for developing cancer in the patient medical record.

84. C: Observing and recording the patient's heart rhythm via ECG is the specific intervention necessary to monitor for the development of dysrhythmias postcardiac catheterization. All of the other interventions listed are correct postcardiac catheterization care but not specific to dysrhythmias. The nurse will keep the patient flat to assist with incision healing, take regular vital signs such as heart rate and blood pressure, and monitor for bleeding and hematoma at the incision site to evaluate the patient's overall stability.

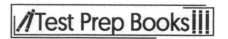

85. B: The nurse should hone in on the cardiac system by assessing the strength and rate of the patient's pulses, comparing them bilaterally. If the rate is above normal and the quality is weak, the nurse knows that the patient's heart is working extra hard, and the reason needs to be discovered. Assessing things like pitting edema, the patient's motor and sensory function, and muscular strength are not the most precise actions the nurse can take to quickly get to the bottom of the patient's symptomology. The nurse will use sound nursing judgment to determine which assessments to make on a patient and when.

86. B: A patient who is undergoing a minimally invasive procedure such as a mole removal will only need a local anesthetic such as topical lidocaine. A regional nerve block affects only one part of the body, usually targeting the epidural, spinal, or paravertebral regions. General anesthesia is used for major surgeries in which the patient needs to be rendered completely unconscious to perform the procedure.

87. C: The nurse may assess the rate of heart beats but not necessarily from chest tube drainage. The three common parameters for assessing drainage are consistency, quantity, and color. These are all ways to monitor and record chest output.

88. A: Based on the abdominal location of the radiation therapy, it is likely that the patient will experience gastrointestinal symptoms, including diarrhea, nausea, and vomiting, as a side effect. Fatigue, trembling, and muscle aches are possible with radiation therapy but not specific to the organs of the abdomen.

89. D: The oral glucose tolerance test is performed between the twenty-fourth and twenty-eighth week of pregnancy to screen for gestational diabetes. Hyperemesis gravidarum is a severe form of morning sickness that occurs in the first trimester but sometimes continues until the third trimester. Preeclampsia is detected through blood pressure monitoring. Iron-deficiency anemia may be detected first through symptoms of fatigue, weakness, and dizziness and then confirmed with a blood test showing a low hemoglobin and hematocrit count. These components of the red blood cells are responsible for carrying oxygen to the organs and tissues of the body and can drop during pregnancy.

90. B: The classic signs of infection are redness, heat, and swelling. If the wound is cool to the touch but appears normal otherwise, that is not suggestive of a developing infection. It may be a sign of decreased blood flow to the site, but the nurse should do a full assessment before jumping to that conclusion.

91. C: The incubation period is the point in time where the organism has already invaded the person's body through a portal of entry, is multiplying, and is getting ready to manifest the first symptoms of infection. The colonization occurs right after entry into the body where the organism takes up residence in the host and prepares to multiply. The prodromal period is when the person develops general signs or symptoms (such as fatigue, headache, fever, etc.) before developing more specific signs and symptoms that help point towards a diagnosis. The convalescent period is when the person is recovering from the illness.

92. C: Neutrophils are the major component of the white blood cells. When their count is elevated, that means the white blood cells are hard at work fighting an infectious process. The nurse would need to investigate this conclusion further, possibly getting an order to draw some blood cultures if appropriate. Blood urea nitrogen is a waste product of the body. An elevated level would suggest failing kidneys but not an infection. Hematocrit is a component of red blood cells and is not part of the body's immune system. A high sodium level is an electrolyte abnormality that may have to do with the renal system or overall patient fluid status but not an infectious process.

93. D: A right-heart catheter, also called a Swan-Ganz catheter or pulmonary artery catheter, is threaded through a patient's central veins into the superior vena cava, terminating at the pulmonary artery. This type of catheter is used for hemodynamic monitoring, giving information about the patient's preload and cardiac output. A PICC line, or peripherally inserted central catheter, can be used for medication and fluid administration but does not give information about hemodynamics. A port-a-cath is another type of central line used for similar purposes as the PICC line and can be kept in the patient for an extended period. A dialysis catheter is a long-term access device for patients receiving regular treatments of dialysis but is not used for hemodynamic monitoring.

94. A: The cardiac index reflects the quantity of blood pumped by the heart per minute per meter squared of the patient's body surface area. Cardiac output measures how much blood the heart pumps out per minute in liters. The mean arterial pressure, or MAP, shows the relationship between the amount of blood pumped out of the heart and the resistance the vascular system puts up against it. The stroke volume measures how much blood the heart pumps in milliliters per beat.

95. D: A calcium channel blocker can lower the pulmonary vascular resistance in a patient. Diuretics, morphine, and nitrates all have potent lowering effects on the systemic vascular resistance, as opposed to the pulmonary vasculature. Knowing the hemodynamic effects certain medications have is helpful in anticipating unwanted side effects and potential drug interactions.

96. B: The patient's cardiac output is very low, suggesting a possible bleed or hypotensive crisis. Normal cardiac output falls between 4 and 8 L/min. All the other values listed are within normal range. Normal mean arterial pressure is between 70 and 100 mmHg. Normal central venous pressure is between 2 and 6 mmHg. Normal pulmonary capillary wedge pressure is between 4 and 12 mmHg.

97. D: The nurse will see the patient who is complaining of shortness of breath first. Airway, breathing, and circulation are always the highest priority for the nurse to address, as they can quickly become life-threatening situations. Maintaining proper respiration is a vital function to the patient's well-being, and stabilization is necessary immediately. The woman who is nauseous and needs antiemetics such as Zofran is the second priority, as she is actively ill and there is something the nurse can do to help her symptoms. The nurse's third priority will be the patient who needs to sign the informed consent. The nurse needs to ensure she gets that signed before the patient leaves the floor, although there are nurses in the cardiac catheterization lab who can obtain the consent if need be. The patient who has a question about discharge is the last priority, as there is no immediate threat to his health and the doctor will need to see the patient before he is discharged anyway.

98. B: A chest radiograph is the test of choice to confirm the placement of a nasogastric tube. The x-ray will show whether the catheter tip is in the gastric body or not. Aspiration of stomach contents, not laryngeal secretions, with a pH test is another, less preferred way to confirm placement. The pH test may be misleading, as there may be gastric contents farther up the esophageal canal and not necessarily within the stomach in some patients with weakened sphincters. An abdominal ultrasound may show the catheter tip, but it is not the preferred method of evaluating placement. Manual palpation of the gastric body is not a way to confirm placement, as it would be very difficult to actually feel the catheter within the stomach.

99. A: A leakage of air into the pleural cavity outside of the lungs is called a *pneumothorax*. This may happen as a complication of central line placement for TPN. Hemothorax results when blood is leaked into the pleural cavity. *Hydrothorax* refers to a leakage of water into the pleural cavity. Pneumonia is an

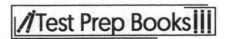

infection that forms in the lungs as the result of an infectious organism and may cause fluid to accumulate in the bases of the lungs.

100. D: Kegel exercises are performed to strengthen the pelvic floor and prevent urinary incontinence, among many other benefits. They are not specifically targeted at preventing postpartum hemorrhage, however. All three of the other options are correct. Massaging the uterine fundus will encourage uterine contractions, which will help prevent excessive bleeding. A boggy fundus is a worrisome sign. The nurse wants to feel a firm uterus, signaling healthy contractions. Monitoring vital signs, especially heart rate and blood pressure, will keep the nurse informed about the woman's hemodynamic stability. The nurse will encourage the patient to empty her bladder regularly, as bladder distention can displace the uterus and interfere with proper uterine contractions.

NCLEX Practice Test #2

1. What does the Patient Self Determination Act of the United States offer protection for?
    a. Patient rights to healthcare decisions that are made without coercion and are protected
    b. Patient rights to influenced decisions by nurses
    c. Patient rights to confidentiality in portal systems
    d. Patient rights to electronic prescriptions

2. Which form of consent does an unconscious patient provide when brought into the emergency department after an accident?
    a. Denied consent
    b. Explicit consent
    c. Implied consent
    d. Expressed consent

3. As the nurse advocates for the patient seeking emergency services, they explain that the patient has a right to receive care regardless of their ability to pay. What law is the nurse referencing in this scenario?
    a. Emergency Healthcare Act
    b. Emergency Medical Treatment and Active Labor Act
    c. The Stark Law
    d. False Claims Act

4. Which nonpharmacological aid should the nurse suggest for a patient with sensory processing disorder who is struggling to rest?
    a. Aromatherapy
    b. Weighted blanket
    c. Heating pad
    d. Television

5. The nurse is providing patient education to a client newly diagnosed with diabetes. Which organ does the nurse explain is responsible for secreting insulin to regulate blood glucose levels?
    a. Liver
    b. Kidney
    c. Pancreas
    d. Spleen

6. The nurse is conducting a community wellness course designed for patients pre-cholecystectomy. What substance does the nurse explain is stored in the gallbladder after being produced by the liver?
    a. Blood
    b. Marrow
    c. Bile
    d. Calcitonin

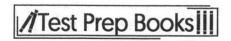

7. The nurse considers which of the following risk factors reported by the patient during the initial assessment to potentially be a trigger for the patient's current presentation of pain in the great toe? Select all that apply.

    a. Increased legumes in the diet

    b. Glass of wine daily with dinner

    c. Increased roughage in the diet

    d. Increased seafood in the diet

    e. Added weekly serving of liver

    f. Fruit juice with breakfast

8. After the nurse assesses the patient's vital signs and finds an elevated heart rate, elevated respirations, and low blood pressure, which position should the nurse place the patient in?

    a. Fowler's

    b. Right-lateral recumbent

    c. Passive leg raise

    d. Prone

9. Which heart rate does the nurse consider within normal range for the two-week-old patient?

    a. 54 beats per minute

    b. 171 beats per minute

    c. 198 beats per minute

    d. 62 beats per minute

10. Which phase of the cardiac cycle involves atrial contraction and is represented by the P wave of the electrocardiogram?

    a. Phase One

    b. Phase Two

    c. Phase Three

    d. Phase Four

11. Which pair is at the greatest risk for the development of domestic violence?

    a. Wealthy husband and wife who work very few hours and exhibit irritability during downtime

    b. Female toddler and father who was abused as a child

    c. Young adult brother and sister struggling with poverty

    d. Economically-disadvantaged husband and wife with limited access to healthcare

12. After noting significant stress in the patient recovering from a motor vehicle accident, the homecare case manager recognizes the patient is exhibiting irritability, frustration, and poor concentration. The nurse also assesses that the patient's vital signs have improved since the previous home visit last week. Which stage of the general adaptation syndrome is the patient presently functioning in?

    a. Homeostasis

    b. Alarm

    c. Resistance

    d. Exhaustion

13. During discharge education, the nurse recognizes that the patient has a clear understanding of most of the considerations for taking the prescribed Doxycycline for Lyme disease treatment. What statement made by the patient alerts the nurse that some additional teaching is necessary?

a. "I will take my medication with a full glass of water."
b. "I will not take iron supplements within two hours of this medication."
c. "I can continue breastfeeding while on this medication."
d. "I need to use a nonhormonal birth control to prevent pregnancy."

14. Before the patient undergoes a liver biopsy, which vitamin-based medication does the nurse administer?

a. Vitamin K
b. Vitamin D
c. Vitamin E
d. Vitamin A

15. After a patient presents to the emergency department with a chief complaint of chest pain, which priority action should the nurse complete FIRST?

a. Assess vital signs
b. Ask questions regarding the radiation of pain
c. Start an IV with normal saline
d. Page the cardiologist

16. During an inpatient hospitalization, a patient is struggling with an acute exacerbation of Meniere's disease. Which device would be most helpful to this patient during this time?

a. Leg lifter
b. Shower chair
c. Button hook
d. Voice box

17. When starting a benzodiazepine medication to treat Generalized Anxiety Disorder (GAD), what side effect should be reported to the prescriber right away?

a. Sedation
b. Agitation
c. Unsteadiness
d. Dizziness

18. A patient struggling with Sjogren's syndrome is prescribed Plaquenil® (hydroxychloroquine), an anti-malarial medication useful for treating a variety of autoimmune diseases. Which side effect is of GREATEST concern with this medication?

a. Bowel blockage
b. Hepatic toxicity
c. Mood changes
d. Retinal toxicity

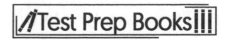

19. In reviewing diagnostic testing orders for a current patient, which antibody test does the nurse expect to see ordered for a patient struggling with symptoms of celiac disease?
    a. Antinuclear antibody
    b. Anti-thyroid peroxidase
    c. Anti-tissue transglutaminase IgA
    d. Anti-topoisomerase I antibody

20. A patient diagnosed with metastatic cancer is prescribed weekly therapeutic massage sessions for pain management. While engaging in patient education regarding complementary and alternative medicine, which therapeutic domain does the nurse explain that this treatment aligns with?
    a. Mind-body
    b. Energy
    c. Manipulative
    d. Biological

21. While working with a patient struggling with schizophrenia and paranoid symptoms, which non-pharmacological therapeutic aid should the nurse suggest to support symptom management?
    a. Book
    b. Television
    c. Instrumental music
    d. Food

22. A patient with metastatic prostate cancer that has spread to the pelvic and lower extremity bones is reporting symptoms of pain secondary to hormone deprivation therapy. What does the nurse encourage as the most helpful for symptom management at this time?
    a. Increase fluid consumption
    b. Cycling
    c. Music therapy
    d. Strength training

23. The nurse is reviewing the interpretation of the cardiac rhythm strip as sinus bradycardia. For this interpretation to be accurate, which heart rate must correlate with these findings?
    a. Below 60 beats per minute
    b. Above 150 beats per minute
    c. From 90–120 beats per minute
    d. From 121–150 beats per minute

24. The nurse responds to a 71-year-old patient presenting to the emergency department with signs and symptoms of septic shock. The patient was discharged from the medical-surgical floor last week after being treated for pneumonia. What findings support a septic shock diagnosis? Select all that apply.
    a. Metabolic acidosis
    b. Respiratory alkalosis
    c. Narrowing pulse pressure
    d. Increased cardiac output
    e. Hypertension

25. During patient intake, the two admission nurses are completing a full body assessment before the patient is introduced into the psychiatric milieu. What should the nurses do after discovering illicit drugs in a small bag concealed in the patient's hair bun?

a. Confiscate the drugs and report this finding to the police to let them decide how to proceed with the patient.
b. Confiscate the drugs and page the nursing supervisor to elevate this concern.
c. Send the illicit drugs home with the patient's spouse.
d. Place the drugs in the patient's belonging bag that the security team monitors and releases back to the patient upon discharge.

26. What score represents the degree to which a patient's psychological symptoms impact their daily life?

a. Apgar score
b. AIMS score
c. GAF score
d. Withdrawal protocol score

27. What defense mechanism, characterized by unconsciously inhibiting thoughts and transferring symptoms, is associated with conversion disorder?

a. Projection
b. Repression
c. Reaction formation
d. Intellectualization

28. A fifteen-year-old male patient is prescribed Haldol® (haloperidol) while inpatient at a psychiatric hospital. The nurse is concerned after the patient complains of nipple discharge from the left breast with subsequent focused assessment findings revealing swelling, pain, and tenderness. What side effect of this medication is the nurse concerned the patient may be experiencing?

a. Stevens-Johnson syndrome
b. Nystagmus
c. Gynecomastia
d. Schizoaffective disorder

29. Which psychotropic medication class necessitates a tyramine-avoidant diet?

a. Selective serotonin reuptake Inhibitors
b. Atypical antipsychotics
c. Tricyclic antidepressants
d. Monoamine oxidase inhibitors

30. The nurse reviews the provider's order, which reads "750 mL of D5W to infuse over 7 hours." The drop factor is 10 gtts/mL. What drip rate should the nurse set this infusion at?

a. 18 gtts/min
b. 420 gtts/min
c. 36 gtts/min
d. 75 gtts/min

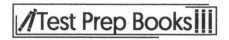

31. During the nurse-to-nurse report, the patient is described as struggling with aphasia. Which description correlates to this finding?
    a. Unable to perform movements
    b. Difficulty sitting still
    c. Difficulty swallowing
    d. Unable to understand or produce speech

32. What color stool does the nurse expect to note from a patient struggling with a bile duct blockage?
    a. White
    b. Green
    c. Black
    d. Red

33. The community health nurse is facilitating an educational class on assistive devices and answers a question regarding the proper length of a cane. Which response by the nurse correctly answers this question?
    a. "Canes should be the length that feels most comfortable for each individual."
    b. "The length of the cane should support the elbow to be only slightly flexed."
    c. "It is best for the cane to be the length that encourages full flexion of the elbow."
    d. "A properly fitted cane allows you to lean forward with full extension of the elbow during ambulation."

34. In receiving a new patient upon admission to an inpatient room, the nurse delegates appropriate tasks to the unlicensed assistive personnel (UAP). What equipment is appropriate for the UAP to safely start on the patient?
    a. Cervical traction
    b. Ventilator
    c. Hemovac drain
    d. Sequential compression device

35. After reviewing a patient's lab work, the nurse recognizes that the patient's antinuclear antibody (ANA) titer is 1:640 with a speckled pattern. What specialist consult does the nurse expect to see ordered next for diagnostic testing?
    a. Dermatology
    b. Cardiology
    c. Rheumatology
    d. Gastroenterology

36. While working with a patient scheduled for an upcoming procedure, the nurse provides education to prepare the patient on what to expect during the test. Which statement made by the nurse accurately describes electromyography?
    a. "A needle will be inserted into your muscle to extract a small sample of tissue."
    b. "A probe will be inserted through your skull."
    c. "A needle will be inserted into your skin at strategic points."
    d. "A needle electrode will be inserted into your muscle."

37. Which type of consent provides the nurse with the opportunity to conduct cardiopulmonary resuscitation on an unaccompanied unconscious patient?

    a. Expressed consent

    b. Opt-out consent

    c. Implied consent

    d. Informed consent

38. While analyzing a patient's coagulation test results, the nurse reviews the prothrombin time test. Which finding aligns with a normal result indicative of proper clotting time prior to the patient's scheduled surgery?

    a. 5 seconds

    b. 14 seconds

    c. 40 seconds

    d. 51 seconds

39. The nurse is delegating the morning weight for a patient with anorexia nervosa and generalized anxiety disorder to the unlicensed assistive personnel (UAP). Which actions by the UAP does the nurse observe that support a thorough understanding of how to accurately obtain this finding? Select all that apply.

    a. Weigh in paper gown

    b. Weigh immediately following breakfast

    c. Weigh in the hall

    d. Weigh with patient's back toward reading

    e. Weigh after a void

40. When reducing the risk of infection transmission, which personal protective equipment (PPE) should the nurse don first?

    a. Gloves

    b. Mask

    c. Gown

    d. Goggles

41. After suspecting celiac disease due to symptom presentation and antibody testing, which tissue test should be performed to diagnose this autoimmune disease?

    a. Small intestine biopsy

    b. Large intestine biopsy

    c. Stomach biopsy

    d. Rectal biopsy

42. During an abdominal physical assessment of a patient with gastrointestinal distress, which action should the nurse perform second?

    a. Percussion

    b. Auscultation

    c. Inspection

    d. Palpation

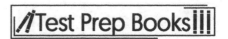

43. During a respiratory physical assessment of a patient with shortness of breath, which action should the nurse perform second?
    a. Inspection
    b. Percussion
    c. Palpation
    d. Auscultation

44. Which fasting blood sugar level is considered within normal range for a healthy client?
    a. 54 mg/dL
    b. 82 mg/dL
    c. 110 mg/dL
    d. 123 mg/dL

45. Which stage of disease is a patient noted to be experiencing when they are asymptomatic following exposure to a pathogenic organism?
    a. Incubation period
    b. Prodromal period
    c. Acute period
    d. Convalescence period

46. Which routine treatment for cystic fibrosis facilitates movement of secretions from small to large airways for subsequent expulsion?
    a. Antibiotics
    b. The six-foot rule
    c. Pulmonary function tests
    d. Chest physiotherapy

47. The nurse caring for a patient post lung lobectomy detects a chest tube air leak when assessing the water-seal chamber after surgery. Which response by the nurse is appropriate at this time?
    a. Call the provider to report the concern.
    b. Document the finding in the patient's chart and continue to monitor.
    c. Elevate this finding to the nursing supervisor.
    d. Initiate a rapid response to obtain support.

48. The nurse is educating a 43-year-old patient regarding their fracture, which has resulted in the fragmentation of the bones in their right hand after a motor vehicle accident. Which type of fracture represents this finding?
    a. Compound fracture
    b. Oblique fracture
    c. Comminuted fracture
    d. Greenstick fracture

49. Which statement made by the nurse encourages a therapeutic engagement with the patient awaiting test results post mastectomy?
    a. "Tell me more about how you feel."
    b. "If the margins aren't clear, you should explore your feelings with your therapist."
    c. "I have worked with many patients faced with your situation."
    d. "If it were me, I would wait until I knew more before deciding what to do next."

50. While working with a female patient 25 years older than the male nurse, the nurse notices that the patient repeatedly shames him and questions his intentions during interventions. After elevating this concern, the nurse case manager discussed this occurrence with the patient. During the discussion, the patient reported that the nurse reminds her of her son, who has ongoing struggles with honesty and maintaining commitments. What is this skewed engagement an example of?

    a. Regression
    b. Countertransference
    c. Transference
    d. Repression

51. When completing an assessment, the nurse notes that the patient has muscular movement only when assisted by gravity. How should the nurse document this finding using the Muscular Strength Scale from 0-5?

    a. 0/5
    b. 1/5
    c. 2/5
    d. 3/5

52. The nurse is completing a pain assessment on an adolescent patient with rheumatoid arthritis who recently suffered a blunt hit to the femur during a field hockey game, and due to the stress of the event, is now experiencing a painful autoimmune flare. Which term describes an exacerbation of pain experienced in addition to long-term underlying pain?

    a. Acute
    b. Chronic-on-acute
    c. Chronic
    d. Acute-on-chronic

53. While providing patient education, the nurse explains that the patient's medication dosage will need to be adjusted to find the most therapeutic level. What is this measured medication practice an example of?

    a. Medication compliance
    b. Medication reconciliation
    c. Medication titration
    d. Medication administration

54. The registered nurse (RN) delegated the first step of the medication reconciliation process to the licensed practical nurse (LPN). Which action by the LPN signified understanding of this step?

    a. Ensured that all medication dosages are within therapeutic range by reviewing lab work
    b. Called the prescriber to clarify an order's dosage when handwriting is illegible
    c. Collected a complete medication history
    d. Documented each medication change and ensured it aligned with all other medication material

55. Which medication does the nurse expect the patient with hyperthyroidism, an overactive thyroid condition, to be prescribed for disease management?

    a. Synthroid® (levothyroxine)
    b. Armour® Thyroid (thyroid desiccated)
    c. Cytomel® (liothyronine sodium)
    d. Tapazole® (methimazole)

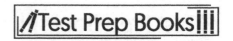

56. While caring for a patient with thyroid disease, the nurse provides education during a primary care appointment to review medication options for thyroid hormone replacement and diet. Which dietary mineral does the nurse encourage the patient to monitor their consumption of?
    a. Iodine
    b. Cobalt
    c. Copper
    d. Manganese

57. What diet is best for the patient diagnosed with phenylketonuria (PKU)?
    a. Low protein
    b. High protein
    c. Low folic acid
    d. High folic acid

58. The home health nurse is meeting with a client after finishing lunch and notices that the client's meal was contraindicated for their condition. Which meal option caused the nurse to feel concerned that the patient with gout does not fully understand appropriate nutritional selection for their condition?
    a. Rice pasta with coconut oil
    b. Liver and onions without bun
    c. Baked potato, plain without cheese
    d. Celery with peanut butter

59. After finishing a tube feeding, which position should the nurse delegate the licensed practical nurse (LPN) to place the patient in?
    a. Semi-Fowler's
    b. Prone
    c. Left side with head of bed flat
    d. Right side with head of bed elevated

60. How should the nurse document the finding of a patient's elevated respiratory rate?
    a. Tachypnea
    b. Orthopnea
    c. Tachycardia
    d. Hyperthermia

61. Which thyroid-stimulating hormone (TSH) level drawn at a preconception appointment would indicate that the patient might need to take thyroid hormone medication to support a healthy pregnancy?
    a. 5.2 mU/L
    b. 2.8 mU/L
    c. 1.7 mU/L
    d. 0.2 mU/L

62. During an appointment with primary care, the patient undergoes lab work to screen for type II diabetes mellitus with the need for insulin management, as the previously drawn hemoglobin A1C from one year ago was supportive of a pre-diabetes diagnosis. Which hemoglobin A1C result alerts the nurse that the patient may now have type II diabetes mellitus and an additional round of testing should be done to confirm?

    a. 3.8 percent
    b. 4.2 percent
    c. 5.9 percent
    d. 6.8 percent

63. The psychiatric nurse is working with a patient who is identified as struggling with a panic attack during inpatient hospitalization. Which as needed (prn) medication does the nurse offer the patient to support symptom management at this time?

    a. Clonidine
    b. Lamotrigine
    c. Fluoxetine
    d. Clonazepam

64. After multiple failed medication trials, which medication may be considered to support psychotic symptom management for a patient struggling with schizoaffective disorder?

    a. Clozapine
    b. Lithobid
    c. Alprazolam
    d. Sertraline

65. A nurse identifies that many collaborative peers have contributed to a possible sentinel event. Does the accredited hospital have to report the sentinel event to The Joint Commission after the nurse elevates their report of the incident?

    a. Yes, always report it.
    b. No, these are always internal only.
    c. Yes, in some cases.
    d. No, but it is encouraged.

66. Which law does the nurse abide by when protecting the patient's personal health information (PHI) while providing a report for continuing care?

    a. Health Information Portability and Accountability Act
    b. Emergency Medical Treatment and Active Labor Act
    c. False Claims Act
    d. Hospital Readmissions Reduction Program

67. The patient must make a decision regarding the next steps in their plan of treatment and in doing so, is weighing out two significantly different care options. Which ethical provision does the nurse practice when ensuring that the patient has the right to make self-directed decisions?

    a. Beneficence
    b. Autonomy
    c. Non-Maleficence
    d. Justice

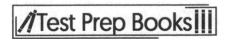

68. Which equipment should the nurse delegate to the unlicensed assistive personnel (UAP) to appropriately chart the outcome of?
    a. Glucometer
    b. Ventilator
    c. Cervical traction devices
    d. Continuous passive motion machine

69. While completing a physical assessment for suspected aortoiliac occlusive disease on a 68-year-old patient, which locations should the nurse assess blood pressure and pulse to detect a blockage? Select all that apply.
    a. Thigh
    b. Arm
    c. Calf
    d. Foot
    e. Wrist

70. The nurse is part of a collaborative team supporting a patient to improve their health status secondary to a multiple myeloma diagnosis. While engaging in a bisphosphonate treatment plan, which imaging needs to be completed to assess progress?
    a. CT Scan
    b. Ultrasound
    c. MRI
    d. Bone scan

71. Which hormone's primary function is to influence the kidneys to balance the amount of water excreted in urine?
    a. Follicle-stimulating hormone
    b. Antidiuretic hormone
    c. Adrenocorticotrophic hormone
    d. Luteinizing hormone

72. The community health nurse is facilitating a Parkinson's disease support group. Which neurotransmitter does the nurse describe as clinically deficient and responsible for symptoms such as tremor, slowness, and stiffness in the patient struggling with Parkinson's disease?
    a. Dopamine
    b. Serotonin
    c. Glutamate
    d. Acetylcholine

73. While working with a patient struggling with anorexia nervosa during an inpatient hospitalization, the charge nurse is assigning tasks. Which task delegated to the mental health worker, an unlicensed assistive member of the team, should have been assigned to a nurse?
    a. Observing the patient during mealtime to determine the percentage of the meal consumed
    b. Standing outside the patient's bathroom door during use after the meal
    c. Delivering the oral Ensure® nutritional supplement to the patient
    d. Providing patient education about the physical effects of this psychiatric condition

74. While the nurse case manager is participating in the psychiatric treatment team meeting, they inquire about the discharges scheduled for the next day. Which patient does the nurse case manager advocate to be rescheduled for discharge several days out?

    a. The patient who had their last round of electroconvulsive therapy this morning

    b. The patient who needs a prior authorization to fill their medication post discharge

    c. The patient who started Clozaril® (clozapine) yesterday

    d. The patient complaining of a headache after missing lunch today

75. The nurse is reviewing new medication orders for a patient with multiple diagnoses, including pernicious anemia. As the nurse has a clear understanding of this type of anemia, which treatment do they suspect to see ordered via subcutaneous injection for this patient?

    a. Iron

    b. Vitamin B-12

    c. Packed RBCs

    d. Stem cells

76. What is the nursing priority for test monitoring during the first day of delivery of total parenteral nutrition (TPN) to a pediatric patient?

    a. Glucose

    b. Vitamin B-12

    c. Calcium

    d. Vitamin D

77. Why is intravenous gamma globulin being administered to the pediatric patient with acquired immune deficiency syndrome (AIDS)?

    a. To increase the absorption of nutritional intake

    b. To inhibit the transmission of AIDS from the patient to others

    c. To reduce nausea and vomiting

    d. To prevent bacterial infections

78. Which medication is delivered via infusion as a treatment for bone metastases for the patient with cancer?

    a. Taxotere® (docetaxel)

    b. Zometa® (zoledronic acid)

    c. Doxil® (doxorubicin)

    d. Xeloda® (capecitabine)

79. The nurse is educating a patient regarding their anemic state. Which organ is the source of the patient's bone failure to produce red blood cells?

    a. Stomach

    b. Kidney

    c. Gallbladder

    d. Hypothalamus

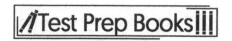

80. Which second-level stage of Maslow's hierarchy of needs must the nurse also support while meeting the patient's priority physiological needs?
    a. Safety
    b. Love and belonging
    c. Esteem
    d. Self-actualization

81. Which accessory organ(s) contribute to digestive activities? Select all that apply.
    a. Salivary Glands
    b. Liver
    c. Large Intestine
    d. Pancreas
    e. Gallbladder

82. Which respiratory rate alerts the nurse to a potential problem in a six-month-old infant?
    a. 24 breaths/minute
    b. 31 breaths/minute
    c. 43 breaths/minute
    d. 56 breaths/minute

83. During an annual physical with primary care, the nurse is reviewing osteoclast and osteoblast functions while providing education to a 78-year-old patient struggling with osteoporosis. Which hormone does the nurse explain increases osteoclast activity?
    a. Insulin
    b. Renin
    c. Parathyroid hormone
    d. Serotonin

84. During a level of consciousness assessment, the nurse finds no articulated verbal response with limited moaning, accompanied by arousal only after vigorous stimulation. How should the nurse document these findings?
    a. "The patient is lethargic."
    b. "The patient is obtunded."
    c. "The patient is stuporous."
    d. "The patient is comatose."

85. The critical care nurse is engaged in a nurse-to-nurse report with the medical-surgical step-down nurse and describes the patient's pitting edema as 2+. Which description aligns with the receiving nurse's understanding of a 2+ finding for planning care?
    a. Barely detectable indentation.
    b. Indentation takes 15 seconds to rebound.
    c. Indentation takes 30 seconds to rebound.
    d. Indentation takes greater than 30 seconds to rebound.

86. While functioning as a preceptor to orient a graduate nurse, the senior nurse is observing the assessment for pitting edema in a patient with emphysema. Which location assessed for skin indentation demonstrates a thorough understanding of this skill by the graduate nurse?

a. Radius
b. Femur
c. Ulna
d. Tibia

87. The nurse delegates two-hour post-meal finger sticks to the unlicensed assistive personnel (UAP) for patients with type II diabetes mellitus. Which blood glucose level(s) concerns the nurse? Select all that apply.

a. 60 mg/dL
b. 100 mg/dL
c. 125 mg/dL
d. 140 mg/dL
e. 195 mg/dL

88. Following a vasectomy, a patient presents to urgent care with a chief complaint of blood in their semen. Which response by the nurse is appropriate at this time?

a. "As you are one week post-operative, this is a normal finding and should resolve soon."
b. "This is a warning sign that the vasectomy may be ineffective in producing sterilization."
c. "As you are experiencing this adverse effect, it is likely that you will continue to experience blood in your semen for your lifetime."
d. "I have paged your surgeon because this is a sign that you are hemorrhaging inside your scrotum."

89. The nurse is caring for a patient with congestive heart failure and is reviewing their medications with them during medication teaching. The patient expresses concern about their potassium level after recalling an issue with low potassium when prescribed a diuretic in the past. Which medication does the nurse explain is a potassium-sparing diuretic during this teaching?

a. Lasix® (furosemide)
b. Demadex® (toresemide)
c. Aldactone® (spironolactone)
d. Microzide® (hydrochlorothiazide)

90. Which medication is a monoamine oxidase inhibitor (MAOI) antidepressant?

a. Celexa® (citalopram)
b. Lexapro® (escitalopram)
c. Prozac® (fluoxetine)
d. Parnate® (tranylcypromine)

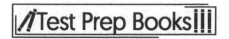

91. The emergency crisis nurse is meeting with a patient to complete a psychiatric evaluation to assess the patient's current condition and determine next steps for treatment. During the assessment, the patient explains that they have discontinued their Zoloft® (sertraline) medication without the guidance of their psychiatrist. Which condition does the nurse first suspect that the patient may be experiencing as a result of the abrupt discontinuation of this medication?
   a. Serotonin syndrome
   b. Neuroleptic malignant syndrome
   c. Prader-Willi syndrome
   d. MAOI syndrome

92. Which patient care intervention is appropriate for the nurse to delegate to the mental health worker, an unlicensed assistive member of the team?
   a. Completing an AIMS exam
   b. Recording patient behavior on the seclusion flowchart
   c. Evaluating the patient responses to the Clozaril® (clozapine) protocol questionnaire
   d. Documenting the findings of a patient fall screening

93. What should the nurse do FIRST when working with a patient who has a tracheostomy and does not use a speaking valve to communicate?
   a. Provide a speaking valve so that the patient can verbally engage
   b. Encourage the patient to write the words they would like to communicate
   c. Request that the patient draw basic pictures on a drawing board
   d. Assess the patient's preferred method of communication

94. Which complementary and alternative medicine (CAM) technique for stress management involves promoting the body's natural healing response via energy fields stimulated by placing the practitioner's hands on or close to the patient's body?
   a. Reiki
   b. Myofascial release
   C. Shiatsu massage
   d. Biofeedback

95. A 72-year-old patient has been admitted post total knee arthroplasty. The patient tells the nurse, "I have been struggling to find meaning lately and have been reaching out to friends to tell the story of my late husband's sudden passing 6 months ago." Which stage of the Kubler-Ross Grief Cycle is this patient's statement aligned with?
   a. Denial
   b. Anger
   c. Bargaining
   d. Depression

96. Before completing a rape kit examination, the sexual assault nurse examiner (SANE) recognizes the need for the patient to give written consent for the examination. What should the nurse do to ensure consent?

    a. Sensitively explain the procedure and ask the patient to sign the consent form.

    b. Tell the physician that the patient already asked questions, so a verbal consent can be used to proceed instead.

    c. Request that the patient's sister, who accompanied them to the examination, sign the consent, as the patient is currently distracted over the precipitating event.

    d. Ensure that the physician explains the procedure in detail and observe that the patient signs the consent form.

97. While discussing psychotropic medication and providing education on dosing and frequency, a patient tells the nurse that they did not refuse to take their Lamictal® (lamotrigine) the day before, as another nurse had documented. Which legislative act decrees that the patient retains the right to correct their medical record?

    a. Health Insurance Protection and Portability Act

    b. False Claims Act

    c. Medical Record Amendment Act

    d. Health Care Quality Improvement Act

98. During the morning community meeting for the adult intensive outpatient program, the clients are identifying their personal goals for the week. Which goal identified by the client struggling with substance abuse does the nurse recognize as realistic?

    a. Use the substance of choice in moderation.

    b. Stop needing to connect with their sponsor.

    c. Avoid places where they typically have used substances in the past.

    d. Use self-control to prevent all cravings.

99. While discussing precipitating events that led to inpatient hospitalization, the young adult patient struggling with major depressive disorder states, "My mother hasn't loved me since I was a little kid." Which response by the nurse encourages therapeutic engagement?

    a. "Have you asked your sister if she knows whether or not your mother loves you?"

    b. "I am sure your mother still loves you and is proud of you."

    c. "Focusing on your mother not loving you will make you feel worse."

    d. "What has led you to believe that?"

100. While discussing signs and symptoms of urinary tract infections, the nurse encourages the patient to report painful urination if the symptom arises. Which term is used to describe this finding?

    a. Anuria

    b. Oliguria

    c. Dysuria

    d. Polyuria

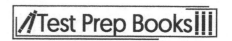

101. While reviewing patient dietary plans, the nurse observes an order for a low sodium diet and quickly becomes concerned. Which patient diagnosis paired with this diet alerts the nurse to a potential order error?
   a. Postural orthostatic tachycardia syndrome
   b. Congestive heart failure
   c. Chronic kidney disease
   d. Pulmonary hypertension

102. The nurse case manager is interfacing with physical therapy regarding patient education on the use of a newly prescribed walker. Which of the following safety guidelines should the patient be educated on to safely use their new walker?
   a. Grooved rubber tips that cover the bottom of the walker's legs should not be used.
   b. Waxed floors support grip while ambulating.
   c. Step up onto curbs with the strong leg before the weak leg.
   d. Carry the walker up a set of stairs on the nonaffected side.

103. While completing oral care on an unconscious patient in the intensive care unit, which position should the nurse place the patient in?
   a. Prone
   b. Supine
   c. Fowler's
   d. Side-lying

104. After presenting to the emergency department with flu-like symptoms, the nurse takes the patient's vital signs. What stage of the nursing process is the nurse functioning in during this interaction?
   a. Planning
   b. Assessment
   c. Diagnosis
   d. Implementation

105. The licensed practical nurse (LPN) is gathering data from a patient that presented to urgent care with prolonged diarrhea and vomiting. The patient reports struggling with weakness, fatigue, heart palpitations, and muscle aches. Which potassium level does the registered nurse (RN) expect to review on the metabolic panel results, considering the symptoms present in the LPN's notes?
   a. 3.0 mEq/L
   b. 3.5 mEq/L
   c. 4.0 mEq/L
   d. 4.5 mEq/L

106. After the patient complains of right upper quadrant pain, which organ does the nurse examine further?
   a. Liver
   b. Stomach
   c. Pancreas
   d. Appendix

107. Procardia® (nifedipine) has been prescribed for a patient in preterm labor. Which response by the nurse correctly describes why this medication has been ordered?

a. "Since this medication blocks calcium, it should help to relax your uterine muscles."

b. "We are hoping to control your pain with this medication."

c. "This medication is designed to raise your blood pressure, which will help you feel better."

d. "This medication will help increase the frequency of your contractions to help expedite the delivery."

108. Which symptom presentation closely aligns with refeeding syndrome for the patient who is receiving total enteral nutrition (TEN)?

a. Nausea and vomiting

b. Weakness, shallow respirations, seizures

c. Peripheral edema, crackles in lungs, bounding pulse

d. Elevated temperature, shortness of breath, increased pulse

109. Which supplement does the nurse plan to administer to the patient struggling with alcohol withdrawal upon admission to the hospital?

a. Niacin

b. Thiamine

c. Riboflavin

d. Folate

110. Which medication alerts the nurse to contact the prescriber to verify the order due to contraindication for a patient with benign prostatic hypertrophy?

a. Fluoxetine

b. Acetaminophen

c. Levothyroxine

d. Ipratropium bromide

111. Which priority intervention should the nurse engage in first after assessing clear nasal drainage in a patient with a head injury?

a. Assess the patient's temperature

b. Check the drainage for the presence of glucose with strip test

c. Send a culture of the drainage to the lab

d. Encourage the patient to blow their nose

112. An adolescent patient presents to the emergency department with a report of sustaining a head injury during a sporting event prior to arrival. Which assessment findings alert the nurse to the patient experiencing Cushing's triad?

a. Bradypnea, tachycardia, widening pulse pressure

b. Tachypnea, bradycardia, narrowing pulse pressure

c. Bradypnea, bradycardia, widening pulse pressure

d. Tachypnea, tachycardia, narrowing pulse pressure

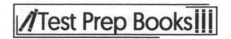

113. The nurse is completing an initial assessment of a patient presenting to the emergency department post motor vehicle accident. The treatment team suspects that the patient may be suffering from head trauma given the details of the report from emergency transport. Which signs and symptoms does the nurse identify that directly support a diagnosis of increased intracranial pressure? Select all that apply.
   a. Nausea
   b. Vomiting
   c. Headache
   d. Blurred vision
   e. Lethargy

114. The nurse is administering a blood transfusion to a patient with liver disease. Which signs and symptoms encourage the nurse to stop the transfusion due to a transfusion reaction? Select all that apply.
   a. Back pain
   b. Shortness of breath
   c. Skin flushing
   d. Hematoma at needle insertion site
   e. Damp IV dressing

115. When administering total parenteral nutrition (TPN), what should the nurse direct the patient to do while changing the bag or bottle?
   a. Valsalva maneuver
   b. Deep breathing
   c. Count to ten, then swallow
   d. Plug ears

116. The nurse is educating the patient regarding nutritional intake and explaining potential side effects of total parenteral nutrition (TPN). While discussing these implications, the nurse used a medical term that this form of nutrition is also known as, which confused the patient. What term did the nurse interchangeably use?
   a. Oral nutritional supplementation
   b. Parenteral hyperalimentation
   c. PEG tube nutrition
   d. Peripheral parenteral nutrition

117. A patient presents to urgent care complaining of pain. After closer examination, a diagnosis of two broken ribs is made and the patient is prescribed opiates for pain management. What additional medication does the nurse expect to see ordered at this time to combat a common side effect of this drug class?
   a. Dolophine® (methadone)
   b. Biaxin® (clarithromycin)
   c. Tegretol® (carbamazepine)
   d. Colace® (docusate sodium)

118. Before administering Catapres® (clonidine), which action does the nurse delegate to the unlicensed assistive personnel (UAP)?
   a. Assist the patient with eating their meal
   b. Ask the patient for the time of their last bowel movement
   c. Take the patient's vital signs
   d. Deliver a heated blanket to the patient's lower extremities

119. What should the nurse administer as a large initial infusion to quickly raise a patient's drug plasma level?
   a. Intermittent intravenous bolus
   b. Loading dose
   c. Onset bolus dose
   d. Maintenance dose

120. A 16-year-old patient presents to the emergency department with a previous diagnosis of anorexia nervosa by her outpatient provider. She is 64 inches tall and weighs 92 pounds. After further discussion, she reveals that she has been consuming only one meal per day for the past two weeks. While reviewing the patient's laboratory results to assess for potential electrolyte imbalances, which potassium result is a cause for concern?
   a. 3.9 mEq/L
   b. 2.7 mEq/L
   c. 4.5 mEq/L
   d. 5.0 mEq/L

121. A 52-year-old menopausal woman reports to urgent care complaining of confusion and muscle aches. While reviewing the patient's laboratory results to assess for a potential calcium imbalance, which calcium result(s) does the nurse identify as outside of normal range? Select all that apply.
   a. 8.5 mg/dL
   b. 9.2 mg/dL
   c. 7.8 mg/dL
   d. 10.3 mg/dL
   e. 11.2 mg/dL

122. In adapting to a terminal diagnosis, the patient inquires about activities that target symptoms of sadness, mourning, and grief. Which therapeutic intervention does the nurse suggest to reduce the risk of these symptoms becoming increasingly debilitating for the patient during this time?
   a. Donate belongings to someone in need
   b. Contribute to a development project in the backyard
   c. Attend weekly radical acceptance groups
   d. Plan a trip with family for next year

123. While caring for a patient with renal failure who is on dialysis, which secondary diagnosis does the nurse educate that the patient is MOST at risk for developing?
   a. Systemic lupus erythematous
   b. Migraine headaches
   c. Anemia
   d. Crohn's disease

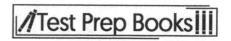

124. Which patient-centered goal is the primary responsibility of the nurse case manager to support?
 a. A reduced length of stay
 b. The ability to care for self
 c. Readmission to the unit post discharge
 d. Connection with support system

125. A nurse is looking to provide information regarding a patient to another nurse utilizing audiotape technology. What is this process referred to as?
 a. Consultation
 b. Case management
 c. Documentation
 d. Report

126. The nurse is viewing a record that contains diverse information from all providers involved in the patient's care. What type of communication system is the nurse using?
 a. Electronic health record (EHR)
 b. Electronic medication administration record (EMAR)
 c. Electronic medical record (EMR)
 d. Personal health record (PHR)

127. Upon retiring from practice after forty years, the nurse shares with their novice colleagues that they have experienced numerous healthcare documentation methods throughout their career. What is new technology that replaces a previously established technology identified as?
 a. Protocol
 b. Disruptive
 c. Gateway
 d. Recovery

128. In guiding practice, the nurse is aware of the nursing science and philosophy of law. What is this practice referred to as?
 a. Fundamentals of nursing
 b. Basic human rights
 c. Nursing process
 d. Nursing jurisprudence

129. What is the activity of providing patient-centered care via a modified scientific method of sequential steps called?
 a. Nursing process
 b. Ethical guidance
 c. Health maintenance
 d. Cultural competence

130. What is the most fundamental stage of Maslow's Hierarchy of Needs that the nurse should consider when prioritizing a client's wellbeing?
 a. Love and belonging
 b. Safety
 c. Physiological
 d. Self-Actualization

131. According to Erikson's Psychosocial Development Theory, how should the nurse educate new parents to respond to their newborn infant's needs?
    a. Wait for the infant to signal all needs
    b. Allow the infant to signal some needs
    c. Anticipate all infant needs
    d. Provide a delayed response to the infant's signal

132. A parent of a 24-month-old child asks the nurse about age-related development considerations during a well visit. What process can most 24-month-old children engage in successfully during mealtime?
    a. Eating with a fork
    b. Cutting with a kid-friendly knife
    c. Drinking from a cup
    d. Pouring into a cup

133. When the client arrived at the psychiatric clinic for their antipsychotic medication, what symptom did the nurse note that supported a concern for tardive dyskinesia?
    a. Tongue thrusting
    b. Headache
    c. Blurred vision
    d. Fever

134. According to Naegele's Rule, what is the estimated date of confinement (EDC) for a pregnant woman who's last menstrual cycle started on 9/18/2019?
    a. 6/18/2020
    b. 6/26/2010
    c. 6/11/2020
    d. 6/30/2020

135. While working with expectant parents to discuss the pending home birth for their first child, the nurse is educating on what to expect during the periods of reactivity. How long does the first period of reactivity last for a newborn right after birth?
    a. 30 minutes
    b. 60 minutes
    c. 120 minutes
    d. 240 minutes

136. While completing an assessment of a pregnant woman in her third trimester, the nurse takes this opportunity to educate the patient on what will be reviewed in her pending labs. What common pregnancy condition occurs in this trimester?
    a. Hypercalcemia
    b. Metabolic alkalosis
    c. Physiologic anemia
    d. Mastocytosis

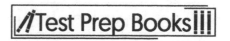

137. During a home visit, the nurse notices that the 68-year-old client is struggling to follow the images and diagrams on the educational handout. What symptom prompts the nurse to encourage the patient to have an eye examination for possible macular degeneration?
    a. Flashes of light
    b. Distorted straight lines
    c. Poor peripheral vision
    d. Reduced depth perception

138. What food is the cause for concern when the nurse questions the diet of the patient with histamine intolerance?
    a. Sauerkraut
    b. Fresh fish
    c. Sweet potato
    d. Blueberry

139. The nurse case manager requests extra paid days from the third party payer for the patient's length of stay in order to continue providing covered treatment. What is this process an example of?
    a. Concurrent review
    b. Prior authorization
    c. Retrospective review
    d. Prospective review

140. When must the discharge planning process start for each patient?
    a. The day before discharge is scheduled to occur
    b. The morning of the planned discharge
    c. After the discharge order has been written
    d. As soon as admission begins

141. All EXCEPT which of the following must be documented for physical restraints?
    a. Reason for intervention
    b. Restraint type
    c. Patient consent
    d. Patient behavior

142. A 23-year-old patient presents to the emergency department with a fever of 103.4 degrees Fahrenheit, tachycardia, tachypnea, hypertension, and muscle rigidity. Upon speaking with the patient, the nurse observes an altered mental status. In reviewing the patient's chart, the nurse notes that a psychiatric evaluation was completed the previous week, at which time the patient reported struggling with a previous diagnosis of schizophrenia. What condition does the nurse suspect the patient is experiencing at this time?
    a. Tardive dyskinesia
    b. Extrapyramidal side effects
    c. Neuroleptic malignant syndrome
    d. Parkinson's disease

143. The nurse ensures to provide truthful engagements with their patients, which is ethically substantiated by what principle?
    a. Fidelity
    b. Veracity
    c. Autonomy
    d. Distributive justice

144. While completing a respiratory assessment on a patient diagnosed with emphysema five years ago, what finding does the nurse expect to note?
    a. Dull percussion
    b. Resonant percussion
    c. Hyper-resonant percussion
    d. Flat percussion

145. When does the case management role begin for the patient with a psychiatric illness?
    a. Upon presentation to the emergency department
    b. Upon status conversion from involuntary to voluntary
    c. Upon primary diagnosis
    d. Upon status conversion from voluntary to involuntary

146. While caring for a patient with a high thyroid-stimulating hormone (TSH) level and a diagnosis of hypothyroidism, which symptom does the nurse NOT expect the patient to report?
    a. Muscle cramps
    b. Weight loss
    c. Fatigue
    d. Coarse hair

147. A patient presents for a scheduled upper GI endoscopy and explains that they have been experiencing black, tarry stools for the past three days. What does the nurse suspect may be causing the patient's melena?
    a. Consumption of iron supplements
    b. Gastrointestinal bleed
    c. Excess beets in the diet
    d. Charcoal from the oral preparatory solution

148. The nurse is utilizing the Five Rights of Delegation when assigning care. The nurse is aware that the rights include the right person, circumstance, communication, evaluation and which other right?
    a. Tool
    b. Time
    c. Team
    d. Task

149. After delegating care to the Licensed practical nurse (LPN), the Registered nurse (RN) is called in to the nurse manager's office to discuss appropriate delegation of tasks. Which delegated intervention should NOT have been assigned to the LPN?
    a. Administer Lasix® (furosemide) via intravenous push
    b. Hang the subsequent bag of normal saline for infusion
    c. Perform a wet-to-dry dressing change
    d. Insert a Foley catheter

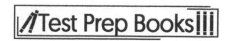

150. Which term is used to describe quality of care over time?
    a. Standard of care
    b. Quality improvement
    c. Continuity of care
    d. Risk management

151. When prioritizing care, which needs group does the nurse identify to be the most basic?
    a. Oxygen, nutrition, elimination
    b. Employment, freedom from danger
    c. Affection, belongingness, connection
    d. Learning, creating, understanding

152. When discussing patient care, how much patient information should a provider disclose?
    a. All information in the chart
    b. The minimum information necessary
    c. Only information about the body system the other provider specializes in
    d. Only information about the current visit

153. Upon discharge, the patient asks the nurse if they are permitted to obtain a copy of their record. Which act enables a patient to request a copy of their medical record?
    a. Affordable Healthcare Act
    b. Health Information Technology for Economic and Clinical Health Act
    c. Indian Healthcare Improvement Act
    d. Health Information Portability and Accountability Act

154. Does the utilization review (UR) nurse have access to medical records in order to complete concurrent patient reviews?
    a. Yes, this process is supported via UR access to records.
    b. No, the utilization review nurse is not a direct member of the treatment team.
    c. No, the UR nurse only has access when obtaining prior authorization for medication.
    d. Yes, but the patient must sign a release for the UR nurse specifically.

155. After the nurse overhears the nurse practitioner attempting to convince the patient to agree to a procedure, they promptly share this event with their nurse manager. The nurse manager reinforces that the patient has a right to make medical decisions without provider influence, which is ethically enforced under what principle?
    a. Beneficence
    b. Nonmaleficence
    c. Autonomy
    d. Justice

156. Before the nurse delegates tasks to other members of the team, they evaluate the role of each member. Which overarching legal directive defines role responsibilities?
    a. State rule
    b. Federal rule
    c. Hospital protocol
    d. Management delegation

157. The nurse is confronted with an ethical dilemma when a patient with methicillin resistant staphylococcus aureus (MRSA) of the nares is assigned a bed next to a patient with pneumonia in a double-occupancy room. In considering potential airborne transmission of the MRSA to the patient with pneumonia, the nurse does not agree with this bed assignment. After expressing this concern to the charge nurse with no resulting change, who should the nurse elevate this concern to next?

    a. Respiratory therapist
    b. Infection control practitioner
    c. Nursing supervisor
    d. Bed captain

158. The nurse is providing a unit-based in-service on safe, transcultural care. In exploring various culturally competent considerations, what process does the nurse describe when discussing the transfer of values and practices from one group to another?

    a. Integration
    b. Assimilation
    c. Separation
    d. Marginalization

159. Which approach to doffing personal protective equipment (PPE) supports infection control?

    a. Removing PPE at the nursing station
    b. Removing PPE at the bedside immediately following use
    c. Removing PPE in the patient's bathroom
    d. Removing PPE at the patient's doorway

160. When should the nurse remove the respirator after working with a patient on airborne precautions?

    a. Outside the medication room after closing the door
    b. Inside the patient's room before opening the patient's door
    c. Outside the patient's room after closing the patient's door
    d. Inside the patient's bathroom after closing the door

161. During a behavioral code, the nursing team responds to a patient who is trying to spit on them. What personal protective equipment (PPE) does the team decide to don during physical intervention for protection?

    a. Gloves and gown
    b. Gown
    c. Gloves and goggles
    d. Gown, gloves, mask with eye shield

162. While educating a group of new nurses during hospital orientation, the nurse educator explains how to properly don personal protective equipment (PPE). What order does the educator use when donning the PPE?

    a. Gloves, mask, goggles, gown
    b. Gloves, gown, mask, goggles
    c. Gown, mask, goggles, gloves
    d. Goggles, mask, gown, gloves

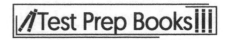

163. What statement made by the patient verbalizes understanding of safety precautions to take at home after being discharged from the hospital on oxygen for respiratory management?
    a. "I should switch from aerosol deodorant to a stick."
    b. "My cigarettes are safe to smoke as long as I smoke one at a time."
    c. "I must use an oven mitt while cooking on my gas stove."
    d. "I should switch from electric candles to flame-based ones."

164. The nurse case manager is discussing discharge planning with a 74-year-old patient. What statement made by the patient elicits the greatest concern?
    a. "I use automatic nightlights in my hallway and bathroom."
    b. "My morning medication makes me feel unsteady on my feet, so I sit much of the morning."
    c. "I set my thermostat at 70 degree Fahrenheit because I get chilly."
    d. "My son lives next door, but he works most days."

165. The nurse is supporting community clients during a wellness education group and discovers conflict within the discussion. In advocating for conflict resolution to promote success, in what order does the nurse apply the stages of conflict?
    a. Latent, perceive, felt, manifest
    b. Felt, manifest, perceive, latent
    c. Manifest, perceive, felt, latent
    d. Felt, perceive, latent, manifest

166. The nurse researcher is engaging in a study regarding perinatal care for a community needs assessment. What must take place before using patient data?
    a. Patient de-identification
    b. Provider consent
    c. Prior authorization from managed care
    d. Patient authorization, even when de-identified

167. While advocating for the patient's individualized nutritional needs after reviewing the results of recent lab work, the nurse meets with the dietician to discuss the patient's hyponatremia. A unique meal plan is instituted. The nurse is aware that all EXCEPT which of following risk factors are commonly associated with this imbalance?
    a. Diarrhea
    b. Vomiting
    c. Diplopia
    d. Polydipsia

168. While providing safety education to a group of patients diagnosed with personality disorders and struggling with urges to self-harm, which form of psychotherapy does the nurse integrate techniques from?
    a. Psychodynamic therapy
    b. Dialectal behavioral therapy
    c. Play therapy
    d. Humanistic therapy

169. Which potential complication should the nurse educate the patient on regarding their newly placed colostomy?
    a. Renal calculi
    b. Dehiscence
    c. Nocturnal enuresis
    d. Pernicious anemia

170. The nurse is educating a group of community members on life planning to include advance directives. What is the nurse describing when they discuss appointing someone to be financially responsible for one's healthcare decisions?
    a. Healthcare proxy
    b. Healthcare power of attorney
    c. Healthcare agent
    d. Healthcare provider

171. During a prenatal educational group session, the community health nurse discusses infant care and growth considerations. In order to support the parents-to-be in understanding newborn health and mortality, what does the nurse share is the leading cause of death during the first month of life?
    a. Failure to thrive
    b. Congenital cardiac defect
    c. Infection
    d. Sudden infant death syndrome

172. During a patient-and-family-centered group at the psychiatric hospital, the nurse educator discusses anxiety disorders and identity development. Which development phase involves the GREATEST onset of psychiatric eating disorders?
    a. Infancy
    b. Young adulthood
    c. Late adulthood
    d. Adolescence

173. The nurse is working with a patient before a scheduled surgical procedure and administers the preoperative sedative medication ordered in the patient's chart. After administering the medication, the nurse notices that the patient has not signed the surgical consent form. What should the nurse do first?
    a. Call the nursing supervisor
    b. Page the surgeon
    c. Ask the health care proxy to sign for consent
    d. Initiate a code

174. The psychiatric nurse is completing an assessment on a 58-year old female patient who just received electroconvulsive therapy (ECT). Which statement by the patient warrants concern?
    a. "I don't remember my name."
    b. "Did I have a bowel movement this morning?"
    c. "My leg is aching."
    d. "Can I have medication for my headache?"

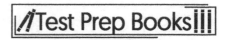

175. The nurse is advocating for updates to the patient's interdisciplinary treatment plan during the morning team meeting. In discussing behavior from the previous night, the nurse describes that the patient was exhibiting detachment from self in present reality. What is this mechanism referred to as?
    a. Disconnection
    b. Dissociation
    c. Displacement
    d. Disillusion

176. The nurse manager is ensuring that everyone on their team meets proficiency guidelines. What is the minimum care that a nurse must provide to meet proficiency called?
    a. Standard of care
    b. Level of care
    c. Quality of care
    d. Continuity of care

177. Which religion should the nursing supervisor take into account when working with the bed captain to assign patient rooms upon hospital admission?
    a. Catholicism
    b. Judaism
    c. Buddhism
    d. Islam

178. Which communication technique informs a patient whether or not their expressed statement was accurately received as intended?
    a. Probing
    b. Restating
    c. Silence
    d. Focusing

179. The triage nurse is assessing a patient's pain post motor vehicle accident. What does the PQRST method of pain assessment consist of?
    a. Presentation, Quality, Risk, Severity, Timing
    b. Presentation, Quality, Region, Source, Task
    c. Provoke, Quality, Region, Severity, Timing
    d. Provoke, Quality, Risk, Source, Task

180. Which diagnosis is chiefly responsible for hospital admission?
    a. Discharge diagnosis
    b. Secondary diagnosis
    c. Primary diagnosis
    d. Principle diagnosis

181. The registered nurse witnesses the licensed practical nurse (LPN) take a radial pulse on an infant patient and decides that education on pediatric pulse sites is necessary. What site should the LPN have used to take this patient's pulse?
    a. Brachial
    b. Femoral
    c. Pedal
    d. Popliteal

182. While the provider is educating a Japanese-American patient regarding a medication change, the patient continuously nods their head throughout the instruction. What does the patient's nodding signify?
    a. Cultural value of communication
    b. Agreement to take the medication
    c. Acceptance of the treatment plan change
    d. Understanding of the entirety of the instruction

183. Which response by the unlicensed assistive personnel functioning in the role of cardiac monitor technician would warrant the nurse to intervene and educate?
    a. Monitoring cardiac telemetry
    b. Printing rhythm strips
    c. Interpreting cardiac rhythm
    d. Notifying the team of no discernible activity

184. Which action witnessed by the nurse of the unlicensed assistive personnel warrants further education?
    a. Applied lotion to the patient's arms after a bed bath
    b. Took vital signs on the ipsilateral arm post right-sided mastectomy
    c. Cut food into small pieces before feeding patient
    d. Rolled patient onto their side during linen change

185. After receiving a counseling by the nurse manager regarding the nurse's poor time management skills, the nurse evaluates how to change their practice. What disciplinary action comes next if the nurse fails to correct this deficit?
    a. Termination
    b. Suspension
    c. Oral warning
    d. Written warning

186. What intervention should the nurse do first after receiving a pediatric admission with meningococcal meningitis?
    a. Obtain intravenous access
    b. Initiate droplet precautions
    c. Assess vital signs
    d. Initiate standard precautions

187. While working with a patient who is three days postop from a coronary artery bypass graft (CABG), the nurse notices that the patient looks pale and feels cold while ambulating in their room. What action does the nurse take first to prevent a fall?
    a. Assist the patient back to bed
    b. Encourage the patient to eat a snack
    c. Increase the flow rate on the patient's nasal cannula
    d. Assess the patient's vital signs

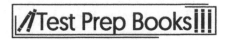

188. What process includes managing outcomes, corrective action plans, and variance trends?
   a. Performance improvement
   b. Information technology
   c. Utilization review
   d. Case management

189. What type of variance occurs when unwarranted tests are ordered and standard tests are neglected?
   a. Managed care
   b. Practitioner
   c. Dispensary
   d. Patient

190. A patient is prescribed Atrovent (ipratropium bromide) for symptom management, however the nurse notices that the patient carries a diagnosis that conflicts with its use. Which health problem contraindicates the use of this drug?
   a. Benign prostatic hypertrophy
   b. Bronchitis
   c. Emphysema
   d. Rheumatoid arthritis

191. While delivering a blood transfusion, the patient complains of a headache and double vision. Which action should the nurse take first?
   a. Call a rapid response
   b. Slow the infusion rate
   c. Stop the transfusion
   d. Assess vital signs

192. While providing care to an infant patient, the nurse reviews the chart to find a history of intussusception, which is a contraindication for what vaccination?
   a. Rotavirus
   b. Polio
   c. Pneumococcal
   d. Haemophilus influenza type B

193. The nurse witnesses the emergency department (ED) technician place the patient presenting with signs and symptoms of hypovolemic shock in the reverse Trendelenburg position. What should the nurse do first?
   a. Educate the ED technician on proper positioning
   b. Reposition the patient in the modified Trendelenburg position
   c. Praise the ED technician for successfully positioning the patient
   d. Report the ED technician as incompetent to the nursing supervisor

194. The public health nurse is providing community education on the connection between sexually transmitted infections and other ailments. In advocating for testing, which disease does the nurse explain is often associated with chlamydia and gonorrhea?
    a. Rheumatoid arthritis
    b. Celiac disease
    c. Pelvic inflammatory disease
    d. Systemic lupus erythematous

195. What is the FIRST thing that the nursing team should do to prevent harm to patients and staff by a patient with a strong history of aggressive behavior?
    a. Seclude the patient
    b. Establish trust and rapport
    c. Administer a sedative by mouth
    d. Use 4-point restraints

196. The nurse is applying Hildegard Peplau's Theory of Interpersonal Relations to an engagement with a patient's family in the emergency department to deescalate a threat. Which phase of the theory defines the problem?
    a. Exploitation
    b. Identification
    c. Orientation
    d. Resolution

197. While applying Patricia Benner's Model of Novice to Expert, what level is the graduate nurse's rule-governed behavior safely functioning at?
    a. Novice
    b. Expert
    c. Competent
    d. Proficient

198. What color of wound prompts the licensed practical nurse to ask the registered nurse to assess for the need for debridement?
    a. Pink
    b. Red
    c. Yellow
    d. Black

199. The interdisciplinary team is collaborating to engage in a "5 Whys Analysis" after a near-miss event took place. What is the team's main focus in opting to conduct this review?
    a. Determine the root cause of the event
    b. Decide who is responsible for the error
    c. Explore which agency should conduct the investigation
    d. Analyze how to navigate the disciplinary process

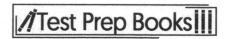

200. The nurse is working with a patient who communicates in a different language while attempting to complete a medication reconciliation form. In order to ensure that the nurse is safely and accurately completing the form, how should the nurse proceed to engage with the patient?

    a. Request support from a healthcare interpreter before continuing

    b. Ask the bilingual spouse to translate the discussion

    c. Draw pictures on the clipboard of what is being asked

    d. Defer this task to the unlicensed assistive personnel who has more time

NCLEX Answer Explanations #2

1. A: The Patient Self Determination Act of the United States, passed in 1990, sets forth that a patient is able to make decisions regarding the specifics of their treatment and the extent of nontreatment. While a patient is encouraged to decide what is best for them, they must be supported to do so without coercion or intimidation. Choices *B*, *C*, and *D* do not reflect protections found within this act.

2. C: When an unconscious patient is brought in for emergency care, they are agreeing to the care by way of implied consent. However, it is important to note that implied consent could never overrule a patient's denial to receive care. Therefore, Choice *A* is incorrect. A patient would need to be conscious and verbal to provide explicit or expressed consent, so Choices *B* and *D* are incorrect. A patient's action and conduct to willingly receive the medical care, even if not expressed verbally, functions as the basis for implied consent.

3. B: The Emergency Medical Treatment and Active Labor Act (EMTALA) was enacted in 1986 in order to protect an individual's right to receive emergency care regardless of their ability to pay for services. The patient has a right to be stabilized and treated. Choice *A* is fictitious, and Choices *C* and *D* do not involve protection of emergent care regardless of ability to pay.

4. B: Choice *B*, a weighted blanket, encourages calming of the body's fight-or-flight response and reduces the overflow of information flooding the nervous system. Choices *A*, *C*, and *D* should be avoided, as they may exacerbate stressed and stimulated senses and further contribute to poor sleep.

5. C: Choice *C*, the pancreas, is responsible for secreting insulin, which maintains proper blood glucose levels. Choices *A*, *B*, and *D*, while important organs for supporting various homeostatic processes, do not secrete insulin.

6. C: Choice *C*, bile, is produced by the liver and then stored in the gallbladder. The nurse's role in facilitating a community wellness course designed for patients pre-cholecystectomy is to foster consideration of the role of the gallbladder and encourage understanding of the procedure to remove it with aftercare considerations as applicable. Choices *A*, *B*, and *D* represent key bodily substances, but none are produced by the liver and stored in the gallbladder.

7. B, D, E, & F: Choices *B*, *D*, *E*, *F* all represent risk factors for triggering gout, an inflammatory condition with a hallmark sign of pain in the great toe. When high levels of uric acid circulate in the blood, urate crystals can accumulate in the joints, particularly that of the big toe. Uric acid is produced when the body breaks down purines, which are found in certain foods such as organ meats, steak, seafood, fruit juices, and alcoholic beverages. Choices *A* and *C* do not correlate to the patient's current symptom presentation and would not be suggestive risk factors at this time.

8. C: Choice *C*, passive leg raise, supports proper positioning for a patient with vital signs indicative of shock. The patient is supine with the legs elevated 8-12 inches. It is the nurse's priority to enhance circulation and assess the need for additional interventions. Choice *A* aligns with a raised upper body, while Choice *B* is side lying, and Choice *D* is face down, none of which support improved vital signs and symptom management of shock for the patient at this time.

9. B: Choice *B* indicates a normal assessment finding for a two-week-old patient. Choices *A*, *C*, and *D* are outside of the normal range for the age of this patient, as the heart rate should be between 70 and 190

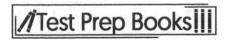

beats per minute. This rate is applicable for the first month of life. At one month of age, the normal heart rate adjusts to 80 to 160 beats per minute.

10. A: Choice *A*, phase one, correlates with atrial contraction, which is represented by the P wave of the electrocardiogram. Atrial contraction accounts for approximately ten percent of ventricular filling at rest. Choice *B* aligns with isovolumetric contraction, Choice *C* represents rapid ventricular ejection, and Choice *D* correlates with slow ventricular ejection, all subsequent processes of the cardiac cycle.

11. B: Males with a history of being physically abused are at risk of becoming abusive, and young children and females are at risk of being abused, so Choice *B* is correct. The people described in Choices *A*, *C*, and *D* are not at heightened risk because socioeconomic class is not directly correlated with increased risk for domestic violence.

12. C: Choices *A*, *B*, *C*, and *D* all represent stages of the general adaptation syndrome. However, only Choice *C*, resistance, is correlated with the symptoms of irritability, frustration, and poor concentration, along with an improvement in vital signs. As the patient moves past the alarm stage and into the resistance stage, the blood pressure and pulse reduce to more normalized levels. Alarm (Choice *B*) is considered the second stage, as it directly follows the homeostatic period (Choice *A*), and then is continued by resistance (Choice *C*) and exhaustion (Choice *D*).

13. C: The patient should not continue breastfeeding, Choice *C*, as breastfeeding is contraindicated with this medication because the medicine could affect bone and tooth development in the infant. Doxycycline should be taken with a full glass of water, and iron supplements should not be consumed within two hours of this medication to support maximum absorption and disease treatment. Therefore, Choices *A* and *B* are incorrect because the statements indicate that the patient understands these factors. The patient needs to use a nonhormonal birth control method to prevent pregnancy, which would put a developing fetus at risk. Doxycycline can reduce the efficacy of hormonal birth control pills. Therefore, Choice *D* is incorrect.

14. A: Choice *A*, Vitamin K, is a fat-soluble vitamin-based medication that is administered prior to liver biopsy procedures to reduce the risk of bleeding because Vitamin K aids in clotting. While the risk of bleeding exists with this procedure, cirrhosis and malignant disease heighten the risk for bleeding even more. Choice *B*, Choice *C*, and Choice *D* all represent fat-soluble vitamin-based medications, though they are not specifically indicated for liver biopsies.

15. A: The nurse must first assess the patient's vital signs before continuing on with subsequent actions. Therefore, Choice *A* is correct. Choice *B*, Choice *C*, and Choice *D* are all relevant interventions, though lack the priority in the case of the patient complaining of chest pain upon presentation to the emergency department. Once the vital signs have been assessed, the nurse should follow the nursing process to proceed with further care options.

16. B: The patient with Meniere's disease, an inner ear vestibular condition, struggles with symptoms of tinnitus and severe vertigo. A shower chair, Choice *B*, is crucial for this patient in order to prevent falls while showering. The patient should be encouraged to use the shower chair during every shower, and if available, grab bars as well, as symptoms can exacerbate in the shower and may lead to unsteady balance. A leg lifter is not a necessary device to offer this patient at this time, as it does not correlate with the patient's condition; thus, Choice *A* is incorrect. Button hooks and voice boxes, Choices *C* and Choice *D*, while supportive, do not align with symptoms of this condition.

17. B: Agitation, Choice *B*, is a chief concern when witnessed with the use of this drug class, as it could signify a paradoxical reaction due to cortical inhibition and excessive enhancement of the neurotransmitter gamma-aminobutyric acid (GABA). This symptom must be reported to the prescriber right away. Additional symptoms that may present in conjunction with agitation include aggression and violence. Sedation is a common side effect of the benzodiazepine drug class, so Choice *A* is not an alarm signal. Choice *C* and Choice *D*, unsteadiness and dizziness, represent typical side effects of this drug class and are not sources of immediate concern.

18. D: Retinal toxicity is a significant reaction to this medication and alerts the provider to a need to look into other treatment options for the patient with Sjogren's syndrome. Retinal toxicity, while rare, contraindicates further use of this drug. Therefore, Choice *D* is correct. Mood changes is a common side effects of Plaquenil® (hydroxychloroquine) and does not pose an immediate cause for concern. Bowel blockages and liver toxicity are not associated with use of this medication, though their appearance in any patient should warrant immediate concern.

19. C: Anti-tissue transglutaminase IgA, Choice *C*, is considered a reliable test for celiac disease diagnosis, often in conjunction with a small intestinal biopsy, so the nurse should expect to see this antibody test ordered when this autoimmune disease is considered. Antinuclear antibody, Choice *A*, is a nonspecific test for rheumatologic autoimmune disorders. Anti-thyroid peroxidase, Choice *B*, is useful for identifying autoimmune thyroid disease. Anti-topoisomerase I antibody, Choice *D*, aids in diagnosis of autoimmune scleroderma.

20. C: Therapeutic massage, along with other interventions such as chiropractic and osteopathic manipulation, is a manipulative treatment. Therefore, the correct answer is Choice *C*. The mind-body domain, Choice *A*, aligns with interventions such as meditation and dance. Interventions such as Reiki fall under the umbrella of energy interventions, so Choice *B* is incorrect. The biological domain, Choice *D*, includes herbal preparations and dietary supplements among other things.

21. C: Instrumental music, Choice *C*, encourages symptom management in reducing psychotic and paranoid symptoms for a patient struggling with schizophrenia, as instrumental music does not contribute to disturbed thought patterns and soothes the ill mind. Books, television, and food all carry the capacity to encourage worsening symptoms and should be avoided. Patients with schizophrenia may worry that their food is poisoned or be influenced to expand on delusional or paranoid thinking when influenced by stories in a book or on television.

22. D: HDT contributes to muscle wasting, which leads to pain. Strength training, Choice *D*, supports a comprehensive approach to strength building, which encourages a reduction in pain caused by hormone deprivation therapy (HDT). Increased fluid consumption (Choice *A*) and music therapy (Choice *C*) do not have a direct impact on reducing pain. Cycling (Choice *B*) may exacerbate pain for this patient, as applying pressure to the bones in the pelvis via cycling is contraindicated for this patient.

23. A: A diagnosis of bradycardia indicates the patient is experiencing a heart rate below 60 beats per minute, so Choice *A* is correct. Choices *B*, *C*, and *D* are within normal to high limits. The normal resting heart rate for adults is between 60 and 100 beats per minute.

24. A, B: During septic shock, metabolic acidosis and respiratory alkalosis are expected findings, along with a symptom presentation of shortness of breath, temperature changes, confusion, and diaphoresis. Thus, Choices *A* and *B* are correct. Choice *C* is incorrect, as the patient would likely experience a widening pulse pressure, not one that is narrowing. Choice *D* is incorrect, as the patient would display a

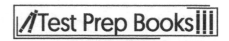

decreased cardiac output. Choice *E* is incorrect, as the patient would typically present with hypotension in this case.

25. B: When illicit drugs are discovered during the physical assessment of a patient, the nurses must page the nursing supervisor to elevate the concern, so Choice *B* is correct. The supervisor will then remove the drugs from the unit with security personnel and they will be destroyed. It would not be appropriate for the nurses to send the drugs home with the patient's spouse (Choice *C*) or plan to return them to the patient at discharge (Choice *D*). Additionally, contacting police to report this finding as a crime would not be legally supported (Choice *A*).

26. C: During a psychiatric evaluation, the clinician will determine the degree to which a patient's psychological symptoms impact their daily life. This score is then represented in the evaluation as a GAF score, which stands for Global Assessment of Functioning (Choice *C*). An Apgar score measures a neonate's general condition at birth (Choice *A*), and an AIMS score measures side effects of antipsychotic medication use (Choice *B*). The withdrawal protocol (Choice *D*) concerns symptoms that, in a patient struggling with substance abuse, must be controlled with medication, typically a benzodiazepine.

27. B: Conversion disorder is the transformation of emotional distress into physical manifestations. These physical manifestations initially appear to be linked to the nervous system, but they have no medical explanation and really originate in the psyche. Conversion disorder is often associated with repression (Choice *B*), a defense mechanism that is characterized by inhibiting or forgetting thoughts the patient does not want to acknowledge. Conversion disorder represents the expression of the disavowed thoughts in the form of transferred symptoms. Projection, reaction formation, and intellectualization while they are defense mechanisms, are not associated with conversion disorder. Therefore, Choices *A*, *C*, and *D* are incorrect.

28. C: Choice *C*, gynecomastia, describes the patient's current symptom presentation and is a side effect of Haldol® (haloperidol) and other psychotropic use. This condition is caused by a secondary hormonal imbalance in which estrogen is elevated. Choice *A* and Choice *B* are both associated with psychotropic use; however, they do not correlate with the patient assessment at this time. Stevens-Johnson syndrome is a rare disorder of the skin and membranes, whereas nystagmus involves uncontrollable ocular movements. Schizoaffective disorder (Choice *D*) represents a psychiatric illness that may encourage the prescription of this medication, though not the side effects of its use.

29. D: Choice *D*, monoamine oxidase inhibitors, demands a tyramine-avoidant diet, as these medications block monoamine oxidase, an enzyme necessary to breakdown tyramine. Choices *A*, *B*, and *C*, while all psychotropic medication classes, do not require the patient to avoid tyramine in their diet. In severe cases, a hypertensive crisis may result when monoamine metabolism is inhibited.

30. A: Choice *A*, 18 gtts/min, represents the appropriate drip rate for this patient's infusion. Choice *B*, Choice *C*, and Choice *D* represent common mistakes in drip rate miscalculation that must be avoided to prevent injury to the patient. Dividing the total volume in milliliters by the time in minutes, then multiplying that quotient by the drop factor in drops per milliliter calculates the drip rate. The drop factor can be found on the tubing package.

31. D: Choice *D* correlates with aphasia, as the patient is unable to understand or produce speech. Aphasia is often witnessed with brain trauma or severe neurological conditions affecting the communication areas of the brain. This condition is also considered a language disorder. Choice *A* describes a patient with apraxia. Choice *B* describes a patient with akathisia. Choice *C* involves dysphagia.

32. A: A reduction in bile can also produce stool that is tan or clay-colored. As less bile is present, the stool becomes paler in color. Thus, Choice *A*, white stool, is seen when a patient is struggling with a bile duct blockage. Green stool, Choice *B,* is indicative of a high vegetable intake or antibiotic use. Black stool, Choice *C,* can be seen with upper gastrointestinal bleeds or iron supplementation, whereas red stool, Choice *D,* can be observed with lower gastrointestinal bleeds or foods with red dyes.

33. B: Choice *B* represents the correct way to measure and use a cane. The length of the cane should ensure that the patient is able to slightly flex the elbow to allow for proper body mechanics and safety. Choice *A* is subjective and should be avoided. Choice *C* should be avoided, as full flexion does not represent properly supported posture or ambulation. Choice *D* must be avoided because full extension of the arm with a forward lean is unsafe and does not support a steady gait.

34. D: The unlicensed assistive personnel (UAP) is able to assist with patient equipment by supporting placement of the sequential compression devices (SCDs). It would not be within the UAP's scope to apply cervical traction (Choice *A*), a hemovac drain (Choice *C*), or a ventilator (Choice *B*).

35. C: A high titer of 1:640 paired with a speckled pattern may be indicative of rheumatologic autoimmune diseases; thus, Choice *C* is the appropriate specialty for continued assessment and additional laboratory testing for this patient at this time. Choices *A*, *B*, and *D*, while potentially appropriate referrals for the future, do not represent applicable specialties for the patient to consult with next.

36. D: Choice *D* describes what to expect during an electromyography procedure. The needle electrode is inserted to record electrical activity and assess for nerve and muscle dysfunction or transmission issues. Choice *A* reflects the process of a muscle biopsy. Choice *B* aligns with intracranial pressure monitoring. Choice *C* describes acupuncture.

37. C: Implied consent, Choice *C,* allows for the nurse to properly administer cardiopulmonary resuscitation to an unconscious patient. Implied consent is not expressly granted, though it is supported by the circumstance and inaction against the intervention. Choices *A*, *B*, and *D* are not appropriate because regardless of the terms of each type of consent, the patient is unable to consciously, therefore competently, engage in them, rendering them invalid.

38. B: Prothrombin, a protein produced by the liver, supports the proper clotting of blood. Choice *B,* 14 seconds, represents a normal prothrombin time test that is indicative of appropriate clotting-function prior to surgery. While test times range between laboratories, Choices *A*, *C*, and *D* are regarded as outside of normal limits.

39. A, D, E: Choices *A*, *D*, and *E* represent appropriate actions by the unlicensed assistive personnel (UAP) while obtaining a morning weight for the patient struggling with anorexia nervosa and generalized anxiety disorder. The patient should be weighed in a paper gown to promote accuracy of the obtained body weight via the same scale each weigh-in. The patient should be weighed with their back to the scale to reduce anxiety symptoms, and the UAP should chart the findings. The treatment team can discuss the findings in a therapeutic way with the patient. The patient should be weighed after a morning void to reduce the incidence of water loading pre-weight, which could skew the result. Choice *B* should be avoided, as weighing the patient post breakfast would alter the result with an inflated finding.

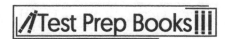

Choice *C* should be avoided, as the patient should not be weighed in the hall. Instead, the patient should be weighed in a place of privacy.

40. C: The first piece of personal protective equipment the nurse should don is a gown, Choice *C*. Choice *A*, gloves, are donned next, followed by Choice *B*, mask, and ultimately, Choice *D*, goggles, are donned last. The nurse must follow this sequence to ensure protection against infection transmission.

41. A: Choice *A* represents the tissue test that is considered the gold standard for celiac disease diagnosis. Tissue biopsies are taken from the small intestine to assess for villous atrophy present with this autoimmune disease. Choices *B*, *C*, and *D* tissue tests do not support a celiac disease diagnosis.

42. B: Auscultation, Choice *B*, is the second step of an abdominal physical assessment. The nurse should first perform Choice *C*, inspection, then Choice *B*, auscultation, followed by Choice *A*, percussion, and finally Choice *D*, palpation. This sequence of techniques is unique to an abdominal physical assessment to promote accuracy in findings by not interfering with the results.

43. C: Palpate, Choice *C*, represents the second step of a respiratory physical assessment. The nurse should first perform Choice *A*, inspect, then Choice *C*, palpate, followed by Choice *B*, percuss, and finally Choice *D*, auscultate. This sequence of techniques is standard for physical assessments—except when performing an abdominal assessment—to promote accuracy in findings.

44. B: Choice *B* represents a fasting blood sugar level that is within normal range, which is considered to be between 60-99 mg/dL. Choice *A* is a below normal finding. Choice *C* and Choice *D* are above normal findings and indicate the possible presence of pre-diabetes.

45. A: The incubation period, Choice *A*, is the stage of disease where the individual often does not yet realize that they have been exposed to a pathogenic organism, as they are asymptomatic. This stage makes up the period of time from exposure to when symptoms become apparent. The prodromal period, Choice *B*, represents the stage during which symptoms are first noted and may be vague in presentation. The acute period, Choice *C*, represents the stage of disease that has progressed to include a worsening of symptoms that are specific to pathogen and illness. The convalescence period, Choice *D*, signifies the stage involving a gradual reduction of symptoms and recovery of health after illness.

46. D: Chest physiotherapy, Choice *D*, is a supportive treatment routinely used for the care of individuals with cystic fibrosis to facilitate movement of secretions from small to large airways. Once the secretions have mobilized, they are much more readily expressed via coughing. Chest physiotherapy involves postural drainage, followed by percussion and vibration to loosen thick mucus and mobilize secretions. Choice *A*, antibiotics, while used for those with cystic fibrosis who develop infections, are not prescribed for routine care to mobile secretions. The six-foot rule, Choice *B*, signifies the practice of two individuals with cystic fibrosis maintaining a minimum 6-foot distance between one another to reduce the likelihood of spreading respiratory infections. Pulmonary function tests, Choice *C*, are done to assess pulmonary function.

47. B: Choice *B* represents an appropriate response to this finding, as it is normal for air to leak until the lung incision heals and is sealed. Choices *A*, *C*, and *D* all involve the nurse elevating this finding as a point of concern, which would be inappropriate at this time. The nurse should document this normal finding, and then continue to monitor the patient's chamber and incision.

48. C: In a comminuted fracture, Choice *C*, the bones break into multiple fragments, as they would have done during the motor vehicle accident. Comminuted fractures typically occur in the hands and feet in response to severe trauma. The nurse would educate the patient regarding the specific fracture that they are suffering from and plan treatment options in response. A compound fracture, Choice A, involves a fracture where the bones break through the skin. An oblique fracture, Choice B, involves a fracture that breaks at an angle. A greenstick fracture, Choice D, involves a fracture where the bones do not break all the way through.

49. A: While encouraging a therapeutic engagement with a patient awaiting test results post mastectomy, the nurse should produce a statement that encourages the patient to explore their feelings, such as that in Choice A. The statements in Choices B, C, and D are nurse-centered, not patient-centered, and should be avoided.

50. C: Choice C, transference, is observed when one member of an interaction transfers thoughts or feelings that were originally about one person onto someone else. In this case, the patient is reminded of her son while interacting with the nurse, and she transfers the negative association she has with her son onto the nurse. Choice B, countertransference, occurs when the clinician displaces their feelings onto the client. Choice A, regression, involves reverting to an earlier version of the self, while Choice D, repression, manifests itself through reducing emotions.

51. C: The Muscular Strength Scale supports proper assessment and documentation of muscular strength and use, allowing patterns of weakness to be noted. The scale ranges from no muscle contraction, which is 0/5 (Choice A), to normal strength, 5/5. The patient exhibiting muscular movement only when assisted by gravity correlates with a rating of 2/5 (Choice C). Choice B represents muscle flicker without movement, and Choice D represents movement against gravity, but not resistance.

52. D: A patient exhibiting a new pain in addition to previously-established pain is considered to be suffering with acute-on-chronic pain (Choice D). New, short-term pain is identified as acute pain (Choice A), unlike pain that is chronic (Choice C). Choice B, chronic-on-acute pain, is not a term that is used. Distinctions in pain are key to proper documentation and intervention in support of quality care and comfort.

53. C: Medication titration, Choice C, involves titrating the dosage to reach a therapeutic level, as it encourages careful consideration to achieve the maximum benefit without adverse reaction. Medication compliance, Choice A, involves patient agreement and fulfillment of medication intake. Medication reconciliation, Choice B, describes the process of creating a list of medications taken. Medication administration, Choice D, involves the practice of delivering medication for intake.

54. C: Choice C represents an accurate understanding of the first step, verification, as an accurate medication history is obtained. Choice A and Choice B represent a misunderstanding by the licensed practical nurse (LPN), as these actions align with clarification, which is the second step of the medication reconciliation process. Choice D aligns with the third and final step of the process, reconciliation.

55. D: Tapazole® (methimazole), Choice D, is a medication used for disease management in hyperthyroidism, an overactive thyroid condition. This condition occurs when the thyroid gland secretes an abundance of hormone and medication is used to reduce this process. Some symptoms of hyperthyroidism include weight loss, rapid heartbeat, diaphoresis, and irritability. Choices A, B, and C are all medications used to treat the underactive thyroid condition known as hypothyroidism.

56. A: Iodine, Choice A, is essential for synthesizing thyroid hormone, which may be deficient in those with hypothyroidism. This condition may develop as an individual's iodine levels reduce. Hypothyroidism may result from iodine deficiency, especially in regions with limited iodine intake. Choice B, Choice C,

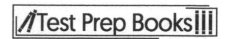

and Choice *D*, while important dietary minerals to ensure adequate consumption of, are not of significant correlation to thyroid disease; therefore, they would not be the nurse's priority in providing patient education at this time.

57. A: A low protein diet, Choice *A*, is the best diet for the patient diagnosed with phenylketonuria, as protein processing is affected in this condition. A high protein diet, Choice *B*, should be avoided. The amino acids found within protein can exacerbate symptoms and lead to risky disease management. Folic acid levels are not closely correlated with phenylketonuria management. Thus, Choices *C* and *D* are incorrect.

58. B: Choice *B* would cause concern, as liver is a type of organ meat. The patient with gout must avoid food high in purines, such as organ meat, to successfully reduce the occurrence of attacks. Choice *A* does not include contraindicated foods. Choices *C* and *D* are meal options considered to be low in purines and safe for those struggling with gout.

59. D: Placing the patient on their right side with the head of the bed elevated enables the food to be properly digested and reduces the risk for aspiration. Choices *A*, *B*, and *C* present significant risks to aspiration after tube feeding and must be avoided.

60. A: Tachypnea, Choice *A*, describes an elevated respiratory rate. Tachypnea can be witnessed in a variety of patient presentations and must be carefully assessed. Rapid breathing is not always overt or labored, so taking the time to count respirations and complete a thorough examination is key. Orthopnea, Choice *B*, represents labored breathing, while tachycardia, Choice *C*, correlates to a rapid heart rate. Hyperthermia, Choice *D*, involves an elevated body temperature.

61. A: The normal range for TSH levels is 0.4-4.0 mU/L. Choice *A* reflects a thyroid-stimulating hormone (TSH) level that is indicative of hypothyroidism and may need to be treated with thyroid hormone medication to support a healthy pregnancy. Choices *B* and *C* reflect TSH levels that are within the normal range and would not require treatment at this time. Choice *D* correlates with hyperthyroidism, which would not require additional thyroid hormone for symptom management.

62. D: Choice *D* correlates with type II diabetes mellitus and alerts the nurse that an additional round of testing should be conducted to confirm this diagnosis and proceed with an appropriate insulin treatment plan. Choices *A* and *B* represent normal hemoglobin A1C results. Choice *C* correlates to a pre-diabetes diagnosis with the need for follow-up testing in one year. A hemoglobin A1C below 5.7 percent is normal, while a result of 5.7 to 6.4 percent is indicative of pre-diabetes. Type II diabetes mellitus is considered when the hemoglobin A1C result is 6.5 percent and above.

63. D: Clonazepam, Choice *D*, is a proper medication to offer to the patient at this time in support of symptom management during a panic attack. Clonidine, Choice *A*, supports the management of hyperactivity, and is also used in the management of hypertension. Lamotrigine, Choice *B*, encourages mood stabilization. Fluoxetine, Choice *C*, promotes the management of depression.

64. A: Clozapine, Choice *A*, may be considered for treatment-resistant psychotic disorders, such as schizoaffective disorder, which did not successfully respond to previous medication trials. While Choices *B*, *C*, and *D* all signify psychotropic medication options, they target a variety of other symptom presentations. Lithobid, Choice *B*, is considered for mood stabilization with patients experiencing episodes of mania. Alprazolam, Choice *C*, is considered for anxiety, and Sertraline, Choice *D*, is considered for depression.

65. D: Choice *D* correctly aligns with the Joint Commission's standards, as sentinel events are not mandatory to report but are encouraged. Choices *A*, *B*, and *C* are inaccurate interpretations of the Joint Commission's role in accredited organization reporting of sentinel events.

66. A: The Health Information Portability and Accountability Act, Choice *A*, includes protection of patient-related personal health information (PHI) and must be preserved by the nurse engaging in a report for continued care planning. The Emergency Medical Treatment and Active Labor Act, Choice *B*, protects the patient's right to emergency care. The False Claims Act, Choice *C*, protects governmental programs from fraud. The Hospital Readmissions Reduction Program, Choice *D*, protects quality care by encouraging improved treatment with reduced readmissions.

67. B: Autonomy, Choice *B*, protects the patient's right to self-directed, independent decisions. Once the patient has received the information they need to make an informed selection of treatment, the patient, or proxy when indicated, autonomously makes the final decision for care. Beneficence, Choice *A*, morally encourages the nurse to do right by the patient. Non-maleficence, Choice *C*, supports not causing harm to the patient. Justice, Choice *D*, stimulates ethical fairness for the patient.

68. A: Of the choices provided, a glucometer, Choice *A*, is a piece of equipment that provides a result that falls within the scope that unlicensed assistive personnel (UAP) are able to chart on. UAP often use glucometers to take point-of-care finger-stick blood sugar readings and chart the findings. Ventilators, cervical traction devices, and continuous passive motion machines (Choices *B*, *C*, and *D*) contain equipment that produce results outside of the scope of the UAP to chart on and should not be delegated to the UAP. The nurse must monitor and chart the findings of these treatment options.

69. A, C, D: Choices *A*, *C*, and *D* all represent the locations where the nurse should assess the patient's blood pressure and pulse to detect a blockage for a patient with suspected aortoiliac occlusive disease. This disease affects the iliac and femoral arteries. The blood pressure and pulse are taken in the thigh, calf, and foot to assess for inadequate blood flow that happens during a blockage. Choices *B* and *E* do not support the assessment of this lower body condition and therefore are not relevant for the nurse's physical assessment of the patient at this time.

70. D: A bone scan, Choice *D*, must be completed to assess for progress after initiating a bisphosphonate medication regimen to strengthen bone health. CT scans, ultrasound, and MRIs, while potentially helpful imaging for various aspects of disease management, do not specifically address the patient's treatment with bisphosphonates and are not necessary at this time. Bisphosphonates are prescribed for patients with multiple myeloma to reduce pain and vertebral fractures. Bone scans examine their effectiveness.

71. B: Antidiuretic hormone is a hormone that primarily functions to encourage the kidneys to balance the amount of water excreted in the urine. This hormone supports healthy blood pressure and volume. Follicle-stimulating hormone, Choice *A*, is involved with pubertal development in both males and females. Adrenocorticotrophic hormone, secreted by the anterior pituitary gland, regulates the production of cortisol and androgen. Thus, Choice *C* is incorrect. Luteinizing hormone, Choice *D*, influences ovulation and the production of testosterone.

72. A: Dopamine, Choice *A*, is significantly reduced in patients struggling with Parkinson's disease. Dopamine deficiency is responsible for the clinical presentation of many symptoms, such as tremor, balance issues, slowness, and stiffness. Choices *B*, *C*, and *D* are all neurotransmitters, but none of these are the primary deficiency in this disease.

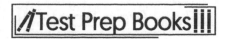

73. D: The mental health worker, an unlicensed assistive member of the treatment team, should not be providing patient education regarding the physical effects of anorexia nervosa (Choice *D*). This task is one that the charge nurse must appropriately delegate to the nurse. Observing the patient during mealtime (Choice *A*), standing outside the bathroom during use (Choice *B*), and delivering Ensure® (Choice *C*) are within the scope of practice for an unlicensed team member and can be appropriately and safely delegated to them.

74. C: The patient who started Clozaril® (clozapine) yesterday should not be scheduled for discharge tomorrow, as this medication must be closely followed and blood work must be monitored for therapeutic level and neutropenia before scheduling a safe discharge home. Choices *A*, *B*, and *D* represent patients who can all be safely discharged tomorrow, since their treatment considerations do not require additional time to support. Electroconvulsive therapy does not necessitate continued observation, a prior authorization can be completed the same day, and a headache after missing a meal is a normal finding.

75. B: Only vitamin B-12, Choice *B,* should be an expected subcutaneous treatment for the patient with pernicious anemia. However, iron, packed RBCs, and stem cells are involved in various other forms of anemia. Multiple forms of anemia exist including iron-deficiency anemia, hemolytic anemia, and aplastic anemia, to name a few. In this case, the patient is suffering from pernicious anemia, an autoimmune condition in which the body is unable to absorb the vitamin B-12 consumed in one's diet, leading to deficiency. Vitamin B-12 injections are required to form healthy red blood cells.

76. A: Glucose, Choice *A*, is the priority for test monitoring for the nurse delivering total parenteral nutrition (TPN) to a pediatric patient on day one. During the first one to two days of delivery, serum glucose levels must be closely monitored to ensure hyperglycemia does not occur from the high-glucose content of this treatment. Levels of vitamin B-12, calcium, and vitamin D are important to monitor for appropriate nutrition and overall wellness, though are not the priority for the nurse during this time period with this treatment and would be more appropriately monitored with longevity.

77. D: Intravenous gamma globulin is delivered to young patients to prevent bacterial infections from forming, and it is also used to treat these infections once occurring. Choice *A*, Choice *B*, and Choice *C* do not directly correlate with the administration of this therapy. While these choices all represent potential concerns of this patient and their caregivers at this time, they are not directly influenced or supported by this particular treatment.

78. B: Zometa® (zoledronic acid), Choice *B*, is prescribed when a patient is struggling with metastatic stages of cancer affecting the bone. This medication is designed to slow the progression and negative effects and is known as a bisphosphonate. It reduces the amount of calcium released from bone. Taxotere® (docetaxel), Choice *A*, is a medication used for metastatic prostate cancer. Doxil® (doxorubicin), Choice *C*, and Xeloda® (capecitabine), Choice *D*, are medications used for metastatic breast cancer.

79. B: The kidney, Choice *B,* is the source of the patient's bone failure to produce red blood cells leading to their current anemic state. The kidney is responsible for stimulating this activity. The organs in Choices *A*, *C*, and *D* do not directly affect the bone's failure to produce red blood cells.

80. A: Maslow's hierarchy of needs includes the following five stages: physiological, safety, love and belonging, esteem, and self-actualization. Choice *A* encourages the nurse to simultaneously consider the patient's need for safety while tending to their most basic physiological needs. Choices *B*, *C*, and *D*, while important, do not represent the second-level stage for prioritizing care.

233

81. A, B, D, E: Salivary glands, the liver, the pancreas, and the gallbladder are all accessory organs that contribute to digestive activities. The large intestine, Choice *C,* is not an accessory organ, as it is part of the digestive tract.

82. A: The normal range for respiratory rate for this age is 30-60 breaths/minute; thus, Choice *A* alerts the nurse to a potential problem in the six-month-old infant. Choices *B*, *C*, and *D* all fall within normal range and are not causes for concern at this time.

83. C: Parathyroid hormone is responsible for increasing osteoclast activity. If the body makes too much parathyroid hormone, calcium will be taken from bones, and the individual will develop osteoporosis. Therefore, Choice *C* is correct. Choices *A*, *B*, and *D* do not directly contribute to osteoclast function. Insulin, Choice *A,* influences blood glucose levels. Renin, Choice *B,* acts on blood pressure control. Serotonin, Choice *D,* regulates mood, sleep, digestion, and libido.

84. C: Choice *C* identifies a stuporous patient exhibiting no articulated verbal response with limited moaning, accompanied by arousal only after vigorous stimulation. Lethargic, Choice *A,* describes a patient who appears drowsy and arouses with gentle stimulation. Obtunded, Choice *B,* describes a patient who responds to repeated external stimulation to maintain attention. A patient that is comatose, Choice *D,* indicates they have no discernable response to stimulation. The levels of consciousness proceed with increasing severity from confused, to lethargic, to obtunded, to stuporous, and finally to comatose.

85. B: Choice *B* is observed with a 2+ response to pitting edema, which takes 15 seconds for the mild indentation to rebound. Choice *A* is observed with a 1+ response to pitting edema, which is an impression that is barely detectable. Choice *C* is observed with a 3+ response to pitting edema, which takes 30 seconds for the moderate indentation to rebound. Choice *D* is observed with a 4+ response to pitting edema, which takes greater than 30 seconds for the severe indentation to rebound.

86. D: Choice *D* identifies the appropriate location for the nurse to assess the patient for pitting edema. The nurse should press on the skin over the tibia bone, then slide fingers over that area to observe the level of indentation and time it takes for the indentation to rebound. This process should be repeated again further up the tibia until edema is no longer noted. The radius, femur, and ulna would not provide accurate assessments of indentation to identify pitting edema for this patient and should be excluded from this focused assessment.

87. A, E: Choices *A* and *E* indicate blood glucose levels outside of normal range. The normal range for a finger stick two hours post meal is 70-180 mg/dl. Choice *A* is below normal range. Choice *E* is above normal range. Choices *B*, *C*, and *D* are within normal range and are not causes for concern for patients with type II diabetes mellitus two hours post meal.

88. A: Choice *A* is the appropriate response from the nurse to the patient presenting to urgent care one week post-operative following a vasectomy. It is a normal finding for the patient to experience blood in their semen as the site heals. Choice *B* is incorrect, as the patient should not expect for sterilization to be ineffective secondary to this finding. Choice *C* is incorrect, as blood in the semen is not an adverse effect and does not indicate a lifetime of this issue. Choice *D* is incorrect, as blood in the semen is not cause for concern of hemorrhaging. Additional side effects noted soon after vasectomy include scrotal bruising, mild pain, and swelling.

89. C: Aldactone® (spironolactone), Choice *C,* is a potassium-sparing diuretic and supports the patient's concern regarding their potassium level at this time. This medication does not encourage the excretion

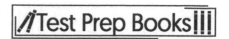

of potassium via urine. Lasix® (furosemide) and Demadex® (toresemide) are loop diuretics and Aldactone® (spironolactone) is a thiazide diuretic. These medications do not specifically target conserving potassium in the body to address the patient's concern arising from their history. Therefore, Choices A, B, and D are incorrect.

90. D: Parnate® (tranylcypromine), Choice D, is in the monoamine oxidase inhibitor (MAOI) class of antidepressants. The MAOI drug class blocks the actions of monoamine oxidase enzymes to support an improvement in depressive symptoms. Choice A, Choice B, and Choice C represent medications that belong to the selective serotonin reuptake inhibitor (SSRI) drug class of antidepressants.

91. A: Zoloft® (sertraline), a selective serotonin reuptake inhibitor (SSRI), can cause serotonin syndrome (Choice A) when discontinued, especially if it is done abruptly. Patients with this syndrome exhibits symptoms of agitation, restlessness, confusion, and elevated vital signs, especially a high fever. Neuroleptic malignant syndrome, Choice B is a life-threatening syndrome that is associated mostly commonly with antipsychotic medication use and is very rarely considered a possibility with SSRIs. Prader-Willi syndrome, Choice C, is a syndromes with genetic origins and is not directly caused by the discontinuation of SSRIs. MAOI syndrome, Choice D, is not an identified syndrome, and Zoloft® (sertraline) is not an MAOI.

92. B: The mental health worker, an unlicensed assistive member of the treatment team, can record patient behavior on the seclusion flowchart (Choice B). This is within the scope of the mental health worker's practice. It would be out of scope for them to complete an AIMS examination to assess for side effects of antipsychotic medication use (Choice A), evaluate patient responses to medication questions (Choice C), or document post-fall screening details (Choice D).

93. D: The first priority for the nurse is to assess the patient's preferred method of communication (Choice D). This practice supports a solid foundation for a therapeutic engagement that is patient-centered and sensitive to unique needs. It would not be appropriate for the nurse to focus on their own preferred method of communication (Choices A, B, and C) over that of the patient's.

94. A: Choices A, B, C, and D all represent complementary and alternative medicine (CAM) techniques. However, only Choice A, reiki, involves promoting the body's natural healing response via energy fields stimulated by placing the practitioner's hands on or close to the body. In Choice B, myofascial release, pressure is applied to myofascial connective tissue. Choice C, shiatsu massage, involves using the hands to apply pressure to various areas of the body's surface. Choice D, biofeedback, uses electrical sensors to attune the body for self-control of physiological functions.

95. C: The Kubler-Ross Grief Cycle includes denial (Choice A), anger (Choice B), bargaining (Choice C), depression (Choice D), and acceptance. An individual struggling to find meaning and frequently retelling the story of their grief is experiencing the bargaining stage (Choice C). The bargaining stage can also be associated with an individual attempting to reconcile the event by contributing positively to their days in hopes the event will be undone. While some people experience these stages in succession, others experience them outside of this linear order or skip some stages altogether.

96. D: The sexual assault nurse examiner (SANE) is responsible for ensuring that proper protocol is followed for obtaining the patient's legal written consent for the examination. Before administering the rape kit examination, the nurse must ensure that the physician has thoroughly explained the procedure and that the patient themselves has signed the form (Choice D). An accompanying support person, such as a family member (Choice C), cannot sign the form for the patient. The nurse cannot legally obtain informed consent for the examination (Choice *A*), nor can the process continue based on verbal questioning (Choice *B*).

97. A: The Health Insurance Protection and Portability Act, Choice *A*, provides the patient with the right to amend their record with correct information when incorrect information was previously recorded. The False Claims Act (Choice *B*) has to do with organizations providing inaccurate information, typically to governmental agencies, in order to receive inflated compensation or financial support. The Medical Record Amendment Act, Choice *C*, is fictitious, and the Health Care Quality Improvement Act, Choice *D*, does not set forth patient rights regarding amending their medical record under these circumstances.

98. C: For an individual struggling with substance abuse, avoiding places where they have typically used substances in the past is a realistic goal for intensive outpatient therapy (Choice *C*). It would not be realistic for the client to use their substance of abuse in moderation (Choice *A*), stop requiring connection with their sponsor (Choice *B*), or prevent all cravings via self-control (Choice *D*) during the week they are engaged in intensive treatment for substance abuse.

99. D: In order to encourage therapeutic engagement with the patient, the nurse should ask an inquiring question that is directly correlated with the statement the patient just made (Choice *D*). In this way, the patient is supported to further explore and share their feelings about the situation. Asking if someone else can verify their feelings (Choice *A*), attesting that the mother still loves the patient (Choice *B*), and warning the patient about feeling worse (Choice *C*), are all ways of minimizing the patient's feelings or perceptions. These should be avoided when attempting to foster therapeutic engagement.

100. C: Dysuria, Choice *C,* is the term for painful urination, a common symptom of urinary tract infections. Bacteria cause inflammation, which leads to the development of painful urination accompanied by a burning sensation. Anuria, Choice *A,* refers to a lack of urine. Oliguria, Choice *B,* refers to the production of a small amount of urine. Polyuria, Choice *D,* describes the production or passage of an excessive amount of urine.

101. A: Choice *A* is cause for concern for an order for a low sodium diet and must be avoided to prevent episodes of severe hypotension and an exacerbation of symptoms. Patients struggling with postural orthostatic tachycardia syndrome are at high risk for hypotension and should avoid interventions that may lead to the reduction of fluid retention with increased excretion by the body. Choices *B*, *C*, and *D,* on the other hand, align with the need for a sodium-restricted diet to encourage fluid excretion for symptom management.

102. C: Choice *C* supports proper use of the new walker. The patient should be educated to step up onto curbs with their strong leg first. The weak leg can then follow as balance is regained atop the curb. Choice *A* is incorrect because it discourages the use of grooved rubber tips; however, they should be placed on the bottom of the walker's legs to improve floor grip and patient balance. Choice *B* is incorrect because it encourages the use of waxed flooring, though this would be unsafe as it could lead to patient falls. Choice *D* should be discouraged, as patients should not carry their walker up stairs.

103. D: Side-lying, Choice *D,* is the best position for the patient during oral care because it encourages an easy flow of fluids outside of the mouth as necessary. The nurse can also use suction to remove secretions during this intervention. Placing the patient in any of the positions noted in Choices *A*, *B*, or *C* could pose a significant risk to the unconscious patient during oral care, as the patient may aspirate, which could lead to pneumonia.

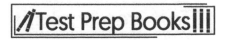

104. B: Taking vital signs aligns with the assessment stage of the nursing process, so Choice *B* is correct. Choices *A, C,* and *D* are later stages to be engaged in after assessing the patient, which in this case involves taking their vital signs. The pneumonic ADPIE can be used to remember the stages of this process: Assessment, Diagnosis, Planning, Implementation, and Evaluation.

105. A: Choice *A* is indicative of hypokalemia—low potassium in the blood—which the patient's symptoms correlate with. Choices *B, C,* and *D* are considered normal potassium blood levels. Additional symptoms that manifest with hypokalemia include digestive problems, numbness and tingling, and mood changes.

106. A: Dividing the abdomen into quadrants and regions allows for thorough assessment and subsequent diagnosis of the source of pain and discomfort. The liver, Choice *A* is located in the right upper quadrant. The stomach and pancreas, Choices *B* and *C,* are located in the left upper quadrant. The appendix, Choice *D,* is located in the right lower quadrant.

107. A: Choice *A* describes why this medication would be ordered for a patient in preterm labor. It is important to relax the uterine muscles and reduce contractions. This medication works by blocking calcium and has indications for use outside of pregnancy and labor. Choice *B* is an ineffective response because this medication is not indicated for pain management. Choice *C* is ineffective, as this medication would lower, rather than raise, blood pressure. Choice *D* is incorrect because not only is that not the function of the medication, but in most cases, increasing the frequency of contractions for a mother in preterm labor would not be desirable.

108. B: Choice *B* clearly describes the symptom presentation of a patient experiencing refeeding syndrome. In addition to weakness, shallow respirations, and seizures, this patient may exhibit confusion and an increased risk for bleeding. Choice *A* correlates with abdominal distention, while Choice *C* correlates with circulatory overload secondary to fluid and electrolyte imbalance. Choice *D* represents a response to a dislodged enteral tube or one that has been misplaced.

109. B: Thiamine, Choice *B,* represents a supplement given to a patient struggling with alcohol withdrawal, typically during the first few days of their inpatient hospitalization. Thiamine is often deficient in the patient experiencing frequent and excessive alcohol consumption. Choices *A, C,* and *D,* while important B vitamins, do not directly correlate with the patient's treatment needs at this time and therefore are not routinely administered as part of the treatment plan for alcohol withdrawal.

110. D: Ipratropium bromide, Choice *D,* is contraindicated for the patient with benign prostatic hypertrophy (BPH) as the use of this medication could encourage the development of urinary retention. Choices *A, B,* and *C* are considered compatible medications for individuals struggling with BPH and do not warrant a phone call to the prescriber for order verification.

111. B: Choice *B* is the priority, as the nurse must learn whether or not the fluid is cerebrospinal fluid (CSF), which would show positive for glucose on a strip test done at the bedside. Choice *A* would be an important next step for the nurse, as a fever could indicate infection in the patient leaking CSF. Choices *C* and *D* are not applicable interventions for this patient at this time. Choice *C* is not necessary as a priority intervention, as the nurse is able to assess for glucose at the bedside instead of sending a sample to the lab. Choice *D* is contraindicated and should be discouraged if the nurse identifies the drainage to be CSF.

112. C: Bradypnea, bradycardia, widening pulse pressure accurately aligns with a patient presentation of Cushing's triad post head injury. These assessment findings indicate that the patient is likely experiencing increased intracranial pressure at this time. Therefore, Choice *C* is correct. Choices *A*, *B*, and *D* do not represent assessment findings indicative of this physiological nervous system response.

113. B, C, D, E: Choices *B*, *C*, *D*, and *E* all represent early warning signs of increased intracranial pressure in the patient suffering from a head injury. Nausea, Choice *A*, is not a typical finding, as a key assessment notation for this diagnosis is vomiting in the absence of nausea.

114. A, B, C: Back pain, shortness of breath, and skin flushing (Choices *A*, *B*, and *C*) encourage the nurse to stop the transfusion due to a transfusion reaction. If the nurse suspects that the patient may be experiencing a transfusion reaction, the priority intervention is to stop the transfusion immediately. Blurred vision and lethargy (Choices *D* and *E*), while problematic, do not correlate with a transfusion reaction; rather, these signs indicate infiltration or vein injury.

115. A: The patient should perform the Valsalva maneuver, Choice *A*, while the nurse is performing bag or bottle changes or replacing tubing for total parenteral nutrition (TPN). This maneuver involves a moderately forceful expression of exhalation while one's mouth is closed and nose is pinched. It is encouraged to reduce the likelihood of an air embolus. Choices *B*, Choice *C*, and Choice *D* should not be encouraged, as they would not support a reduced likelihood of air embolus during this time.

116. B: Parenteral hyperalimentation, Choice *B*, is a term used interchangeably with total parenteral nutrition (TPN). TPN is designed to be an individual's complete source of nutrition. Oral nutritional supplementation, Choice *A*, describes nutrition consumed by mouth. PEG nutrition, Choice *C*, describes nutrition delivered via a percutaneous endoscopic gastrostomy tube directly to the digestive system. Peripheral parenteral nutrition, Choice *D*, involves nutrition that is complementary to another form of intake.

117. D: Colace® (docusate sodium), Choice *D*, can be prescribed alongside opiates to ease constipation, a common side effect of this drug class. Choice *A* represents a medication that is prescribed for opioid addiction and would not be prescribed at the time of opioid prescription for symptom management. Choice *B* and Choice *C* are both contraindicated for use while taking opiates and should be avoided at this time.

118. C: The nurse should ensure that the patient's vital signs are taken before administering Catapres® (clonidine), Choice *C*, as this medication often reduces blood pressure and pulse. While this medication is indicated to treat hypertension, it also is used outside of this indication, such as in the management of attention deficit hyperactivity disorder, anxiety, and sleep. Taking patient vital signs is an appropriate task to delegate to the unlicensed assistive personnel (UAP). Assisting the patient with eating their meal and asking about the time of their last bowel movement (Choices *A* and *B*), while important interventions in daily patient care, do not directly influence the administration of Catapres® (clonidine); therefore, they are not current priorities. Delivering a heated blanket, Choice *D*, does not directly impact the administration of this medication and is typically reserved to support circulatory concerns.

119. B: The loading dose, Choice *B*, is administered at the original dose to start the patient off with a quickly accumulated level to reach therapeutic effect quickly. Once the loading dose is administered, the patient then continues on with maintenance doses, Choice *D*, to maintain the therapeutic plasma concentration. Intermittent intravenous bolus, Choice *A*, is administered occasionally, as a larger plasma concentration is desired, oftentimes at the drug's half-life. An onset bolus dose, Choice *C*, is not a term that is used.

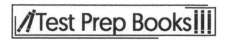

120. B: Choice *B* is cause for concern because it is below the normal range and alerts the nurse that the patient is experiencing hypokalemia, low circulating potassium in the blood. Choices *A*, *C*, and *D* are within normal range and are not causes for concern at this time. The normal range for serum potassium is 3.5–5.0 mEq/L.

121. C, E: Choice *C* and Choice *E* are causes for concern because they fall outside of the normal range. Choice *C* is below normal and alerts the nurse that the patient is experiencing hypocalcemia, low circulating calcium in the blood. Choice *E* is above normal and alerts the nurse that the patient is experiencing hypercalcemia, excessive circulating calcium in the blood. Choices *A*, *B*, and *D* are within normal range and are not causes for concern at this time. The normal range for serum calcium is 8.5–10.5 mg/dl.

122. C: Choice *C* directly influences symptoms of sadness, mourning, and grief by encouraging the client to work toward acceptance of their terminal diagnosis. Choice *A* should not be encouraged and, in fact, may be a sign of significant depression or suicidal ideation in this client. Choices *B* and *D* represent establishing engagements with long-term plans—time this patient might not have—which could further contribute to symptom exacerbation and is unlikely to produce a reduction of sadness, mourning, and grief.

123. C: Patients in renal failure who are on dialysis are at a heightened risk for developing anemia. As the kidneys are responsible for signaling the bones to make red blood cells, if they fail to function properly, the body may lack sufficient red blood cells and the patient will develop signs and symptoms of anemia. The patient is not MOST at risk for developing systemic lupus erythematous (Choice *A*), migraine headaches (Choice *B*), or Crohn's disease (Choice *D*).

124. B: The primary responsibility of the nurse case manager is to support the patient's ability to care for self. The nurse case manager is responsible for supporting positive patient outcomes and promoting quality of care across the continuum. Choices *A, C,* and *D* do not represent the primary responsibility.

125. D: The verbal handoff from nurse-to-nurse between shifts is referred to as a report. When the nurse uses an audiotape device to record critical components and an overall review of the shift for each patient, they are preparing a verbal recap of the care given for the next shift to consider. Choices *A, B,* and *C* do not involve leaving patient information on audiotape for another nurse to review.

126. A: The electronic health record (EHR) is a document containing charted documentation from multiple providers across specialties supporting patient care. Choice *C*, the medical record (EMR), is a charting system used by one provider, while the patient uses a personal health record (PHR) system (Choice *D*). Choice *B*, electronic medication administration record (EMAR), involves documentation of medication only.

127. B: Disruptive technology involves a modern technique that replaces and renders a previous technology obsolete. The current use of electronic health record (EHR) and electronic medical record (EMR) systems are examples of disruptive technologies. Choices *A, C,* and *D* do not involve technology that replaced previous technology.

128. D: Nurses must practice with consideration to nursing science and philosophy of law. These laws stem from both state and federal statues and guide practice consideration. Nursing jurisprudence is the act of navigating nursing practice with these considerations as the managing foundation for care. Choice *A* involves basic nursing care. Choice *B* includes basic rights that all humans hold, whereas nursing process, Choice *C*, involves sequential steps of the nursing practice.

129. A: The nursing process contains five sequential steps that function as a guiding system for nursing care. The steps of the nursing process include: Assessment, Diagnosis, Planning, Implementation, and Evaluation. These steps promote a rational method of organizing and implementing care.

130. C: In consideration of Maslow's Hierarchy of Needs, the nurse practices with attention to client wellbeing and prioritizes care accordingly. The hierarchy includes the following five stages: physiological; safety; love and belonging; esteem; and self-actualization. Physiological concerns make up the most fundamental stage of this theory and signify the most basic human needs for care.

131. B: Erikson's Psychosocial Development Theory involves eight stages centered on healthy development from infancy to late adulthood. The theory, designed by Erik and Joan Erikson in the twentieth century, encourages parents to allow the infant to signal some needs before responding, and then promptly respond with support.

132. C: Drinking from a cup is considered an age-appropriate developmental milestone of the 24-month-old child. Eating with a fork (Choice A), pouring into a cup (Choice D), and cutting with a kid-friendly knife (Choice B) typically come later in child development.

133. A: Tardive dyskinesia, a serious side effect of antipsychotic medication, produces many involuntary movements including tongue thrusting. Tardive dyskinesia is an involuntary neurologic movement disorder with persistent effect. Headache (Choice B), blurred vision (Choice C), and fever (Choice D) are not symptoms of Tardive dyskinesia.

134. B: Naegele's Rule sets forth that the estimated date of delivery for a newborn can be calculated by adding a year, subtracting three months, and then adding seven days to the mother's date of last menses.

135. A: The first period of reactivity following the birth of a newborn typically lasts 30 minutes. It takes place during the first 30 minutes of life and involves the initial episode of engagement with stimuli. After this activity and alertness ends, the newborn falls into a deep sleep.

136. C: Pregnant women during their third trimester are at risk for developing physiologic anemia. Expanded maternal blood volume during this trimester contributes to the anemia. Choices A, B, and D are not conditions that are commonly associated with third trimester pregnancy.

137. B: Age-related macular degeneration causes numerous symptoms, including the distortion of straight lines. The lines may appear wavy to the individual struggling with this condition. Flashes of light (Choice A), poor peripheral vision (Choice C), and reduced depth perception (Choice D) can be witnessed in other ocular disorders, though are not typical symptoms of macular degeneration.

138. A: The patient with histamine intolerance may struggle to process fermented foods, such as sauerkraut, which is pickled cabbage. Fermented foods promote histamine overload in those with histamine intolerance. The nurse should provide patient education and request a nutritional consult with a dietician. Fresh fish (Choice B), sweet potato (Choice C), and blueberry (Choice D) are considered low-histamine foods.

139. A: The nurse case manager engages with third-party payers during a patient's inpatient stay in order to review current treatment, cost, and plans for additional care. This process, known as concurrent review, is a standard activity of the inpatient stay. Choice B, prior authorization, is specific to

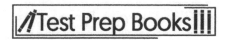

medication or individual intervention. Choice C, retrospective review, takes place after discharge to seek coverage for care. Choice D, prospective review, happens before admission.

140. D: The discharge planning process starts right away at admission for every patient. Each aspect of care is provided with an end-goal in mind. When the patient comes into the care of a healthcare organization, the treatment plan involves interventions with an ultimate anticipated outcome of safe discharge.

141. C: Patient consent is not needed for a physical restraint. In order for a physical restraint to move forward, the reason for the intervention (Choice A), the type of restraint used (Choice B), and the supporting patient behaviors (Choice D) must be documented. The use of this intervention must be thoroughly documented and substantiated.

142. C: Neuroleptic malignant syndrome (NMS), a life-threatening reaction, includes symptoms such as hyperthermia, confusion, tachycardia, tachypnea, muscle rigidity, altered mental status, and variable blood pressure. NMS can occur in response to antipsychotic medication. While Choice A, tardive dyskinesia (TD), and Choice B, extrapyramidal side effects (EPS), can also occur in response to antipsychotic medication use, these conditions possess alternative symptoms. Parkinsonian symptoms can be seen with antipsychotic medication use; however, Choice D, Parkinson's disease, is not linked to this medication class.

143. B: The ethical principle of veracity is grounded in truth. Ethical practice is integrated into all aspects of nursing care. The nurse should be honest and tell the truth to patients and caregivers, as this is the basis to building trust in the relationship and supporting fair, autonomous, informed decision making.

144. C: During a respiratory assessment of a patient with emphysema, it is critical for the nurse to percuss the patient's chest wall. This technique helps to inform what lies beneath, such as air, fluid, or solid mass. The nurse expects to note hyper-resonance upon examination of this patient.

145. C: The patient with psychiatric illness is entitled to receive the benefit of care from the members of the interdisciplinary team—including case management—upon primary diagnosis at initial admission. This support is not reliant on patient's legal status for admission (Choices A, B, and D).

146. B: An elevated level of circulating thyroid-stimulating hormone (TSH) causes symptoms that correlate with hypothyroidism. Choice A, muscle cramps, Choice C, fatigue, and Choice D, coarse hair, are all symptoms of this disease, while weight loss is a symptom of hyperthyroidism. In hyperthyroidism, the nurse would expect to see a low TSH level.

147. B: Black, tarry stool, known as melena, is a sign of a gastrointestinal bleed. The higher up in the gastrointestinal track the bleed is, the darker the blood is in the stool. While Choice C, the consumption of beets, and Choice A, iron supplements, can affect the color of stool, they do not cause melena. Melena would not be seen from consuming a preparatory solution, and upper GI tract endoscopies do not entail an oral preparatory solution (Choice D).

148: D: The Five Rights of Delegation include the right person, circumstance, communication, evaluation, and task. This process of delegation supports the evaluation of time management skills and aligns the appropriate individual with the correct task.

149. A: The licensed practical nurse (LPN) has the authority to perform dressing changes (Choice C), insert Foley catheters (Choice D), and hang subsequent bags of normal saline for infusion (Choice B). The

LPN does not have the ability to push intravenous medications. The registered nurse (RN) should not have delegated the administration of Lasix (furosemide) via intravenous push to the LPN.

150. C: Continuity of care is a longstanding process that involves an ongoing relationship between a patient and their providers, with shared goals to establish the most effective care. Continuity of care retains a focus on maintenance and wellbeing with cost-effective approaches in mind. The key to this relationship is longevity with health-maintenance engagements. Choice *A* signifies minimum standards, while Choice *B* and Choice *D* focus on reducing risks and improving care.

151. A: Basic human needs consist of oxygen, nutrition, hydration, elimination, temperature, rest, sex, and shelter. While Choices *B*, *C*, and *D*, include needs important for stable wellbeing, they are considered secondary to the most basic, physiological needs for survival.

152. B: Healthcare professionals must ensure to provide only the minimum information necessary to safely and properly treat a patient. Additional information, otherwise not applicable to care, should be omitted.

153. D: The Health Information Portability and Accountability Act of 1996 (HIPAA) is a federal law that enables patients to request their medical records. In addition, this law provides protection of personal health information (PHI) from being disclosed without the patient's consent. The HIPAA privacy rule affects physical, administrative, and technical aspects of healthcare business. Choices *A*, *B*, and *C* do not involve obtaining a patient record for self-use.

154. A: The utilization review nurse is part of the interdisciplinary team and is granted access to patient records. The UR nurse accesses medical records in order to secure financial payment from third-party payers by completing concurrent patient reviews that explore the medical services offered and their associated monetary costs.

155. C: The ethical provision of autonomy sets forth that a patient has the right to make autonomous, therefore independent, self-directed decisions. The provider must not influence the patient. Education and information should be provided in order to promote informed consent, whether for or against treatment interventions. Choice *A*, beneficence, promotes the moral imperative of doing right, while Choice *B*, nonmaleficence, is to do no harm. Choice *D*, justice, promotes an ethical fairness to healthcare practices.

156. A: Role responsibilities for each interdisciplinary member of the team are delineated under state rule. While Choice *B*, federal rule, provides general guidelines, state rule defines the specifics regarding healthcare roles and responsibilities. Choice *C*, hospital protocol, and Choice *D*, management delegation, come secondary and cannot overrule state statue.

157. C: Ethical dilemmas in practice happen, and the nurse must be prepared to advocate for the patient. When reporting a concern, the nurse should first report up the chain of command (in this case, to the charge nurse). When the charge nurse failed to respond, the nurse would appropriately elevate this issue to the nursing supervisor. Choices *A*, *B*, and *D* do not follow the nursing chain of command.

158. B: The transfer of values and practices from one cultural group to another is referred to as assimilation. Choice *C*, separation, involves leaving the dominant host culture, while Choice *A*, integration, combines two cultures—the culture of origin and the dominant host culture. Choice *D*, marginalization, occurs when both the culture of origin and the dominant host culture are rejected.

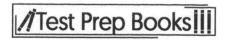

159. D: Personal protective equipment (PPE) must be removed at the patient's doorway. In addition, it would also be appropriate to remove PPE just outside the patient's room. PPE must not be removed at the nursing station (Choice A), at the bedside (Choice B), or in the patient's bathroom (Choice C), as these occurrences would put infection control and safety at risk.

160. C: When working with a patient on airborne precautions, the nurse must remove their respirator outside of the patient's room after closing the patient's door. It would not be appropriate to remove the respirator outside of the medication room (Choice A), inside of the patient's room (Choice B), or in the patient's bathroom (Choice D).

161. D: While working with a patient who is attempting to spit on the staff during a behavioral code, the nurse should instruct the team to apply gowns, gloves, and masks with eye shields. Donning of this personal protective equipment (PPE) fosters safe infection control practices by protecting at-risk surfaces during the code. Choices A, B, and C would not protect all at-risk surfaces.

162. C: Personal protective equipment (PPE) must be systematically applied to promote proper infection control. In effectively applying PPE, the educator first dons their gown, then mask, then goggles, followed by gloves.

163. A: The patient utilizing oxygen for respiratory management should switch from aerosol to stick deodorant, as aerosol cans present a fire risk. To promote safe discharge, the nurse must assess for understanding of proper use of new equipment in the home. Choices B, C, and D do not show safe handling to prevent fire.

164. B: Before discharge, the nurse case manager discusses home care considerations with the patient. When the patient reports that their morning medication causes an unsteady gait, the nurse case manager is alerted to the need to address this safety issue, as the patient is at risk for falls. Choices A, C, and D do not exhibit risk and do not need to be addressed at this time.

165. A: The Stages of Conflict represent a sequential conflict process that includes four stages: latent, perceive, felt, manifest. When participants in conflict are initially engaged, they often perceive themselves to hold incompatible outcomes. Understanding the Stages of Conflict provides the nurse with an opportunity to examine the core process of conflict resolution for success.

166. A: When using patient data for research, authorization (Choices C and D) and consent (Choice B) are not necessary; however, the nurse researcher must ensure to de-identify all patients.

167. C: A patient struggling with hyponatremia is at increased risk for developing vomiting (Choice B), diarrhea (Choice A), and polydipsia (Choice D). Diplopia, double vision, is not commonly associated with this imbalance.

168. B: Dialectical behavioral therapy (DBT), developed in the late 1980s, is a specific type of psychotherapy that is effectively applied to support populations struggling with personality disorders and urges to self-harm. Psychodynamic therapy (Choice A), play therapy (Choice C), and humanistic therapy (Choice D) would not be appropriate for the nurse to use given the context of the situation (nurse-facilitated group) and the patient population involved.

169. B: The nurse must educate the patient regarding the risk for dehiscence of the new colostomy. If the stoma is retracted, it could lead to dehiscence at the mucocutaneous junction. Ultimately, the patient would be at risk for intraperitoneal contamination. Renal calculi (Choice A), nocturnal enuresis

(Choice *C*) and pernicious anemia (Choice *D*) do not require education at this time, as they are not chief concerns associated with a new colostomy.

170. B: The healthcare power of attorney is financially responsible for one's healthcare decisions. When an individual is looking to complete advance directives, consideration for who will approve charges and manage financial concerns is a crucial part of the healthcare planning process. The healthcare proxy (Choice *A*), agent (Choice *C*), and provider (Choice *D*) are not authorized to control finances.

171. D: Sudden infant death syndrome (SIDS) is the leading cause of infant mortality during the first month of life. SIDS involves the unexplained death of an infant, typically during sleep. The cause of SIDS is currently unknown.

172. D: Eating disorders primarily develop during adolescence. Eating disorders are psychological disorders involving extreme disturbances in eating behavior, often accompanied by intrusive thoughts. While disordered eating can develop in infancy (Choice *A*) manifested through failure to thrive, the etiology differs. While young (Choice *B*) and late (Choice *C*) adulthood phases involve numerous disordered eating cases, some with similar etiology (psychological) and others that differ (stemming from physical manifestations), they do not result in the greatest number of initiated cases.

173. A: The nurse should report this issue to the nursing supervisor. This action promotes the elevation of a concern up the discipline (nursing) chain of command. In this specific case, the nursing supervisor may opt to connect with the surgeon (Choice *B*) to formulate a plan for next steps, including consent (Choice *C*). Choice *D*, a code team, is not necessary to determine how to proceed at this time.

174. C: The nurse should be concerned about the patient reporting an aching leg, as this is not a normal finding after electroconvulsive therapy (ECT). Temporary amnesia, headache, mild confusion, and forgetfulness are all normal side effects of ECT and are to be expected; therefore, Choices *A*, *B*, and *D* are incorrect.

175. B: Dissociation is an experience involving a disconnection from the present moment. Triggers for a dissociative episode typically include an overload of stimuli, often connected to a traumatic event.

176. A: In order for a nurse to be deemed competent, a minimum level of proficiency, referred to as standard of care, must be maintained. The nurse must provide care that another reasonable nurse with similar resources would provide. Choices *B*, *C*, and *D* involve where the care takes place, the length of care provision, and the overall quality, but do not define minimum proficiency.

177. D: When working with the bed captain to assign patient rooms upon hospital admission, the nursing supervisor should consider the Muslim (Islam) patient's need to have a room that faces the direction of the Kaaba in the Hejazi city of Mecca. This is the direction that the patient will need to face when praying. The religions found within Choices *A*, *B*, and *C* do not influence room placement.

178. B: While probing (Choice *A*), focusing (Choice *D*), and the use of silence (*C*) are all therapeutic communication techniques, restating specifically involves reiterating what was verbally expressed. This technique provides reassurance to the patient that the nurse is listening and has heard what they have said. It also fosters a therapeutic opportunity to ensure that the message was accurately received.

179. C: When assessing pain, the PQRST method, which stands for provoke, quality, region, severity, and timing, can prove helpful. This technique encourages a comprehensive review of the patient's pain, which leads to appropriate intervention and management.

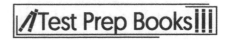

180. D: The principle diagnosis is the chief reason for the patient's inpatient hospitalization, while the primary diagnosis (Choice *C*) is what requires the most resources during their stay. Oftentimes, the principle diagnosis will also turn out to be the primary diagnosis, although this is not always the case. Secondary diagnoses (Choice *B*) either coexist at the time of admission or develop during the hospitalization in addition to the primary and principle diagnoses. The discharge diagnosis (Choice *A*) focuses on the diagnosis the patient leaves the episode with.

181. A: Infant patients require review of brachial pulses to achieve the most accurate results indicative of cardiac functioning. Using one or two fingers inside the infant's arm at the crease of the elbow, the nurse is able to palpate the brachial artery. The pulse placements found in Choices *B*, *C*, and *D* do not support proper infant cardiac functioning, rather are more effective in assessment of child and adult populations.

182. A: The cultural value of interpersonal harmony may be reflected in the head nodding expressed by the Japanese-American patient. The provider must not assume that the patient agrees (Choice *B*) or accepts the treatment change (Choice *C*), nor should they assume that the patient has a full understanding of the intervention (Choice *D*).

183. C: The cardiac monitor technician, an unlicensed assistive member of the team, has the authority to monitor telemetry (Choice *A*), print rhythm strips (Choice *B*), and notify the team when no discernible activity is detected (Choice *D*). The monitor technician should never interpret cardiac rhythm, as that is beyond their scope of practice.

184. B: Vital signs must not be taken on the arm of the affected side (which is termed the ipsilateral side) post-mastectomy. Vital signs should be taken on the contralateral arm to support accurate readings and avoid aggravating possible lymphedema on the affected side, especially during blood pressure readings. Choices *A*, *C*, and *D* are all appropriate actions that do not warrant further education at this time.

185. C: The standard progression of discipline involves counseling, oral warning, written warning (Choice *D*), suspension (Choice *B*), termination (Choice *A*), typically in that order. For grand offenses, the earlier stages of discipline may be omitted. If the nurse fails to correct their behavior resulting in continued poor time management after the counseling, the next disciplinary action to be expected is an oral warning.

186. B: A patient with meningococcal meningitis must be placed on droplet precautions. After completing twenty-four hours of antibiotic therapy, the patient's treatment can transition to standard precautions. Droplet precautions involve the use of a private room. Every individual who enters the room must wear a mask. The nurse must prioritize this intervention before engaging in others. Choices *A* and *C* are not priority interventions, as they should take place after the patient is placed on the appropriate precaution level to prevent the spread of infection. Standard precautions, Choice *D*, are not sufficient.

187. A: The most immediate action the nurse should take after noticing that the patient looks pale and feels cold is to assist the patient back to bed to prevent a fall. Afterward, the nurse can assess the patient's nutrition and hemodynamic status (Choices *B*, *C*, and *D*).

188. A: Performance improvement is an organizational process aimed at improving efficiency and measuring output. This system involves managing outcomes, corrective action plans, and variance trends.

189. B: When unwarranted tests are ordered and standard tests are omitted, the variance is identified to be from the practitioner source. The practitioner is modifying the standard process and is inconsistent with the customary treatment for a given symptom set or diagnosis. Choices *A*, *C*, and *D* do not represent the cause of the variance in this scenario.

190. A: Patients diagnosed with benign prostatic hypertrophy should not use Atrovent (ipratropium bromide). The use of this drug could cause acute urinary retention and must be avoided.

191. C: The nurse must stop the blood transfusion immediately after the patient complains of a headache and double vision. These symptoms may signify a transfusion reaction. Additional intervention, such as assessing vital signs (Choice *D*) and calling a rapid response (Choice *A*) may be indicated; however, these actions would take place after the transfusion has been stopped. Choice *B*, slowing the transfusion, is incorrect, as the correct response, stopping the transfusion, must take place.

192. A: The infant patient with a history of intussusception is not a candidate for the rotavirus vaccine. Intussusception involves a bowel blockage and bowel ischemia stemming from the colon folding into itself. Infants with a history of intussusception are at greater risk of developing intussusception again post rotavirus vaccination. Choices *B*, *C*, and *D* are not contraindicated by intussusception.

193. B: The patient presenting to the emergency department with signs and symptoms of hypovolemic shock should be placed in the modified Trendelenburg position to improve blood pressure and cardiac output. The nurse should educate the technician on proper positioning when time warrants (Choice *A*). The nurse should not praise the technician (Choice *C*), as the placement was incorrect. The nurse may report this incompetent behavior to the supervisor; however, it should happen after the nurse corrects the position and the patient is stabilized (Choice *D*).

194. C: Chlamydia and gonorrhea, sexually transmitted infections, are associated with the development of pelvic inflammatory disease (PID). When bacteria from these infections travel upward to the reproductive organs from the vagina or cervix, pelvic inflammatory disease may develop. The disorders and diseases represented by Choices *A*, *B*, and *D* are not associated with PID.

195. B: When working with a patient who has a strong history of aggressive behavior, the nursing team should start the therapeutic relationship by establishing trust and rapport. The team should strive to maintain a proactive approach to support and anticipate patient needs. The use of medication (Choice *C*), restraints (Choice *D*), and seclusion (Choice *A*), while potential interventions for care, should not happen first or without warrant by the current episode.

196. C: Hildegard Peplau's Theory of Interpersonal Relations includes four sequential phases, which are orientation, identification, exploitation, and resolution. The orientation phase is when the nurse and patient first meet, and the problem is defined. Choice *B*, the identification phase, focuses on appropriate assistance. Next, the exploitation phase (Choice *A*) encompasses using the assistance to address the problem. Finally, the resolution phase (Choice *D*) involves the termination of the relationship now that the problem has been addressed and the patient's needs have been met.

197. A: The graduate nurse is functioning at the most fundamental stage of Patricia Benner's Model of Novice to Expert, the novice stage. With each stage having defined accomplishments and characteristics, the novice stage, as it encompasses the new nurse functioning within simple, objective tasks, is the stage the graduate functions in. As the nurse strives to understand how to use discretionary judgment, which comes in later stages, they successfully transition onward. Nursing theorist Patricia Benner first

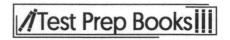

introduced this model in 1982. The five sequential stages include: novice, advanced beginner, competent (Choice *C*), proficient (Choice *D*), and expert (Choice *B*).

198. D: The licensed practical nurse would appropriately report a wound that is black in color to the registered nurse for further assessment, as wounds of this color may need to be debrided and should not be rewrapped by the licensed practical nurse without further review. Pink (Choice *A*), red (Choice *B*), and yellow (Choice *C*) wounds do not signify the need to debride at this point.

199. A: While many findings are often noted within a "5 Why's Analysis," the chief focus of this type of review is to determine the root cause of an event. The root cause informs the team how to move forward with establishing next steps for quality improvement. During this analysis, the interdisciplinary team asks why an event occurs, then asks why to the response of the first question, and so on, until the root cause has been identified.

200. A: When working with a patient who communicates in a different language from that of the nurse, the nurse should request support from a healthcare interpreter to ensure effective interpersonal communication takes place. This process fosters safe, quality care, which would not be seen by implementing Choices *B*, *C*, or *D*, all of which would carry substantial risk for miscommunication and liability.

Index

A&OX3, 160

ABC, 19, 20, 41

ABCs, 19, 181

Abduction, 49, 102

Acceptance, 64, 79, 83

Accident Prevention, 36

Action Phase, 83

Active Range of Motion Exercises, 68, 69, 102, 105

Acuity, 11, 30, 33, 146, 174

Acute Infections, 51

Adduction, 102

Administrative Law, 24, 32, 35

Adrenal, 96, 173, 176

Adrenal Medulla, 174

Adrenaline, 91, 174

Advance Directives, 9, 60, 78

Adverse Effect, 117, 118, 122

Advocacy, 9, 10

Advocate, 9, 10, 11, 12, 18, 30, 33, 65

Aged Population, 59, 60

Airborne Droplets, 50

Airborne Precautions, 50

Alanine Transaminase (ALT), 153, 155

Aldosterone, 174

Alveoli, 172

Ambulating, 42, 105

American Nurses Association's Code of Ethics, 21

Amino Acids, 109

Anaphylaxis, 96, 117, 188

and Low-Density Lipoprotein (LDL), 155

Anger, 63, 79

Antagonistic Drug Interactions, 118

Antepartum Care, 60

Anti-Embolism Stockings, 104

Apnea, 137

Arousal and Reactivity Symptoms, 85

Arterial Blood Gas (ABG), 153

Arteries, 113, 115, 148, 153, 171

Artifact, 140, 142

Ascending Colon, 172

Aspartate Aminotransferase (AST), 153, 155

Aspiration, 68, 69, 131, 134, 156, 157, 165, 166, 192, 195

Assistive Devices, 37, 38, 43, 75, 97, 98, 101, 102

Atherosclerosis, 108

Atrial Fibrillation, 117, 143

Auscultation, 60, 113, 115, 150, 168

Autoclaves, 46

Autogenic Training, 106

Automated Cell Counts, 154

Automated External Defibrillator (AED), 183

Avoidance Symptoms, 85

Bacteria, 45, 49, 50, 51, 100, 118, 154

Bargain, 79

Basic Metabolic Panel (BMP), 153

Bedsores, 103

Biofeedback, 106

Biohazards, 45

Bipolar Disorder, 74, 84, 85, 96, 181

Bladder, 80, 82, 99, 100

Blood Pressure, 22, 36, 94, 96, 106

BMI, 149, 152

Brachial Pulse, 135

Brachytherapy, 46

Bradycardia, 136

Bradypnea, 137

Buccal Medications, 124

Capillaries, 113, 115, 171

Carbohydrates, 108, 109, 110, 174

Cardiac Diet, 106

Cardiac Index, 179, 180, 192, 194

Cardiac Output, 135, 157, 179, 180, 192, 194, 195

Cardiovascular System, 171, 179

Case Manager, 11, 12, 13, 18, 29, 30, 33, 72

CAT Scan, 139

Catabolism, 129

Catheter, 53, 100, 120, 127, 130, 133

C-Diff, 52

Celiac Disease, 110

Central Nervous System, 161, 170

Central Venous Access Devices, 120

Central Venous Pressure (CVP), 179, 180

Certified Nursing Assistants (CNAs), 17, 33

Cervix, 152, 173

Chambers, 120, 136, 138, 171

Charting by Exception, 26

Child Neglect, 71

Cholesterol, 106, 108, 109, 118, 153, 155

Clinical IT (CIT), 23

Clostridium Difficile, 50, 52

Coagulation Testing/International Normalized Ratio (INR), 154

Cocaine, 90, 94, 95, 96

Cognition and Mood Symptoms, 85, 86

Collaboration, 15, 16, 92, 155

Colostomy, 99, 100

Common Law, 24, 32, 35

Complete Blood Count (CBC), 138, 153, 169

Complete Heart Block, 143

Complete Protein, 109

Compound Fracture, 185

Comprehensive Metabolic Panel (CMP), 153

Comprehensive Method, 26

Concussions, 184

Consent, 9, 13, 14, 17

Constipation, 99, 104

Constitutional Law, 24, 32, 35

Contact Precautions, 50

Contact-Guard Assistance (CGA), 38

Continuity of Care Model, 18

Contractures, 68, 105

Contraindication, 117

Corticosterone, 174

Cortisol, 174

Cotton Mouth, 81

Criminal Law, 25, 32, 35

Crisis Plan, 74

CRP, 156

Cryoprecipitate, 119

Crystal, 90

CT, 64, 130, 139, 166

Culture, 9, 27, 76, 77, 80, 91, 111, 154, 156

CVADs, 120, 130

Cyanosis, 175

Deep Vein Thrombosis (DVT), 104

Delirium Tremens (DTs), 89

Denial, 63, 79

Depression, 32, 54, 59, 61

Descending Colon, 172

Diabetic Diet, 106

Diabetic Neuropathy, 111

Diagnostic Test, 73, 138, 139, 157

Diaphragm, 148, 171, 172

Diarrhea, 50, 51, 52, 67

Diastolic Number, 136

Dietary Fiber, 109

Dietary Supplements, 109

Digestive System, 171, 172

Distraction, 74, 106

Do Not Resuscitate (DNR), 9

Droplet Precautions, 50, 56

Drug Interaction, 118, 195

Dysphagia, 156

Dysthymia, 84

E Chart, 146

Echo, 138

Echocardiography, 138

Edema, 110, 160, 165, 167, 179, 189

EHR (Electronic Health Record), 24

Elder Abuse and Neglect, 72

Electrolytes, 109, 133, 152, 153, 175, 176, 178

Eliminate, 18, 22, 99

Emotional, 14, 44, 53

Emotional Awareness, 74

End of Life Care, 60, 77, 78

Endocrine System, 96, 173, 176

Endoscope, 138

Endoscopy, 138, 164, 166

End-Tidal Carbon Dioxide (ETCO2), 159

Epinephrine Pen, 188

Epi-Pen, 188

Ergonomics, 42

Erythrocyte Sedimentation Rate (ESR), 154

Esophagus, 89, 108, 157, 165, 167, 172

Essential Amino Acids, 109

Estrogen, 174

Evidence-Based Practice (EBP), 27, 28

Expected Outcome, 114, 115, 122, 131

Expired Air, 172

Extension, 103

Fair Treatment, 14

Fallopian Tubes, 173

Fats, 108, 110, 155, 174

Fat-Soluble Vitamins, 109

Fight-Or-Flight Response, 85, 174

Financial Abuse, 14

First-Degree Burns, 186

Flashbacks, 85

Flexion, 103

Fluid-Restricted Diet, 107
Formulary, 122, 131, 133
Fresh Frozen Plasma (FFP), 119
Fungal Infections, 50
Gait Belts, 37, 43, 102
Gambling Addiction, 91
General Anesthesia, 128, 161, 167
Glomerular Filtration Rate (GFR), 155
Growth Chart, 152
Halal, 107
Handoff Report, 25, 26
Hazardous Material, 45, 46
Head Circumference, 152
Health Care IT, 23
Health Insurance Portability and Accountability Act (HIPAA), 13, 17, 18
Health Promotion, 63, 72
Heart Rate, 77, 135, 136, 144, 145, 161, 165, 167, 168, 179, 189, 193, 195
Heart-Healthy Diet, 69, 106
Hematocrit (HCT), 154
Hematopoietic System, 171
Hematuria, 100
Hemodynamic Measurement, 180
Hemodynamics, 179, 194
Hemoglobin, 119, 138, 149, 153, 154, 155, 157, 171, 194
Hemoglobin A1c, 155
Heparin, 95, 96, 119
High Fowler's Position, 101
High-Density Lipoprotein (HDL), 108, 155
High-Risk Behaviors, 59, 65, 83, 88
Holter Monitor, 144
Homeostasis, 34, 78, 174, 175, 176, 178
Horse, 90
Hospice, 29, 60, 77, 78
Human Chorionic Gonadotropin, 156
Hydrocortisone, 174
Hypercalcemia, 178
Hypermagnesemia, 178
Hypernatremia, 176
Hyperphosphatemia, 178
Hypersexuality, 90
Hypertensive, 136
Hyperthermia, 137, 161
Hypocalcemia, 153, 178
Hypomagnesemia, 153, 178
Hyponatremia, 153, 176

Hypophosphatemia, 153, 178
Hypothalamus, 173, 174
Hypothermia, 36, 137, 158
Hypoxia, 175, 180
Implanted VAD, 120
Implied Consent, 22, 34
Impressionable-Years Hypothesis, 62
Including Blood Urea Nitrogen (BUN), 153, 155
Incomplete Protein, 109
Incontinence, 81, 82, 99, 104, 111, 195
Increasing Persistence Hypothesis, 62
Information Technology (IT), 22, 23, 24
Informed, 10, 21, 22, 57, 161, 181, 192, 195
Informed Consent, 10, 21, 22, 161, 192, 195
Initial Assessment, 66, 73, 78, 88, 181
Insoluble Fiber, 109
Inspection, 150, 152
Inspiration, 172
Instilled, 125
Instructions for Use (IFU), 48
Insulin, 47, 110, 125, 126, 129, 174, 177, 181
Intake and Output (I&O), 107
Integumentary, 169
Intentional Tort, 25, 32, 35
Intercostal Muscles, 172
Intimate Partner Violence and Abuse, 71
Intramuscular Injections, 123
Intrapartum Care, 60
Ishihara Color Vision Test, 145
Jaeger Card, 146
Joint Commission's Surgical Care Improvement Project (SCIP), 159
Joints, 43, 102, 105, 109, 170
Kidneys, 90, 139, 153, 155, 172, 173, 176, 194
Kosher, 87, 107
Kubler-Ross Grieving Model, 79
Lactase, 107, 110
Lactose, 107, 110
Lactose Intolerant, 107
Large Intestine, 172
Latent Infections, 51
Lateral, 43, 101
Left Ventricular End-Diastolic Pressure (LVEDP), 180
Liability, 25
Life-Long Openness Hypothesis, 62
Ligaments, 170, 173
Local Anesthesia, 161

Low-Density Lipoprotein (LDL), 108
Lymph, 171, 176, 178
Lymphatic System, 171
Lymphatic Vessels, 171
M-A-A-U-A-R, 19, 31, 34
Major Depression, 84
Malignant Hyperthermia (MH), 159
Mammography, 64, 138, 164, 166
Manipulation, 150
Maximum Assistance (MAX), 38
Mean Arterial Pressure (MAP), 179, 180, 195
Melanin, 169
Membrane Potential, 176
Menopause, 173
Mensuration, 150
Mental Abuses, 14
Mental Status Exam, 60
Mindfulness, 74
Mineral/Electrolytes, 109
Minimum Assistance (MIN), 38
Molluscum Contagiosum, 51
Monospot Test, 155
Mood Disorder, 84, 85, 178
Mood Disorder Related to Another Health
    Condition, 84
Moral Agent, 10
Morgue, 82
Musculoskeletal System, 160, 170
Myelin Sheath, 170
Myocardial Infarction (MI), 159
N-Acetylcysteine (NAC), 155
Nasal Cannula, 81, 174, 175, 187, 188
Nasogastric (NG) Tube, 108, 158, 182, 192
Nebulizers, 125
Negative Coping Mechanisms, 44
Nephron, 172, 173
Neurological Assessment, 60, 160
Normal Sinus, 142
Nursing Practice, 9, 25, 66
OneSOURCE, 48
Opposite Action, 74
Oral Medications, 72, 124
Organic, 108, 109
Oriented Times One, 160
Oriented Times Three, 160
Orthostatic Hypotension, 137, 166
Osteoporosis, 64, 170
OTC Medications, 123

Ovaries, 152, 173, 174
Overeating, 86, 91
Overworking, 90
Oxygen Saturation Rate, 149
Packed Red Blood Cells (PRBC), 119
Palliative Care, 29, 60, 77
Palpated, 135
Palpation, 113, 115, 150, 152, 192, 195
Pancreas, 89, 110, 173
PAP Smear, 152
Parathyroid, 173
Parenteral, 117, 120, 121, 127, 128, 131, 134
Partial Thromboplastin Time (PTT), 119
PASS, 41, 57, 61, 162, 172, 173
Passive Range of Motion Exercises, 68, 69, 102,
    105
Pathophysiology, 169, 181, 189
Patient-Centered Medical Home (PCMH), 19, 33
PDCA Cycle, 27
Peak Flow Rate, 147
Pelvic Exam, 152
Penis, 61, 173
Perception, 16, 83
Percussion, 150
Performance Improvement, 26
Periosteum Membrane, 170
Peripheral Nervous System, 170
Peripherally Inserted Central Catheter (PICC)
    Line, 120, 130, 133, 192, 194
Peristalsis, 105, 172
Personal Protective Equipment (PPE), 49, 50,
    56, 57, 162
Pharmacological Therapy, 117, 181
Physical Abuse, 14, 71
PICOT Framework, 27
Pinch-Off Syndrome, 120
Pineal Gland, 174
Pituitary Gland, 174
Pneumothorax, 189, 193, 195
Polydipsia, 161
Polyuria, 161
Positive Coping Mechanisms, 44
Postpartum Hemorrhage, 189, 193, 195
Postpartum Phase, 61
Power of Attorney, 9, 14
Pre-Contemplation, 83
Prehypertensive, 136
Preload, 179, 194

Prescription Drugs, 122, 123
Pressure Sores, 54, 68, 69, 70, 103, 104
Pressure Ulcers, 11, 57, 81, 103, 157
Preterm, 61
Primary Prevention, 63
Progressive Muscle Relaxation, 106
Prone, 101, 111, 127
Prostate Gland, 173
Protected Health Information (PHI), 17
Proteins, 109, 131, 134, 155, 171, 174
Prothrombin Time/International Normalized Ratio (PT/INR), 119
Pulmonary Artery Catheter (PAC), 179
Pulmonary Artery Occlusion Pressure (PAOP), 179
Pulmonary Artery Pressure, 179, 180
Pulmonary Capillary Wedge Pressure (PCWP), 180
Pulmonary Embolism (PE), 104
Pulse Oximetry Device, 149
RACE Acronym, 41
Radial Pulse, 135, 150, 164, 166
Radio Frequency Identification (RFID), 23
Range of Motion Exercises, 69, 102, 104, 112
Rapid Influenza Diagnostic Test (RIDT), 156
Rate of Breathing, 137, 164, 166
Real Time Polymerase Chain Reaction, 156
Rectal Tube, 99, 100, 111, 168
Red Bone Marrow, 171
Referral, 29, 32, 35, 97, 98
Regional Anesthetic, 161
Relapse Stage, 83
Renal Diet, 106
Report, 14, 17, 25, 26
Respiratory System, 172
Restraints, 53, 54, 108
Rhinoviruses, 51
Right of Self-Determination, 13
Right Ventricular End-Diastolic Volume (RVEDV), 179
Right-Heart Catheter, 179, 192, 194
Rock, 90
Safe Lifting Techniques, 43
Saturated Fats, 108
SBAR Method, 26
Scrotum, 173
Sebum, 169, 170
Second-Degree Burns, 186

Self-Actualization, 20, 181
Self-Esteem, 20, 34, 62, 71, 84, 86
Self-Harm, 75, 83, 91
Self-Image, 62, 104
Self-Soothing, 74
Semi-Fowler's Position, 101
Seminal Vesicles, 173
Sensory Organs, 174
Sequential Compression Devices (SCDs), 104, 159
Serum Electrolyte Panel, 152
Sexual Abuse, 14, 54, 71
Sexual Addiction, 90
Sexually-Transmitted Bacterial Infections, 51
Shock, 15, 79, 117, 137, 158, 180, 186, 192
Side Effects, 36, 42, 105, 107, 110
Sinus Bradycardia, 143
Sinus Tachycardia, 142
Skeletal Muscles, 170
Smack, 90
Small Intestine, 100, 110, 124, 172
SMART, 65, 73, 78, 83, 92
Soluble Fiber, 109
Speech-Awareness Recognition (SAT), 146
Speech-Detection Threshold (SDT), 146
Speech-Recognition Threshold (SRT), 146
Sphygmomanometer, 136, 148
Spirometry, 147
Spleen, 171
Stand by Assistance (SBA), 38
Standard Precautions, 49, 50, 57
Statutory Law, 24, 32, 35
Stethoscope, 148, 150
Stomach, 43, 89, 101, 105
Stroke Index, 180
Stroke Volume (SV), 180
Sublingual Medications, 124
Substance Abuse, 32, 35, 71, 89, 93
Substance-Induced Mood Disorder, 84
Supine, 101, 102, 125, 139
Suppositories, 125, 126
Suprathreshold Word Recognition, 146
Swan-Ganz Catheter, 179, 192, 194
Sweat, 169, 170
Swing-Through Crutch Gait, 39
Swing-to Crutch Gait, 39
Synergistic Interaction, 118
Systemic Vascular Resistance Parameter, 180

Systolic Number, 136
Tachycardia, 136, 159
Tachypneic, 137
TED Hose, 104
Tendons, 170
Testes, 173, 174
Testosterone, 174
Therapeutic Communication, 91, 92
Thermoregulation, 137, 158
Third-Degree Burns, 186
Three Foundational Principles of Proper Body
    Mechanics, 43
Three-Point Crutch Gait, 39
Thrombocytopenia, 119, 158, 164, 166
Thymus, 171, 172
Thyroid, 136, 137, 173, 178
Tolerance, 89, 105, 111, 127
Tonsils, 171
Topical Medications, 124
Tort, 25, 35
Total Parenteral Nutrition (TPN), 128, 129, 132,
    134, 189, 193, 195
Transdermal Medications, 125
Transdermal Patches, 124
Transducer, 138
Transfer Belts, 102
Transmission-Based Precautions, 50
Transverse Colon, 172
Trapeze, 102
Tuberculosis Tests/Purified Protein Derivative
    (PPD) Skin Tests, 147
Two-Finger Technique, 136
Two-Point Crutch Gait, 39
Tympanic Membrane, 147

Type a Extinguishers, 41
Type AB, 41
Type ABC, 41
Type B Extinguishers, 41
Type C Extinguishers, 41
Unintentional Tort, 25, 32, 35
Unsaturated Fats, 108
Ureters, 172, 173
Urethra, 100, 172, 173
Urinary Catheter, 99, 100, 111, 158, 168
Urinary System, 172, 173
Uterus, 152, 173, 189, 195
Vagina, 125, 173
Varicella Zoster Virus, 51
Vas Deferens, 173
Vegans, 107
Vegetarians, 107
Veins, 104, 113, 115, 120, 127, 128, 171, 194
Venous Thromboembolism (VTE), 159
Ventricle Fibrillation, 144
Verbal Consent, 22, 34
Vernix Caseosa, 170
Villi, 172
Viruses, 45, 50, 51
Visual Fields, 146
Vital Signs, 16, 17, 22, 26, 33
Vitamins, 63, 109, 129, 171
Water-Soluble Vitamins, 109
Withdrawal, 89, 90, 120, 128
Workaholism, 90
Written Consent, 22, 34
Yellow Bone Marrow, 171
Z-Track Technique, 123, 134

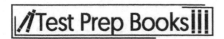

Dear NCLEX-RN Test Taker,

We would like to start by thanking you for purchasing this study guide for your NCLEX-RN exam. We hope that we exceeded your expectations.

Our goal in creating this study guide was to cover all of the topics that you will see on the test. We also strove to make our practice questions as similar as possible to what you will encounter on test day. With that being said, if you found something that you feel was not up to your standards, please send us an email and let us know.

We would also like to let you know about this other book in our catalog that may interest you.

Test Name	Amazon Link
CEN	amazon.com/dp/1628454768

We have study guides in a wide variety of fields. If the one you are looking for isn't listed above, then try searching for it on Amazon or send us an email.

Thanks Again and Happy Testing!
Product Development Team
info@studyguideteam.com

Interested in buying more than 10 copies of our product? Contact us about bulk discounts:

bulkorders@studyguideteam.com

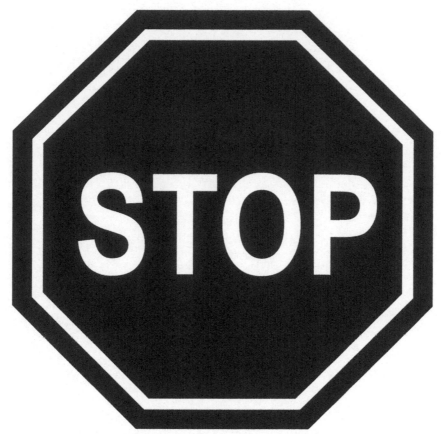

FREE Test Taking Tips DVD Offer

To help us better serve you, we have developed a Test Taking Tips DVD that we would like to give you for FREE. **This DVD covers world-class test taking tips that you can use to be even more successful when you are taking your test.**

All that we ask is that you email us your feedback about your study guide. Please let us know what you thought about it – whether that is good, bad or indifferent.

To get your **FREE Test Taking Tips DVD**, email freedvd@studyguideteam.com with "FREE DVD" in the subject line and the following information in the body of the email:

    a. The title of your study guide.

    b. Your product rating on a scale of 1-5, with 5 being the highest rating.

    c. Your feedback about the study guide. What did you think of it?

    d. Your full name and shipping address to send your free DVD.

If you have any questions or concerns, please don't hesitate to contact us at freedvd@studyguideteam.com.

Thanks again!

Made in the USA
Monee, IL
15 July 2020